Erythrocyte Band 3 Protein

Author

James M. Salhany, Ph.D.

Veterans Administration Medical Center
and
The Departments of Internal Medicine and Biochemistry
University of Nebraska Medical Center
Omaha, Nebraska

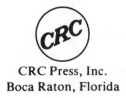

CRC Press, Inc.
Boca Raton, Florida

Library of Congress Cataloging in Publication Data

Erythrocyte band 3 protein.

Includes bibliographies and index.
1. Erythrocytes. 2. Membrane proteins. I. Title. II. Title:
Erythrocyte band three protein.
[DNLM: 1. Band 3 Protein.   WH 400 S164e]
I. Salhany, James H.
QP96.S25   1990   612.1'11 — dc20   89-9735
ISBN 0-8493-6861-8

Direct all inquiries to CRC Press, Inc., 2000 Corporate Blvd., N.W., Boca Raton, Florida, 33431.

© 1990 by CRC Press, Inc.

International Standard Book Number 0-8493-6861-8

Library of Congress Card Number 89-9735
Printed in the United States

PREFACE

"I have diverse times endeavoured to see and to know what parts the blood consists of and at length I have observed, taking some blood out of my hand, that it consists of small round globules driven through a crystalline humidity of water; yet whether all blood be such, I doubt."

Anton van Leeuwenhocek, 1674

There have been many doubts about the structure and function of the red cell and its component parts which have come and gone since van Leeuwenhocek wrote those words over 300 years ago. Many questions remain about the structure and function of certain component parts. There are new questions being raised about the role of the membrane in the integration of the systems necessary to accomplish the very specialized function of oxygen and carbon dioxide transport. Just as the study of hemoglobin has taught us so much about allosteric proteins, we can hope that the study of red cell membrane components will teach us new general principles. This hope of finding broadly applicable biophysical or biochemical laws by studying red cells brings to mind certain passages from one of the early modern sages in the field, Eric Ponder, who wrote the following in his classic treatise "Hemolysis and Related Phenomena":

"I have been told that I tend to speak of the red cell as if it were a microcosm, and as if an understanding of its nature and properties would include an understanding of nearly everything else in the cellular world. To some extent this is true, for there is scarcely a fundamental problem in general physiology which does not have a relation of one kind or another to the problems which have arisen in connection with the erythrocyte.

If the application of biophysical and biochemical methods to the mammalian red cell has continued steadily over a period of more than fifty years, it is largely because the investigators have felt that their results have important general implications. In the meantime, the theoretic treatment of the behavior of a simplified model of the erythrocyte has run far ahead of the more slowly developing ideas regarding its real structure ...

....the investigator's mind is rarely able to conjure up, *de nove,* a picture which even remotely resembles what happens in the living cell, and that observations and experiment reveal situations which, if he were told about them without having seen them, he would dismiss as highly improbable or even absurd. What happens to the simplified idea is that it succeeds for a time and then becomes untenable; it is then replaced by another conception which appears reasonable to investigators who have a different idea of what constitutes simplicity, and one can only hope that the series of replacements is a convergent one."

Eric Ponder, 1948

The present book is about the succession of ideas currently in progress concerning the erythrocyte band 3 protein. I attempt a new synthesis of the data in the literature in order to understand major functional enigmas in the band 3 transport kinetic literature. The purpose of this discussion is to stimulate the further succession of new ideas (and even revive some older ones) concerning the structure and function of this relatively recently discovered protein.

It is impossible to compose a book of any size without the help and cooperation of many people. I am particularly indebted to my wife Christine Sheil-Salhany and my daughter Paula Marie Salhany for their support and many sacrifices in this endeavor. I would like to offer a personal dedication to them and to my parents Mitchell and Mary.

I am especially grateful to Dr. M. F. Sorrell and the Department of Internal Medicine for the support they have given me without which this project could not have been completed. I am also grateful to Dr. Hiroshi Mizukami for providing me with a visiting professorship in the Department of Biological Sciences at Wayne State University in Detroit, where the bulk of the research and composition took place. I am particularly indebted to Dr. Ted Steck for reading the first draft of this book and for his critical comments. His views on both the details of its content and the development of the theme were invaluable. Many fruitful discussions with Dr. Robert Cassoly and Mr. Mark Mercer were both enjoyable and valuable to the development of the final version. The completion of the book depended very significantly on the excellent editorial assistance of Ms. Karen A. Cordes and the able library work of Ms. Vera Bariss. Special thanks to Mr. John Friel for the preparation of the illustrations used in this book.

Many thanks to all who gave figure permissions and sent originals. Unfortunately, I was not able to use all of these due to space limitations.

Finally, I would like to acknowledge my teachers and collaborators who have so strongly influenced me over the last 20 years. They are Jerry A. Peterson, Hiroshi Mizukami, Robert S. Eliot, Alan S. Keitt, Ted Steck, Paul Sigler, Robert Shulman, Seiji Ogawa, John Hopfield, Quentin H. Gibson, Robert Cassoly, Robin Briehl, Joseph Eisinger, Michael F. Sorrell, Katherine C. Gaines, Steve Demma, Jan Swanson, Nurith Shaklai, Elizabeth D. Gaines, Karen A. Cordes, Peter B. Rauenbuehler, and Renee L. Sloan.

I would like to dedicate this book to the late Professors Jens Otto Wieth and Martin Morrison; two individuals who will be remembered as distinguished pioneers in this field.

James M. Salhany, Ph.D.
Omaha, Nebraska
January 30, 1989

THE AUTHOR

James M. Salhany, Ph.D., is a professor of internal medicine and biochemistry in the College of Medicine at the University of Nebraska Medical Center and is a research biophysicist at the Veterans Administration Medical Center in Omaha, NE.

Dr. Salhany received his B.S. in chemistry with honors from the University of Florida in Gainesville, FL in 1972. He then received his Ph.D from the Department of Biophysics of the University of Chicago in 1974, performing his thesis research on the hemoglobin structure-function problem with Dr. R. G. Shulman at the Bell Telephone Laboratories in Murray Hill, NJ. He then remained at Bell labs to perform postdoctoral research on the application of high resolution NMR to intact biological cell systems. Dr. Salhany came to the VA Medical Center and the University of Nebraska Medical Center in August of 1975.

Dr. Salhany has been supported by the Medical Research Service of the Veterans Administration for the last 14 years and was the recipient of an established investigatorship from the American Heart Association for the period from 1980 to 1985. He is a member of the American Chemical Society and the Biophysical Society (USA). His current research interest is the band 3 protein structure-function problems.

TABLE OF CONTENTS

Chapter 4
Cytosolic Associations of Band 3 Protein and the Potential for
Heterotropic Allosteric Control of Anion Exchange 149

Chapter 5
Band 3 Porter: General Considerations 189

Chapter 1

INTRODUCTION AND PERSPECTIVE

I. OVERVIEW

The respiratory functions of blood have been systematically examined since the work of the Belgian philosopher and scientist Jean Baptiste van Helmont in the 16th century.[1] Yet it has only been within the last 100 years that significant progress has been made toward an understanding of the respiratory function of blood on a molecular level. That molecular understanding began with the publication of papers by Bohr and co-workers,[2,3] Haldane and co-workers,[4] and Haurowitz.[5] The Bohr papers established a connection between the oxygen and CO_2 transport functions of blood by showing that increasing CO_2 tension could lower the oxygen affinity (Figure 1). The clear demonstration of the S-shaped nature of the curve also put to rest Hüfner's attempt to fit the hemoglobin oxygen dissociation curve to a simpler, unimolecular mechanism.[6] The Haldane paper[4] showed that deoxygenated blood will take up more CO_2 than oxygenated blood. These linkages are today known to be predominantly related to a change in hemoglobin quaternary structure with oxygenation as established through the X-ray crystallographic work of Perutz.[7,8] The idea that a change in protein structure occurs with oxygenation was first suggested by Haurowitz[5] in his studies on the oxygenation of deoxyhemoglobin crystals.

There is another equally important red cell respiratory process involving CO_2, the molecular basis of which is only now being elucidated. An enzyme exists within the red cell which rapidly catalyzes the hydration and dehydration of CO_2. It is known as carbonic anhydrase (CA) and it was discovered in the early 1930s by Roughton and co-workers.[9,10] The major events of respiration are summarized in Figure 2. Tissue CO_2 freely diffuses into the cell containing CA and deoxygenating hemoglobin. The products of hydration are proton and bicarbonate. The proton is buffered by deoxyhemoglobin, and this accounts for the lowering of the oxygen affinity with increasing CO_2 tension (the Bohr effect). However, bicarbonate buildup is also a problem. Buffering this product would further drive the hydration reaction to completion and increase the CO_2 carrying capacity of blood. The molecular mechanism available to "buffer" the intracellular concentration of bicarbonate is found in a membrane protein known as band 3, which functions to rapidly exchange chloride for bicarbonate (Figure 2). Clearly, such an exchanger can provide the means to dilute the intracellular concentration of bicarbonate by providing an additional extracellular volume for this species. Provision of a larger total volume for bicarbonate favors the CO_2 hydration reaction and increases the amount of CO_2 carried as bicarbonate. At the lung, the entire process shown in Figure 2 is reversed.

The general process of red cell chloride-bicarbonate exchange was originally discovered in cell swelling experiments by Nasse in 1878.[11] Nasse's discovery at such an early date is remarkable in many respects, not the least of which is the fact that it predated by 9 years Arrhenius' discovery of electrolyte dissociation.[12] The discovery of the anion-exchange pathway of the red cell is often attributed to Hamburger[13] and von Limbeck.[14] The exchange process is sometimes called the "Hamburger shift", although it might more appropriately be named the "Nasse shift".

Despite the early realization that an anion transport pathway should exist, it took about 100 years from Nasse's discovery to the actual identification of the specific membrane component responsible for exchanging chloride for bicarbonate. The identity of that component was strongly indicated in experiments by Cabantchik and Rothstein working in Toronto in 1972.[15] Certain inhibitors of the anion-exchange pathway were found to bind specifically to an abundant, 100,000-Da, integral polypeptide of the human red cell known as band 3.[16,17] Recently, Scheuring and co-workers[18] reconstituted the major functional properties of red cell

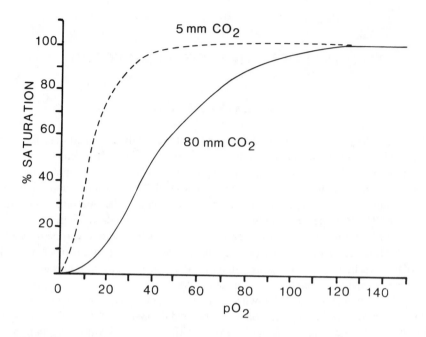

FIGURE 1. Experiment of Bohr, Hasselbalch, and Krogh[2] showing the effect of carbon dioxide tension on the binding of oxygen to blood. Ordinate is percent saturation and abscissa is oxygen tension in mmHg.

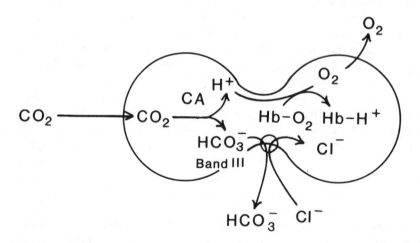

FIGURE 2. Some processes occurring in the red cell during oxygen and carbon dioxide transport. CA is carbonic anhydrase.

sulfate exchange by inserting band 3 into phosphatidylcholine vesicles. Since the general functional characteristics of band 3 were preserved in a system free of contaminating proteins, this work offers the final proof that band 3 contains the red cell anion-exchange function.

The placement of a passive porter in the membrane to exchange chloride for bicarbonate has certain practical implications for respiratory physiology and has general implications for how membrane proteins function as porters. One wonders if band 3 anion exchange is sufficiently rapid to keep pace with all of the demands of the system or whether some molecular compensatory mechanism exists to facilitate band 3-mediated chloride-bicarbonate exchange. If there is such a possibility for modulation, then this raises an even more fundamental question as to how porters work so that modulation could take place. In this chapter evidence is explored suggesting that one may indeed need some mechanism to modulate the band 3 antiport during extreme exercise. Then the structural and functional aspects of porters are examined so that a rational working hypothesis of modulation of porter function may be developed.

II. RELATIONSHIP OF THE RED CELL ANION-EXCHANGE RATE TO CO_2 EVOLUTION AT THE LUNG

Is the red cell anion-exchange mechanism rate limiting to CO_2 transport? Although oxygen release from red cells at 37°C is sufficiently rapid to keep pace with the shortest capillary transit times (about 300 ms), the rate of CO_2 equilibration may be too slow to reach completion within this time frame.[19] In the tissue, CO_2 diffuses through the endothelial membranes and enters the plasma. Blood flow could be sufficient to flush out the system, but the uncatalyzed hydration of CO_2 is too slow to make this an efficient process. Although there is evidence for extravascular CA activity in the lung, intracellular catalysis seems to be the preferred pathway.[20] The uptake of Bohr protons by deoxygenating hemoglobin efficiently buffers most of the protons generated by CO_2 hydration. However, Wieth and co-workers[21] have calculated that considerably less CO_2 would be taken up by blood in the absence of either the Haldane effect or the anion-exchange mechanism.

The possible importance of the anion exchange mechanism in CO_2 transport has been examined through extensive theoretical calculations.[22,23] Crandall and Bidani[22] have made an interesting theoretical study of the specific role of the bicarbonate-chloride exchange on the rate of elimination of CO_2 from blood in pulmonary capillaries. Their analysis was based on an earlier model[23] which took into account the physicochemical events occurring in blood during and after gas exchange. This model can be used to compute the time courses of changes in blood pCO_2, pO_2, and pH. The application quantitatively considers: (1) CO_2 hydration-dehydration in plasma and red cells, (2) the reaction of CO_2 with hemoglobin, (3) the hemoglobin-oxygen dissociation curve, (4) intra- and extracellular proton buffering, (5) the rate of anion exchange across the membrane, (6) transcellular movement of water, and (7) diffusion of gases between alveolar gas and blood. The authors investigated the effect of changes in the bicarbonate permeability on the rate of CO_2 elimination in the lung and on the chemical disequilibrium within blood after it leaves the pulmonary capillaries.

Figure 3 is modified from Crandall and Bidani,[22] and it shows the effect of exercise on the relationship between $P_{bicarbonate}$ (rate of exchange of bicarbonate for chloride) and the release rate of CO_2 at the lung. It is important to note that the bicarbonate exchange rate, indicated by the arrow, was measured *in vitro* with oxygenated blood. In Figure 3B, at rest the normal permeability of the red cell to bicarbonate (10^{-4}, arrow) is sufficiently fast to provide near maximal release of CO_2 at the lung. However, using that same anion-exchange rate and assuming no compensatory change, Figure 3A shows that a limitation does develop with extreme exercise according to these calculations. The normal permeability value for red cells is more nearly at the midpoint of the curve. The authors conclude: "...carbon dioxide exchange could be more efficient if the red cell membrane were more permeable to bicarbonate ions (or if the membrane were not there at all), and that any decrease in the speed of the chloride shift ... results in a large fall in CO_2 elimination."

However, what if the assumption of a constant chloride-bicarbonate exchange rate during exercise is not correct? What if a molecular compensatory mechanism exists for increasing the rate of anion exchange during severe exercise? Several studies have been published showing that inhibitors of anion exchange marginally slow CO_2 efflux in perfused rat lungs[24] or at rest in anesthetized dogs.[25] However, these experiments do not tell if anion exchange is limiting during severe exercise or if a molecular compensatory mechanism might exist to speed up the exchange rate under those conditions. Compensatory mechanisms would require modulation of the rate

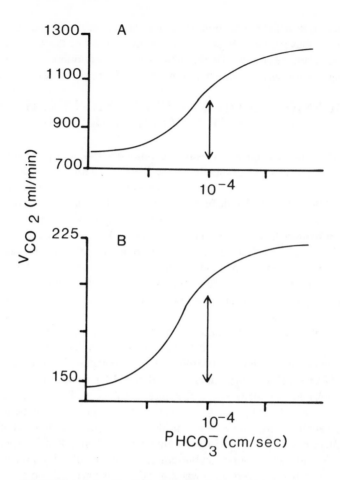

FIGURE 3. Relationship of calculated rate of release of CO_2 at the lung vs. bicarbonate permeability through the red cell anion-exchange protein (band 3) at rest (B) and during severe exercise (A). This figure is a composite of Figures 2 and 7. (From Crandall, E. D. and Bidani, A., *J. Appl. Physiol. Respir. Environ. Exercise Physiol.*, 50, 265, 1981. With permission.)

of anion exchange. Such modulation would have to be coupled to some significant characteristic which changes during severe exercise such as cell pH or, more probably, the amount of deoxyhemoglobin present in the cell. Allosteric regulation at rate-limiting steps is often used for the purpose of control. Homotropic allosterism between two or more porter active sites, when combined with heterotropic allosterism at a modulatory ligand-binding site, could afford a compensatory mechanism to "fine-tune" the putative rate-limiting step of the system.

III. EXPECTATIONS FOR PORTER STRUCTURE

A. INTRODUCTION

The possibility of modulating band 3 anion exchange raises a broader question concerning the basic mechanism by which porters function. Clearly, if the structure of a porter is fixed and rigid, no modulation would be possible. A reading of the current transport literature brings to light some generally held views of porters, almost none of which lend themselves readily to an allosteric modulation theory. The structure of each porter monomer is often seen as forming an independent, single site which offers no simple means for modulation. The concept of an independently functioning monomer has led to some interesting interpretations of primary amino acid sequences determined from DNA sequences. Often as many as 12 membrane-spanning helices are presumed, and attempts to pack these have led to structures ranging from loosely constructed channels to two-channels-per-monomer models. Lodish[26] has questioned the interpretation of the multispanning nature of transport protein monomers. He proposes two rings of helices per monomer, an outer ring in contact with the lipid and an inner ring of shorter helices in contact with the outer ring, but not with the lipid. This inner ring forms the aqueous channel. The general theme is still maintained: one protomer, one independent functional transport site with little hope for modulation.

There must certainly be some passageway for solutes formed by integral proteins. But why should a single protomer make a single channel? Why, indeed, when many porters are oligomeric.[27] The interstitial space between monomers of an oligomer provides an alternative to the single monomeric channel. Such an oligomeric model would be at least consistent with the known structures of proteins in solution (e.g., hemoglobin).[7,8,28] Each monomer could contribute an individual, independent site to a common channel or half of a site.[27] Alternatively, each monomer could have an independent channel, the structure of which was dependent on the quaternary structure of the oligomer with "channel-channel" interactions occurring between subunits. In either case, changes in quaternary structure with ligand binding could modulate activity of the sites within each channel. Quaternary state could, in turn, be controlled by ligand binding to a heterotropic regulatory site on the porter. Evidence is needed to support arguments favoring classic allosterism within porter oligomers.

B. STRUCTURE OF MEMBRANE PROTEINS AND GENERAL FEATURES OF PORTERS AND CHANNELS OTHER THAN BAND 3

The present view of the disposition and structure of membrane proteins recognizes the existence of two fundamental types of proteins: so-called integral proteins which are intercalated in the membrane lipid to varying degrees and so-called peripheral proteins which can be removed from their association with the membrane.[29] Peripheral proteins do not seem to bind directly to the surface of the phospholipid bilayer. There is good evidence that they are, more often than not, associated with an extension of an integral membrane protein or with some other protein which, in turn, binds to an integral protein. Guidotti[29] mentions two types of integral membrane protein which he calls type I and type II forms. Type I proteins have most of their mass and their functional domain extending from the membrane to the extracellular space. The membrane portion serves only to anchor the protein. An example of this would be erythrocyte glycophorin. In type II integral proteins the majority of the protein mass is cytoplasmic and the integral domain is small. An example of this type is cytochrome b_5. Guidotti[29] makes a subdivision of type II which might even be designated as a type III integral membrane protein. In this class, between 50 and 90% of the protein mass is intercalated with the lipid bilayer. Type III integral proteins with large lipid intercalated masses are often involved in membrane transport and are of major concern here.

One of the best-studied and most often-cited structures of a membrane protein is that of bacteriorhodopsin from the purple membrane of *Halobacterium halobium*. This protein naturally occurs in hexagonal arrays, which have been useful in determining its structure.[30] The resolution of the structural determination was 7 Å parallel to the plane of the membrane and 14 Å perpendicular. Although the individual amino acids cannot be located at this resolution, the general outline of the protein can be determined. The models usually shown indicate that the protein contains seven transmembrane rods, arranged as a cylinder with a diameter of 30 Å. The best molecular biophysical and theoretical analyses of the primary structure indicate that the seven rods are alpha-helical in secondary structure. Approximately 70% of the cylinder is integral and its length is about 40 Å. The connecting segments are extramembranous and nonhelical.[30] Recent diffraction studies from Jap and co-workers[31] have indicated that a few of the rods contain some secondary beta-sheet domains. The tentative arrangement of the seven

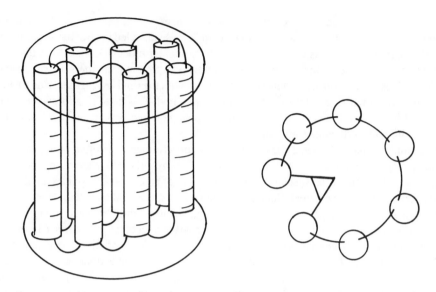

FIGURE 4. Schematic of the arrangement of helices in bacteriorhodopsin viewed axially (left) and perpendicular to the membrane plane (right). The triangle represents the chromophore.

transmembrane segments is shown schematically in Figure 4. A few other integral membrane proteins have been studied but with lower resolution. The analyses generally confirm the cylindrical nature of the membrane-spanning domain.[32]

Although bacteriorhodopsin is one current model for integral membrane protein structure, only a vague structural outline is available of this protein which transports protons when its chromophore is activated by light (Figure 4).[33] Nevertheless, it does show that transport proteins probably contain several membrane-spanning segments. Guidotti's type I proteins with at most one or two membrane-spanning segments do not appear to transport solutes. Although one may expect to see that all transport protein monomers contain at least six membrane-spanning segments (with about 30 amino acids composing one hydrophobic or amphipathic segment), should one expect that a given monomer could form a functional channel? In the case of bacteriorhodopsin an aqueous channel or large pocket inside the protein can be excluded on the basis of neutron diffraction studies in deuterium.[34,35] The density of exchangeable protons is higher in the vicinity of the hydrophilic groups thought to be concentrated within the center of the seven helices (Figure 4), but proof of an aqueous monomeric channel is lacking.

Are dimers or higher oligomers fundamental to solute or even solvent transport? Some anion transport proteins have been described to the level of their primary structure. In certain of these, the state of protomer association is known (Table 1). They include the mitochondrial membrane proteins: ATP/ADP exchanger, P_i carrier, and the uncoupler protein.[36,37] Another class of very interesting proteins for our later consideration is that of the porins.[38-40] Bacteriorhodopsin and the integral domains of murine and human nonerythroid band 3 are also listed for comparison. It is clear that all of these transport proteins exist as protein oligomers.

The phenomenological events occurring in the mitochondria in association with the synthesis of ATP are quite well known. In recent years, much effort has been spent in isolating some of the membrane porters responsible for each event. The most abundant porter of the mitochondria is the ATP/ADP translocase protein.[41] As indicated in Table 1, its monomeric molecular weight is 33kDa. However, when isolated in nonionic detergent solutions, it is found to exist as a dimer.[36] Dimer formation is also a property of the phosphate carrier and of the uncoupler protein. In the case of the ATP/ADP translocase, there is evidence that the dimer is the functional unit and that the protein works according to a "half-of-the-sites" mechanism, where one binding center is thought to require two porter monomers.[36]

TABLE 1
Structural Comparison of Certain Membrane Transport Proteins

Protein	Mol. wt. integral domain (kDa)	Assoc. state found	Hydrophobic and amphipathic seg. per monomer	Function	Ref.
ATP/ADP exchanger	33	Dimer	6	Electrogenic ATP/ADP exchanger	36
Phosphate carrier	35	Dimer?	6	Phosphapte transport	36
Uncoupler protein	33	Dimer	6	H+ carrier	36
Bacteriorhodopsin	26	Multimer	7	Light-driven H+ Pump	33
Protein P *P. aeruginosa* porin	48	Trimer	?	Selective Cl Channel	38
PhoE *E. coli* porin	38	Trimer	?	Anion selective channel	38
Mouse band 3	52	Dimer and other forms	12?	1:1 Anion exchanger	84

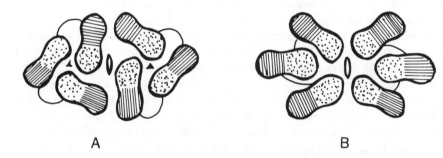

A   B

FIGURE 5. Two possible arrangements of the transmembrane helices of a dimeric carrier in a view perpendicular to the membrane plane. The more hydrophobic helices (hatched) are directed toward the phospholipid environment while the amphipathic helices (stippled) are situated in the centers. In A, each monomer has a central pore accommodating an axis of pseudo threefold symmetry, and the two monomers have a central axis of twofold symmetry. In B, the dimer has one central pore accommodating a central axis of pseudo twofold symmetry. (From Aquila, H., Link, T. A., and Klingenberg, M., *FEBS Lett.,* 212, 1, 1987. With permission.)

The primary sequences of all three mitochondrial porters have been determined.[36,37] They have very similar overall structures and may well have arisen from a common ancestor. They all have the same molecular weight. They are very sensitive to sulfhydryl reagents and lose function in their presence. Hydrophobicity plots of the three proteins were constructed by Runswick and co-workers,[37] and the analysis suggests that each could contain six membrane-spanning segments. The length of the segments (25 amino acids) is consistent with an alpha-helical structure long enough to span the membrane. The regions between the hydrophobic segments are relatively hydrophilic stretches. It has been proposed that they form extramembranous domains. Based on these structural and functional considerations, Aquila and co-workers[36] present two possible common arrangements for the two monomers of each of the three carriers. These structures are shown in Figure 5. Since the translocase shows "half-of-the-sites" reactivity, one could account for this behavior structurally by suggesting that each monomer has a central pore forming a pseudo threefold dimeric axis of symmetry (Figure 5A) with half-site reactivity due to classic homotrophic allosterism. Alternatively, the two monomers may contribute to a dimeric central or common channel with a molecular twofold symmetry (Figure 5B). Here, each monomer should contribute a true half site, much like the 2,3-diphosphoglycerate binding site along the dyad axis of deoxyhemoglobin.[8]

We see in this analysis a persisting impediment to the understanding of the structure of integral membrane proteins which are involved in transport. If there is a monomer with several helices which can form a channel, is a monomeric channel formed or are channels only formed by oligomeric aggregates of the proteins? It will be recalled that in neutron diffraction studies of bacteriorhodopsin, the presence of a central aqueous pore within the monomer could not be confirmed.[34]

Toyoshima and Unwin[42] have recently presented some very interesting pictures of the structure of an ion channel. They studied the nicotinic acetylcholine receptor. This molecule responds transiently to chemical stimuli by opening a water-filled channel through the membrane for cations to diffuse. They report the structure of the channel at 17-Å resolution. The walls of the channel made by the synaptic portion of the receptor extend fully 65 Å from the bilayer. At the cytoplasm, a peripheral protein is attached to the channel. The channel is composed of five receptor subunits symmetrically encircling the 25-Å-wide synaptic entrance. The subunits follow paths that are almost parallel to the axis of the molecule throughout most of the length, proceeding through the lipid bilayer and emerging as five symmetrically disposed densities on the cytoplasmic side. These densities project 15 to 20 Å from the phospholipid head groups and bind the peripheral protein. The subunits form a narrow pore for ion passage which is not resolvable. But clearly, the structural motif is that oligomers form a common channel. A single subunit does not seem to form channels per se.

Another interesting type of membrane transport protein to consider is the so-called porin.[38] Porins form permeability channels for hydrophilic solutes on the outer membrane of Gram-negative bacteria. These channels may be considered the most elementary of transport functional units, namely, they literally provide a "hole in the wall" through which substances diffuse in a manner usually dependent on the size of the diffusing substance. This contrasts significantly with band 3, for example, which moves anions across the membrane by some type of electroneutral exchange mechanism. There are two porins which seem extremely relevant to the study of band 3 by way of contrast. One is called protein P which is an anion (chloride) selective channel with a monomer molecular weight of 48 kDa (Table 1). The second porin is PhoE from *Escherichia coli* which forms when the organism is grown on a phosphate-deficient medium. These both are electrogenic transport proteins.

The interesting point about anion transport by these two porins is that they seem to require trimeric states of aggregation to function (Table 1).[38] These trimeric structures are thought to form large, water-filled pores. Nakae and co-workers[43] have found that porin monomers are inactive when reconstituted into vesicles individually. Once again, oligomeric states of membrane proteins seem to be required for function. Even the relatively simple function of anion diffusion through a pore seems to require a complex structure.

The amino acid sequence of PhoE has been determined by Overbeeke and co-workers.[40] Interestingly, the sequences of the monomers are not particularly hydrophobic. Only a few segments have been found with three consecutive hydrophobic amino acids.[38] This would suggest that the arrangement of the polypeptide chain in the tertiary and quaternary structure is responsible for, and even essential to, pore formation. *E. coli* porin contains a large amount of beta-sheet secondary structure which may support the view that the monomer per se does not form an intercalated pore.

IV. HOW COULD PROTEIN OLIGOMERS FUNCTION AS PORTERS?

The idea that the interstitial space of oligomeric transport proteins could form a channel is an old one. It was first proposed by Jardetzky in a 1966 paper[44] in *Nature* entitled "Simple Allosteric Model for Membrane Pumps". It is clear from the writing that Jardetzky was influenced by Perutz's solution of the structure of hemoglobin and the demonstration that there is a change in quaternary structure with oxygenation.[7,8] Jardetzky's criteria for function of an oligomeric porter were (1) that it must contain a transmembrane channel between subunits large enough to admit a small molecule; (2) that it must assume two different quaternary structures such that the channel is open to one side of the membrane or the other; and (3) that there must be a binding site for the transported species, the affinity of which is different in the two conformations.

In many respects Jardetzky's paper was far ahead of its time. The structure of membrane proteins was then not known. There were to be even further discoveries in the hemoglobin field which would have enhanced his argument. Only 1 year later Chanutin and Curnish[45] and Benesch and Benesch[46] showed that there was oxygen-linked binding of the anion 2,3-diphosphoglycerate to the central cavity of hemoglobin. In deoxyhemoglobin the cavity is open and 2,3-diphosphoglycerate can bind, while oxygenation and the attendant change in quaternary structure occludes that anion binding site of the central cavity.[8] Later experiments showed that there are also protein conformational linkages in the binding of chloride to hemoglobin.[47-50] Even more dramatic is the evidence with crocodilian hemoglobin, where changes have occurred such that the central cavity no longer binds 2,3-diphosphoglycerate but now binds bicarbonate in an oxygen-linked fashion.[51-54] Can anion binding to a protein channel (like the central dyad axis of hemoglobin) be regulated by quaternary structure as suggested by the Jardetzky model? Yes, very definitely. Although hemoglobin is not an integral membrane porter, might the same theme have appealed to the "celestial committee" as they deliberated the problem of how to use protein conformational changes to transport solutes across membranes? Unfortunately, there was no way to test Jardetzky's idea at that time and the paper rested in libraries for several years.

Not until the early 1970s was there any evidence that a porter might exist as an oligomer in the membrane. It came with Steck's[55] demonstration that band 3 could be cross-linked to a dimer by mild air oxidation. However it was not yet known for sure that band 3 was the anion antiport, and there was no public discussion of the relationship between the probable oligomeric structure of band 3, its transport function, and Jardetzky's "simple" model until the late 1970s. At that juncture, Singer began to consider membrane structure and the role of proteins in transport.[56,57] He had independently suggested that protein oligomers could serve as a basis for portage of solutes across membranes. In his, as in Jardetzky's model, the theme was that protomers contribute to the formation of a central cavity which can, through changes in quaternary structure, lead to alternating access of the sites at each membrane surface. Singer[57] carried the theory further by suggesting that a homotropic dimer could exist with two active sites related to the twofold rotation axis (see Figure 5). He states that the existence of such sites might lead to cooperativity in binding and transport activity of either a positive or negative type. Here, for the first time, is a functional prediction relating a realistic protein structural change to a transport kinetic pattern. Cooperativity could go hand in hand with the oligomeric existence of the porter if each monomer had a separate and distinct active site (channel) the activity of which was coupled to the function of its neighbor within the oligomeric unit.

In the early 1980s Klingenberg[27] presented a summary which offered a clear synthesis strongly suggesting that protein oligomers and transport could be related. However, two major factors began to lead the field in a contrary direction. Almost immediately after the publication of Klingenberg's paper, Kyte[58] published a paper contending that most apparent half-site evidence was erroneous. In addition, one of the best characterized porters which exists as a dimer, band 3 protein, showed linear inhibition with covalent binding of a certain class of nonphysiological inhibitors, suggesting that if there is coupling between monomers it was not obligatory to some basic transport function of the porter.[59] But does this mean that homotropic allosteric coupling does not exist naturally? Does conformational coupling exist for porter function with physiological ligands? Only a review of the kinetic patterns can tell. If the Jardetzky-Singer model is correct and porters naturally use multisite allosteric interactions to function, then porter kinetic patterns may be complex, as first predicted by Singer,[57] and the modulation theory of transport can be resurrected from its current position on library shelves.

V. FUNCTIONAL EXPECTATIONS FOR TRANSPORT KINETICS

A. INTRODUCTION

The type of transport kinetic patterns observed provides a framework for discussion of porter mechanisms. These kinetic patterns must ultimately be related to porter structure. There are numerous discussions of transport kinetic equations, and some basic models will be shown here without development. Complete developments have been published and may be found in Stein's book.[60]

The most easily understood transport kinetic pattern is that associated with simple or unmediated diffusion. The flux in this type of transport will be linearly related to solute concentration. Mediated diffusion, on the other hand, involves (1) some basis for selectivity of the transported solute, (2) a higher temperature coefficient than the temperature dependence of free diffusion, and (3) saturation kinetics. Saturation kinetics is very strictly defined in that transport activity describes a rectangular hyperbola and is parameterized according to the Henri-Michaelis-Menten formalism of enzyme kinetics.[61] A typical curve is shown in Figure 6, where V_{max} and K_m are graphically defined.

What does the observation of saturation kinetics mean in transport studies? In general, it means that a finite number of mediation sites exist. Although both simple and mediated diffusion can occur simultaneously, the observation of saturation kinetics generally rules out simple diffusion and suggests the existence of a transport entity within the membrane. Channels (operationally defined as constricted passageways where protein conformational changes play a small part in transport) and porters (defined as constricted passageways where protein conformational changes play a determining role in transport) would both be expected to show saturation kinetics. Thus, saturation kinetics does not distinguish between channel and porter mechanisms, nor does it tell by what mechanism (single site or multiple site) a porter is operating. Additional types of kinetic experiments are required for these distinctions.[60] Ultimately, it is through the relationship of kinetic behavior to mediator structure that the role of integral proteins in solute transport is learned. To focus expectations, consider next the kinetic behavior of protein pores, channels, and porters.

B. BEHAVIOR OF PROTEIN PORES AND CHANNEL-LIKE PORES

The concept of a protein pore for hydrophilic solutes is relatively simple. The protein must, in some manner, create an aqueous passageway to allow the diffusion of the solute without partition. Pores often show size selectivity (sieving). The kinetics of diffusion through the pore should otherwise be simple, barring weak chemical interactions with the pore itself. The structure of porins from Gram-negative bacteria have already been discussed. The outer membrane of these organisms acts as a sieve by allowing those hydrophilic solutes up to a defined exclusion limit to pass through, while excluding larger hydrophilic and all hydrophobic solutes. The porins have been shown to be trimers which form large water-filled channels. One would expect ions to be freely diffusible within the pore. This is clearly the case for the outer membrane protein PhoE of *E. coli*.[39] Although this protein is anion selective, three to ten times more permeable to chloride than to alkali ions,[39] the dependence of the average single-channel conductance on chloride concentration is linear, consistent with free diffusion of the anion within the pore (Figure 7). Also shown in Figure 7 is the same type of plot for *protein P* from the outer membrane of *Pseudomonas aeruginosa*.[62] Although protein P demonstrates anion selectivity, the dependence of the single-channel conductances on chloride concentration shows

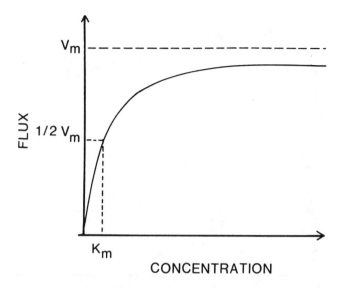

FIGURE 6. Plot of transport flux vs. solute concentration with V_m (maximal velocity) and K_m (concentration for 1/2 maximal velocity) defined. The curve follows the equation:

$$Flux = V_m[S] / (K_m + [S])$$

where S = substrate concentration.

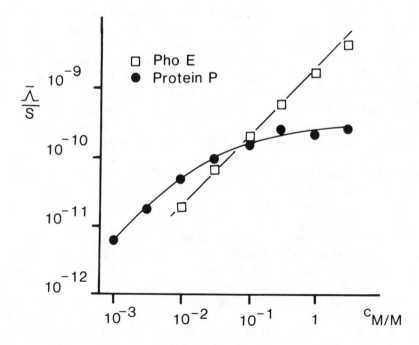

FIGURE 7. Plot of the average single channel conductances vs. the molal chloride concentration for the bacterial porins PhoE (open square) and protein P (closed circle). Note that PhoE shows a linear dependence while protein P shows saturation kinetics. (From Benz, R., *Curr. Top. Membr. Transp.*, 21, 199, 1984. With permission.)

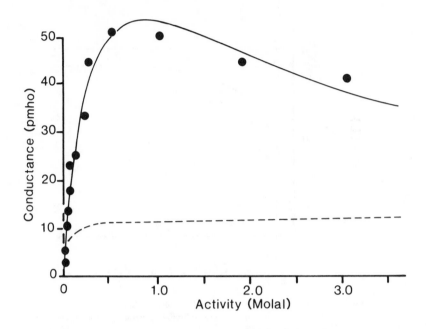

FIGURE 8. Plot of single-channel conductances for Cs⁺ through gramicidin A channel as a
function of the molality of the ion. Note the apparent self-inhibition. The dashed curve shows
expected single-ion model result. (From Finkelstein, A. and Andersen, O. S., *J. Membr. Biol.,*
59, 155, 1981. With permission.)

saturation behavior. Thus, most porins form water-filled pores, but some pores must be larger
than others. The larger ones show weak interactions between solute ion and protein, while the
smaller ones show distinct interactions leading to saturation kinetics. For example, PhoE shows
weak selectivity for anions over cations as mentioned above. Protein P, on the other hand, shows
over 100-fold higher preference for anions as well as saturation phenomena.[39] There is some
evidence which could explain the differences. Apparently, protein P contains a constriction of
around 0.5 to 0.6 nm in diameter within the channel and has a lysine amino group in the vicinity
of this constriction, while PhoE protein shows no evidence of a constriction and its channel
diameter can be estimated to be around 1.2 nm.[39] Since the protein P channel follows saturation
kinetics (Figure 6), the K_m for chloride can be determined; it is about 30 to 50 mM.

C. TRANSPORT KINETIC BEHAVIOR OF CHANNELS

The functional difference between a pore and a channel leads to a consideration of the
development of adequate kinetic models to describe the interactions of the ion as it "conducts"
through the channel. This subject has been thoroughly discussed in several reviews[63-67] and has
its historical roots in the formulation of Hodgkin and Huxley.[68] They demonstrated that the
instantaneous current-voltage relationship is linear. This has led to a generally accepted view of
the ion channel in which transport is divided into three parts: gating, conductance, and driving
force. Gating restricts the membrane to the conduction of the specific ion. Conductance
measures the ion passage through the membrane after the gating process, with the driving force
being the electrochemical potential difference of the ion across the membrane. This view of what
Fishman calls the phenomenological channel in his summary[63] is challenged by data which show
distinct evidence for nonlinear events. The Hodgkin-Huxley channel functions by a linear
mechanism and does not predict alterations in kinetics and conductance at high ion concentrations.[63] Figure 8 shows single-channel conductances for Cs⁺ conductance through the gramicidin A channel as a function of the molality of the ion. There is a clear "self-inhibition"
phenomenon.

What could be the explanation for the nonlinear dependence of single-channel conductance on the activity of the transported ion? There may be ion-ion interactions within the channel which affect the conductance at high concentration.[66] In one model a single ion occupies one of two bound states and prevents another ion from entering the channel. A second model has multiple sites within the channel. Both of these involve a static channel structure.

There are also nonstatic mechanisms to be considered. In one, the second ion binding site is seen as a regulatory binding site which modulates channel protein conformations. A second nonstatic mechanism is that of Läuger[64,65] in which fluctuating channel conformations are taken into account. Läuger's fluctuating barrier model proposes changes in barrier heights and well depths seen by the traversing ion. The ion may itself change the barrier fluctuations through strong coulombic fields around it, leading to a polarized form of the protein. When the protein fluctuations are fast compared to barrier hopping, the equations are the same as without fluctuations, with only a different meaning to the constants. However, when the conformational transitions are slow compared to ion hopping, the ion may leave the original binding site before the protein structure has relaxed. These kinetic effects will lead to complex behavior, evidenced in plots of single-channel conductance vs. the concentration of the ion. Keep in mind that this model is for a single protein channel with a single "binding site". Multiple binding sites or interactions between channels are not needed to explain the type of complexities seen in Figure 8.

Fishman[63] has considered the application of nonlinear rate processes to membrane conduction. He points out several papers in the literature which suggest that there may be interactions between cation channels.[69-72] This implies that the channels either exist as oligomeric structures or polymerize in the membrane plane upon ligand binding. The existence of the acetylcholine channel as an oligomeric structure is established.[42]

D. KINETIC BEHAVIOR OF PORTERS

Thus far it is noted that preconceptions about structure based on transport kinetics alone without structural correlates can be misleading. Also noted was a pore which showed saturation kinetics as if it were a channel. A channel showed kinetic complexities of unproven origin. Now consider expectations for porter kinetics. Saturation kinetics is one expectation, but as already stated there are important additional distinctions to be made. The functional distinction between channels and porters lies in the way the initial influx velocity depends on the *trans* solute concentration (i.e., the solute concentration on the other side of the membrane). Channel kinetics show *trans* inhibition (i.e., that the opposite solute blocks the entrance of the permeating solute).[60] Porter kinetics show *trans* acceleration[60] (the molecular basis for this is the underlying subject of the present book). The usual explanation for *trans* acceleration is that some type of protein conformational change is involved in recycling the site. Acceleration then occurs because the *trans* solute has "brought out" new sites, and this speeds up the entrance of the permeating solute. The common view of porter function is that a single site is involved in the cycle. However, in reality the "carrier" (as it is often called) may be composed of two or more sites which are tightly coupled to behave kinetically as if they were one.

There are two kinetic schemes for the simple carrier. They are illustrated in Figure 9. In the first, two forms of the loaded and of the unloaded carrier are assumed. The second scheme may be structurally more basic in that it supposes two forms of the unloaded carrier but only one loaded form. Lieb and Stein[73] have shown that the two schemes illustrated in Figure 9 are kinetically indistinguishable. Another important aspect of the simple carrier model is that there is a specific set of kinetic experiments which serve to fully characterize the system.[74] One type involves the so-called *zero trans* procedure in which the substrate concentration at the recipient side of the membrane is kept at zero while that at the other face is varied. There are obviously two zero *trans* experiments, one for each side of the membrane. A second type of experiment (done with isotopes) is the so-called *equilibrium exchange,* where the substrate concentration

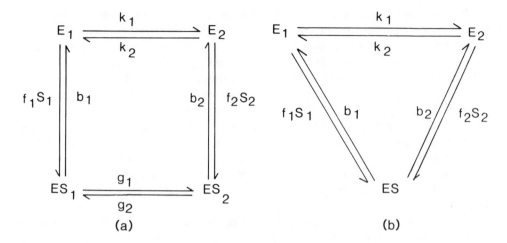

FIGURE 9. Two transport kinetic schemes of the simple carrier. E represents unloaded forms, while ES represents substrate-bound forms of the carrier. Rate constants are indicated next to reaction steps, while subscripts represent forms available to sides 1 or 2 of the membrane. (From Stein, W. D., *Transport and Diffusion Across Cell Membranes*, Academic Press, New York, 1986. With permission.)

is varied on both sides of the membrane with the ratio between the two sides held constant. *Infinite trans* procedures are described where the concentration at *trans* membrane surface is kept saturated. The concentration of labeled substrate at the other face of the membrane is then varied and the unidirectional flux measured. Finally, the so-called *infinite cis* procedure can be performed where net movement of substrate is measured from the *cis* face of the membrane, which is kept saturated, while *trans* substrate is varied.[75] The model of the four-state simple carrier shown in Figure 9 may be either kinetically symmetric or asymmetric, depending on the actual values of the various constants within the cycle.

The simple carrier model describes the movement of a carrier involved in the transport of a single substrate from one side of the membrane to the other. If two different substrates share the same carrier, then a more complex model is required to describe the process. Such a model is illustrated in Figure 10. For a detailed discussion of the meaning of the constants for this two-substrate model, the reader should consult Stein's monograph.[60] The reason this model is shown here is by way of a transition between the simple porter (Figure 9) and the *obligatory exchange porter*.

The model shown in Figure 10 is not an obligatory exchange porter because the carrier may move from one side of the membrane to the other by two pathways: either through transitions of the binary complexes (EPs or ESs) or through transitions of the unloaded carrier forms (E_1 or E_2). Obligatory exchangers can be easily distinguished from the two-substrate countertransport model as shown in Figure 11. This shows the scheme for the exchange-only carrier. The most significant difference is that there is *no* pathway for the interconversion of the unloaded forms of the carrier. The only time the carrier site can move from one side of the membrane to the other is when loaded with substrate. The quantitative analysis of exchange-only (sometimes called "Ping-Pong" after the enzyme kinetic mechanism)[61] systems has been discussed by Stein[60] and by Fröhlich and Gunn.[76]

Besides the lack of interconversion of the unloaded forms in exchange-only models, a single-site obligatory mechanism can be distinguished from a mechanism involving a central ternary complex. In the latter, one site faces "out" and other faces "in", and exchange occurs only when both sites are loaded (not shown). The distinction between central complex and "Ping-Pong" models is made according to the following criteria. When central complexes are not involved, the kinetic pattern of a single-site, Ping-Pong, obligatory exchange porter will show the

(a) (b)

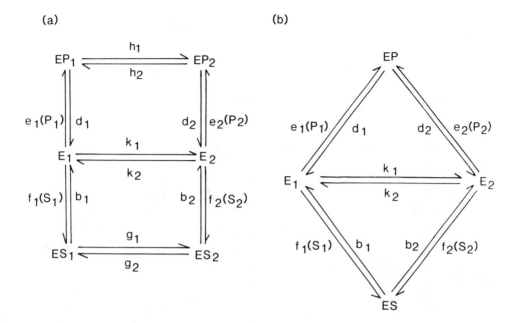

FIGURE 10. Two substrates S and P that share the same carrier. Kinetic schemes for counter transport and competitive inhibition. (From Stein, W. D., *Transport and Diffusion Across Cell Membranes,* Academic Press, New York, 1986. With permission.)

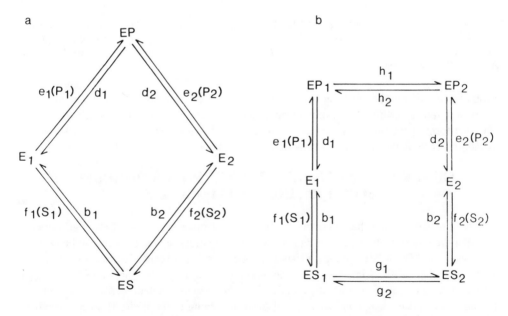

FIGURE 11. Kinetic schemes for an exchange-only carrier: (a) with one form of each carrier-substrate complex, (b) with two forms. Notation as in Figure 10. (From Stein, W. D., *Transport and Diffusion Across Cell Membranes,* Academic Press, New York, 1986. With permission.)

following two characteristics: (1) hyperbolic kinetics over the entire concentration range for velocities measured with respect to both sides of the membrane at a single constant *trans* anion concentration and (2) parallel Lineweaver-Burk plots when the plots are constructed as a function of various constant *trans* anion concentrations.[76] Other distinguishing characteristics

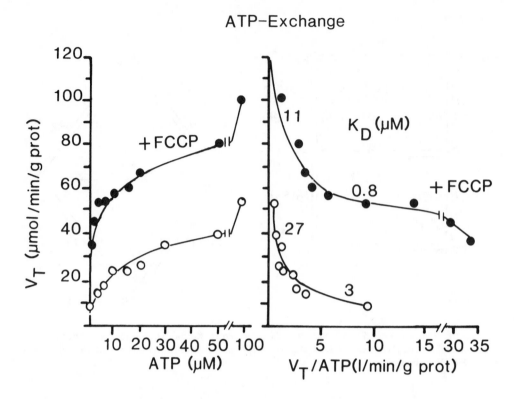

FIGURE 12.   Concentration dependence of ADP/ATP exchange. Influence of uncoupling. Each point corresponds to a first-order rate evaluation of the kinetics at 18°C with rat liver mitochondria. (From Klingenberg, M., in *The Enzymes of Biological Membranes: Membrane Transport,* Vol. 3, Martonosi, A. N., Ed., Plenum Press, New York, 1976, 383. With permission.)

attributed to a single-site model are site recruitment and the potential ability to uncouple the influx step from the efflux step. Although these latter characteristics rule out an exchange model with one form of the unloaded carrier and with two sites, each facing opposite sides of the membrane, they do not rule out all two-site transport models.

VI. GENERAL KINETIC CHARACTERISTICS OF SELECTED PORTERS, INCLUDING BAND 3

What are the kinetic characteristics of band 3 and other obligatory exchange porters? Consider three porters: the ADP/ATP exchanger, the oxoglutarate exchanger, and band 3. As mentioned, the ADP/ATP exchanger exists as a dimer in the membrane. Each monomer may be nonfunctional in the dissociated state, but this does not necessarily mean that the two monomers are functioning in a conformationally coupled fashion when associated. Yet, as seen in Figure 12, the plot of the exchange velocity vs. substrate according to the Eadie-Hofstee formalism shows apparent negative cooperativity. There is no other porter capable of exchanging ATP for ADP, and total coverage of the porter with an irreversible inhibitor stops all transport. These deviations from hyperbolic transport kinetics suggest the existence of site-site interactions which would be consistent with a dimeric functional unit. It is clear that none of the classic models shown in Figures 9 through 11 can simply explain the observation of negative cooperativity.

Another obligatory exchanger which has been very thoroughly kinetically characterized, but the structural disposition of which is not known, is the oxoglutarate exchanger. The kinetics of

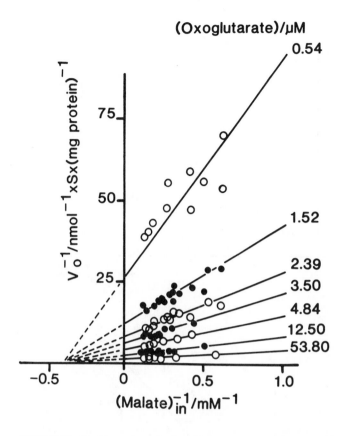

FIGURE 13. Double reciprocal plot of dependence of the rate of oxoglutarate/malate exchange on the internal malate concentration at various oxoglutarate concentrations. (From Sluse, F. E., Sluse-Goffart, C. M., Duyckaerts, C., and Liébecq, C., *Eur. J. Biochem.*, 56, 1, 1975. With permission.)

this porter do not follow "Ping-Pong" expectations[76] as seen by the intersecting lines in Figure 13.[77,78] Intersecting lines indicate that two substrate binding sites are involved as a central complex. However, the system is even more complex, as illustrated in Figure 14 where double reciprocal plots are shown to exhibit multiple plateaus indicative of cooperativity in substrate binding.[77,78] More structural evidence is needed, but the kinetics give little support to a single-site Ping-Pong model.

When band 3 anion exchange was first investigated by Gunn and co-workers,[79] they observed apparent saturation kinetics. However, when experiments were performed over a wider concentration range, by Cass and Dalmark,[80] the kinetic pattern was shown not to follow saturation kinetics. Instead, partial substrate inhibition was observed as illustrated in Figure 15. What does this failure to follow Henri-Michaelis-Menten kinetics mean about the structure and function of the porter? The first impulse is to suggest that physiology somehow "stops" at the top of the curve and that the deviation is artifactual. However, this is definitely not a supportable position. First, both branches of the curve show competitive effects which cannot be explained by simple ionic strength effects.[81] Second, chemical modification of the protein causes an apparent activation of the velocities in the substrate inhibition region, resulting in hyperbolic transport kinetic curves.[82] Although it was originally suggested that there exists an external modifier site,[81] substrate inhibition is only partial and is most strongly dependent on internal anion concentration. [83] Furthermore, the chemical modification which eliminated the partial

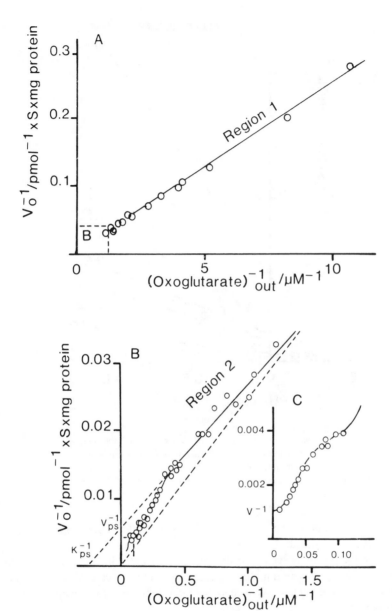

FIGURE 14.   Double reciprocal plot of the initial rate as a function of the
reciprocal of the external-oxoglutarate concentration at 4 mM internal malate.
(A). Region 1 between 0.1 and 0.7 µM oxoglutarate; (B) region 2 between 0.7
and 3.0 µM oxoglutarate. Region C is the higher concentration insert. (From
Sluse, F. E., Sluse-Goffart, C. M., Duyckaerts, C., and Liebecq, C., *Eur. J.
Biochem.,* 56, 1, 1975. With permission.)

substrate inhibition effect was accomplished with an impermeant reagent added to the outer
surface.[82] Kinetic theory states that true noncompetitive modifier sites must drive the velocity
to zero, and this is not observed for chloride or sulfate. Could band 3 be functioning as an
oligomeric, conformationally coupled allosteric porter according to the almost forgotten
Jardetzky-Singer model? What is the evidence to support such an interpretation? What would
be the significance of allosteric conformational coupling to CO_2 transport physiology? These
questions are dealt with in the chapters which follow.

19

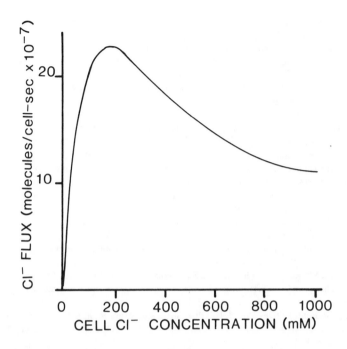

FIGURE 15. Dependence of the chloride equilibrium exchange flux on intracellular chloride concentration at 0°C, pH 7.2. Under these conditions, chloride concentrations inside and outside were nearly equal. The flux reaches a maximum at 200 m*M* chloride and thereafter declines. (From Knauf, P. A., *Curr. Top. Membr. Transp.*, 12, 251, 1979, Academic Press, New York. With permission.)

REFERENCES

1. **Ness, P. M. and Stengle, J. M.,** Historical introduction, in *The Red Blood Cell,* Vol. 1, 2nd ed., Surgenor, D. MacN., Ed., Academic Press, New York, 1974, 1.
2. **Bohr, C., Hasselbalch, K., and Krogh, A.,** Über einen in biologischer Beziehung wichtigen Einfluss, den die Kohlensäurespannung des Blutes auf dessen Sauerstoffbindung übt., *Skand. Arch. Physiol.,* 16, 402, 1904.
3. **Bohr, C.,** Theoretische Behandlung der quantitativen Verhältnisse bei der Sauerstoffaufnahme des Haemoglobins, *Zentralbl. Physiol.,* 17, 682, 1903.
4. **Christiansen, J., Douglas, C. G., and Haldane, J. S.,** The absorption and dissociation of carbon dioxide by human blood, *J. Physiol.(London),* 48, 244, 1914.
5. **Haurowitz, F.,** Das Gleichgewicht zwischen Haemoglobin und Sauerstoff, *Z. Physiol. Chem.,* 254, 266, 1938.
6. **Hüfner, G.,** Über das Gesetz der Dissitiation des Oxyhaemoglobins und über einige sich daran knüpfende wichtige Fragen aus der Biologie, *Arch. Anat. Physiol.,* 5, 187, 1907.
7. **Perutz, M. F.,** The haemoglobin molecule, *Proc. R. Soc. London, Ser. B,* 173, 113, 1969.
8. **Perutz, M. F.,** Stereochemistry of cooperative effects in haemoglobin, *Nature (London),* 228, 726, 1970.
9. **Meldrum, N. U. and Roughton, F. J. W.,** Carbonic anhydrase: its preparation and properties, *J. Physiol. (London),* 80, 113, 1933.
10. **Brinkman, R., Margaria, R., Meldrum, N. U., and Roughton, F. J. W.,** The CO_2 catalyst present in blood, *J. Physiol. (London),* 75, 3P, 1932.
11. **Nasse, H.,** Untersuchungen über den Austritt und Eintritt von Stoffen (Transsudation und Diffusion) durch die Wand der Haargefässe, *Arch. Gesamte Physiol. Menschen Tiere,* 16, 604, 1878.
12. **Arrhenius, S.,** Über die Dissociation der in Wasser gelösten Stoffe, *Z. Physiol. Chem.,* 1, 631, 1887.
13. **Hamburger, H. J.,** Über den Einfluss der Athmung auf die Permeabilität der Blutkörperchen, *Z. Biol.,* 28, 405, 1891.

14. **von Limbeck, R.,** Über den Einfuss des respiratorischen Gaswechsels auf die rothen Blutkörperchen, *Arch. Exp. Pathol. Pharmakol.,* 35, 309, 1895.
15. **Cabantchik, Z. I. and Rothstein, A.,** The nature of the membrane sites controlling anion permeability of human red blood cells as determined by studies with disulfonic stilbene derivatives, *J. Membr. Biol.,* 10, 311, 1972.
16. **Fairbanks, G., Steck, T. L., and Wallach, D. F. H.,** Electrophoretic analysis of the major polypeptides of the human erythrocyte membrane, *Biochemistry,* 10, 2606, 1971.
17. **Steck, T. L.,** The organization of proteins in the human red blood cell membrane, *J. Cell Biol.,* 62, 1, 1974.
18. **Scheuring, U., Kollewe, K., Haase, W., and Schubert, D.,** A new method for the reconstitution of the anion transport system of the human erythrocyte membrane, *J. Membr. Biol.,* 90, 123, 1986.
19. **Otis, A. B.,** Carbon dioxide exchange, *Atti Accad. Med. Lomb.,* 20, 1, 1965.
20. **Bidani, A. and Crandall, E. D.,** Velocity of CO_2 exchanges in the lungs, *Annu. Rev. Physiol.,* 50, 639, 1988.
21. **Wieth, J. O., Andersen, O. S., Brahm, J., Bjerrum, P. J., and Borders, C. L., Jr.,** Chloride-bicarbonate exchange in red blood cells: physiology of transport and chemical modification of binding sites, *Philos. Trans. R. Soc. London, Ser. B,* 299, 383, 1982.
22. **Crandall, E. D. and Bidani, A.,** Effects of red blood cell HCO_3^-/Cl^- exchange kinetics on lung CO_2 transfer: theory, *J. Appl. Physiol. Respir. Environ. Exercise Physiol.,* 50, 265, 1981.
23. **Bidani, A., Crandall, E. D., and Forster, R. E.,** Analysis of postcapillary pH changes in blood in vivo after gas exchange, *J. Appl. Physiol. Respir. Environ. Exercise Physiol.,* 44, 770, 1978.
24. **Crandall, E. D., Mathew, S. J., Fleischer, R. S., Winter, H. I., and Bidani, A.,** Effects of inhibition of RBC HCO_3^-/Cl^- exchange on CO_2 excretion and downstream pH disequilibrium in isolated rat lungs, *J. Clin. Invest.,* 68, 853, 1981.
25. **Brahm, J., Grønlund, J., Hlastala, M. P., Ohlsson, J., and Swenson, E. R.,** Effects of *in vivo* inhibition of red-cell anion exchange and Haldane effect on carbon dioxide output (V_{CO2}) in the dog lung, *J. Physiol. (London),* 390, 245P, 1987.
26. **Lodish, H. F.,** Multi-spanning membrane proteins: how accurate are the models?, *Trends Biochem. Sci.,* 13, 332, 1988.
27. **Klingenberg, M.,** Membrane protein oligomeric structure and transport function, *Nature (London),* 290, 449, 1981.
28. **Baldwin, J. M.,** Structure and function of haemoglobin, *Prog. Biophys. Mol. Biol.,* 29, 225, 1975.
29. **Guidotti, G.,** Membrane proteins. Structure, arrangement and disposition in the membrane, in *Physiology of Membrane Disorders,* Andreoli, T.E., Hoffman, J. F., Fanestil, D.D., and Schultz, S.G., Eds., Plenum Press, New York, 1986, 45.
30. **Henderson, R. and Unwin, P. N. T.,** Three-dimensional model of purple membrane obtained by electron microscopy, *Nature (London),* 257, 28, 1975.
31. **Jap, B. K., Maestre, M. F., Hayward, S. B., and Glaeser, R. M.,** Peptide-chain secondary structure of bacteriorhodopsin, *Biophys. J.,* 43, 81, 1983.
32. **Kleinfeld, A. M.,** Current views of membrane structure, *Curr. Top. Membr. Transp.,* 29, 1, 1987.
33. **Stoeckenius, W. and Bogomolni, R. A.,** Bacteriorhodopsin and related pigments of halobacteria, *Annu. Rev. Biochem.,* 51, 587, 1982.
34. **Zaccai, G. and Gilmore, D. J.,** Areas of hydration in the purple membrane of *halobacterium halobium:* a neutron diffraction study, *J. Mol. Biol.,* 132, 181, 1979.
35. **Rogan, P. K. and Zaccai, G.,** Hydration in purple membrane as a function of relative humidity, *J. Mol. Biol.,* 145, 281, 1981.
36. **Aquila, H., Link, T. A., and Klingenberg, M.,** Solute carriers involved in energy transfer of mitochondria form a homologous protein family, *FEBS Lett.,* 212, 1, 1987.
37. **Runswick, M. J., Powell, S. J., Nyren, P., and Walker, J. E.,** Sequence of the bovine mitochondrial phosphate carrier protein: structural relationship to ADP/ATP translocase and the brown fat mitochondria uncoupling protein, *EMBO J.,* 6, 1367, 1987.
38. **Benz, R.,** Structure and selectivity of porin channels, *Curr. Top. Membr. Transp.,* 21, 199, 1984.
39. **Benz, R., Darveau, R. P., and Hancock, R. E. W.,** Outer-membrane protein PhoE from *Escherichia coli* forms anion-selective pores in lipid-bilayer membranes, *Eur. J. Biochem.,* 140, 319, 1984.
40. **Overbeeke, N., Bergmans, H., van Mansfeld, F., and Lugtenberg, B.,** Complete nucleotide sequence of *PhoE,* the structural gene for the phosphate limitation inducible outer membrane pore protein of *Escherichia coli* K12, *J. Mol. Biol.,* 163, 513, 1983.
41. **Klingenberg, M.,** The ADP/ATP carrier in mitochondrial membranes, in *The Enzymes of Biological Membranes: Membrane Transport,* Vol. 3, Martonosi, A. N., Ed., Plenum Press, New York, 1976, 383.
42. **Toyoshima, C. and Unwin, N.,** Ion channel of acetylcholine receptor reconstructed from images of postsynaptic membranes, *Nature (London),* 336, 247, 1988.
43. **Nakae, T., Ishii, J., and Tokunaga, M.,** Subunit structure of functional porin oligomers that form permeability channels in the outer membrane of *Escherichia coli, J. Biol. Chem.,* 254, 1457, 1979.

44. **Jardetzky, O.,** Simple allosteric model for membrane pumps, *Nature (London),* 211, 969, 1966.

45. **Chanutin, A. and Curnish, R. R.,** Effect of organic and inorganic phosphates on the oxygen equilibrium of human erythrocytes, *Arch. Biochem. Biophys.,* 121, 96, 1967.

46. **Benesch, R. and Benesch, R. E.,** The effect of organic phosphates from the human erythrocyte on the allosteric properties of hemoglobin, *Biochem. Biophys. Res. Commun.,* 26, 162, 1967.

47. **O'Donnell, S., Mandaro, R., Schuster, T. M., and Arnone, A.,** X-ray diffraction and solution studies of specifically carbamylated human hemoglobin A, *J. Biol. Chem.,* 254, 12204, 1979.

48. **Chiancone, E., Norne, J. E., Forsén, S., Antonini, E., and Wyman, J.,** Nuclear magnetic resonance quadrupole relaxation studies of chloride binding to human oxy- and deoxy-haemoglobin, *J. Mol. Biol.,* 70, 675, 1972.

49. **Chiancone, E., Norne, J. E., Forsén, S., Bonaventura, J., Brunori, M., Antonini, E., and Wyman, J.,** Identification of chloride binding sites in hemoglobin by nuclear-magnetic-resonance quadrupole-relaxation studies of hemoglobin digests, *Eur. J. Biochem.,* 55, 385, 1975.

50. **Rollema, H. S., de Bruin, S. H., Janssen, L. H. M., and van Os, G. A. J.,** The effect of potassium chloride on the Bohr effect of human hemoglobin, *J. Biol. Chem.,* 250, 1333, 1975.

51. **Perutz, M. F.,** Species adaptation in a protein molecule, *Adv. Protein Chem.,* 36, 213, 1984.

52. **Bauer, C., Forster, M., Gros, G., Mosca, A., Perrella, M., Rollema, H. S., and Vogel, D.,** Analysis of bicarbonate binding to crocodilian hemoglobin, *J. Biol. Chem.,* 256, 8429, 1981.

53. **Leclercq, F., Schnek, A. G., Braunitzer, G., Stangl, A., and Schrank, B.,** Direct reciprocal allosteric interaction of oxygen and hydrogen carbonate sequence of the haemoglobins of the Caiman *(Caiman crocodylus),* the Nile crocodile *(Crocodylus niloticus)* and the Mississippi crocodile *(Alligator mississippiensis), Hoppe-Seyler's Z. Physiol. Chem.,* 362, 1151, 1981.

54. **Perutz, M. F., Bauer, C., Gros, G., Leclercq, F., Vandecasserie, C., Schnek, A. G., Braunitzer, G., Friday, A. E., and Joysey, K. A.,** Allosteric regulation of crocodilian haemoglobin, *Nature (London),* 291, 682, 1981.

55. **Steck, T. L.,** Cross-linking the major proteins of the isolated erythrocyte membrane, *J. Mol. Biol.,* 66, 295, 1972.

56. **Singer, S. J.,** The molecular organization of membranes, *Annu. Rev. Biochem.,* 43, 805, 1974.

57. **Singer, S. J.,** Thermodynamics, the structure of integral membrane proteins and transport, *J. Supramol. Struct.,* 6, 313, 1977.

58. **Kyte, J.,** Molecular considerations relevant to the mechanism of active transport, *Nature (London),* 292, 201, 1981.

59. **Jennings, M. L.,** Oligomeric structure and the anion transport function of human erythrocyte band 3 protein, *J. Membr. Biol.,* 80, 105, 1984.

60. **Stein, W. D.,** *Transport and Diffusion across Cell Membranes,* Academic Press, New York, 1986.

61. **Segel, I. H.,** *Enzyme Kinetics,* John Wiley & Sons, New York, 1975.

62. **Benz, R., Gimple, M., Poole, K., and Hancock, R. E. W.,** An anion selective channel from the *Pseudomonas aeruginosa* outer membrane, *Biochim. Biophys. Acta,* 730, 387, 1983.

63. **Fishman, H. M.,** Relaxations, fluctuations and ion transfer across membranes, *Prog. Biophys. Mol. Biol.,* 46, 127, 1985.

64. **Läuger, P.,** Kinetic properties of ion carriers and channels, *J. Membr. Biol.,* 57, 163, 1980.

65. **Läuger, P.,** Channels with multiple conformational states: interrelations with carriers and pumps, *Curr. Top. Membr. Transp.,* 21, 309, 1984.

66. **Cooper, K., Jakobsson, E., and Wolynes, P.,** The theory of ion transport through membrane channels, *Prog. Biophys. Mol. Biol.,* 46, 51, 1985.

67. **Fox, J. A.,** Ion channel subconductance states, *J. Membr. Biol.,* 97, 1, 1987.

68. **Hodgkin, A. L. and Huxley, A. F.,** A quantitative description of membrane current and its application to conduction and excitation in nerve, *J. Physiol. (London),* 117, 500, 1952.

69. **Neumcke, B., Schwarz, W., and Stämpfli, R.,** Slow actions of hyperpolarization on sodium channels in the membrane of myelinated nerve, *Biochim. Biophys. Acta,* 558, 113, 1979.

70. **Neumcke, B. and Stämpfli, R.,** Alteration of the conductance of Na$^+$ channels in the nodal membrane of frog nerve by holding potential and tetrodotoxin, *Biochim. Biophys. Acta,* 727, 177, 1983.

71. **Horn, R., Vandenberg, C. A., and Lange, K.,** Statistical analysis of single sodium channels. Effects of N-bromoacetamide, *Biophys. J.,* 45, 323, 1984.

72. **Kiss, T. and Nagy, K.,** Interaction between sodium channels in mouse neuroblastoma cells, *Eur. Biophys. J.,* 12, 13, 1985.

73. **Lieb, W. R. and Stein, W. D.,** Testing and characterizing the simple carrier, *Biochim. Biophys. Acta,* 373, 178, 1974.

74. **Eilam, Y. and Stein, W. D.,** Kinetic studies of transport across red blood cell membranes, in *Methods in Membrane Biology,* Vol. 2, Korn, E. D., Ed., Plenum Press, New York, 1974, 283.

75. **Sen, A. K. and Widdas, W. F.,** Determination of the temperature and pH-dependence of glucose transfer across the human erythrocyte membrane measured by glucose exit, *J. Physiol. (London),* 160, 392, 1962.

76. **Fröhlich, O. and Gunn, R. B.,** Erythrocyte anion transport: the kinetics of a single-site obligatory exchange system, *Biochim. Biophys. Acta,* 864, 169, 1986.

77. **Sluse, F. E., Sluse-Goffart, C. M., Duyckaerts, C., and Liébecq, C.,** Evidence for cooperative effects in the exchange reaction catalysed by the oxoglutarate translocator of rat-heart mitochondria, *Eur. J. Biochem.,* 56, 1, 1975.

78. **Sluse-Goffart, C. M. and Sluse, F. E.,** Kinetics as a tool for the study of transmembrane exchanges exemplified by the study of the oxoglutarate translocator, in *Dynamics of Biochemical Systems,* Damjanovic, S., Keleti, T., and Tron, L., Eds., Elsevier, Amsterdam, 1986, 521.

79. **Gunn, R. B., Dalmark, M., Tosteson, D. C., and Wieth, J. O.,** Characteristics of chloride transport in human red blood cells, *J. Gen. Physiol.,* 61, 185, 1973.

80. **Cass, A. and Dalmark, M.,** Equilibrium dialysis of ions in nystatin-treated red cells, *Nature (London) New Biol.,* 244, 47, 1973.

81. **Dalmark, M.,** Effects of halides and bicarbonate on chloride transport in human red blood cells, *J. Gen. Physiol.,* 67, 223, 1976.

82. **Jennings, M. L., Monaghan, R., Douglas, S. M., and Nicknish, J. S.,** Functions of extracellular lysine residues in the human erythrocyte anion transport protein, *J. Gen. Physiol.,* 86, 653, 1985.

83. **Knauf, P. A. and Mann, N. A.,** Location of the chloride self-inhibitory site of the human erythrocyte anion exchange system, *Am. J. Physiol.,* 251, C1, 1986.

84. **Kopito, R. R. and Lodish, H. F.,** Primary structure and transmembrane orientation of the murine anion exchange protein, *Nature (London),* 316, 234, 1985.

Chapter 2

THE DISPOSITION AND STRUCTURE OF BAND 3 PROTEIN

I. INTRODUCTION

A modulation theory of anion transport would require several unique structural features for both the protein porter and the surrounding membrane. Porter structure must lend itself to modulation. The intimate interactions of the porter with the lipid and with other proteins must not be restrictive. Restrictions, if they occur, must be dynamically reversible since a permanently restricted, rigid porter would not be modulatable.

Allosteric modulation of porter activity could arise from several structural motifs, many of which were thoroughly outlined by Klingenberg.[1] One such motif proposes a porter oligomer with each porter monomer containing an anion-binding site. The anion site could exist within a separate single channel on each monomer. Alternately, each site could contribute to a common channel. In either case, activity per se or inhibitor binding to the active site of the channel would depend on the oligomeric state of association since the monomeric sites are not energetically insulated. Interactions between functionally identical sites of a protein oligomer are classically defined as homotropic allosteric effects. There may also be a variety of so-called heterotropic allosteric interactions for such a porter. One type may involve an ion binding site on the monomer which is not on the transport pathway, but the occupancy of which allosterically activates or *partially* inhibits the transport velocity at the active site. Another type of heterotropic site may be one which binds nonionic entities such as cholesterol or other lipids within the membrane plane. Other proteins may bind either in-plane (if they are integral) or at internal or exofacial sites (if they are cytosolic or plasmic, respectively) and alter porter conformation and transport activity. Cytosolic interactions which could modulate activity may require a structural extension of the porter. This extension should be able to take different conformational states which are of consequence to porter activity. The extension itself would not be expected to be obligatory to the activity at the integral homotropic sites.

As we begin to study the structure of band 3, questions arise. How is band 3 placed in the membrane? What is the state of association of the band 3 monomer? What is the structure of the monomer? Is there a cytosolic extension? Does monomeric structure depend on the state of association? This last question bears on the fundamental issue of whether there may be energetic communication between separate monomeric transport sites on a porter oligomer.[1] To approach these and other questions and set the stage for the discussion of functional data, we first consider the general structure of the red cell membrane where the band 3 porter is found in abundance.

II. THE STRUCTURE OF THE RED CELL MEMBRANE

A. INTRODUCTION

Generalizations about the structure of membranes were being made before they were actually observed under the electron microscope(EM). Membranes were viewed as barriers through which compartmental exchange of substances took place. In 1899, Overton noted that substances soluble in nonpolar solvents permeated cells faster than water soluble-substances.[2] He concluded that cell surfaces might have an oily component. In 1926, Gorter and Grendel[3] proposed that a single lipid bilayer covering the cell surface composed a membrane. Ten years later, Danielli and Harvey[4] made surface-tension measurements and concluded that the surface tension was too low to be explained by a pure lipid bilayer model. These results led Danielli and Davson[5] to propose a model in which a layer of protein molecules was added to each side of the lipid bilayer.

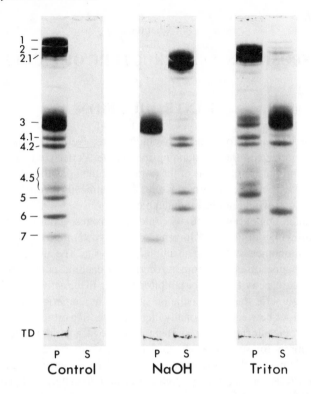

FIGURE 1. Selective solubilization of polypeptides from ghosts by protein perturbants and nonionic detergents. Isolated ghosts were incubated in 5 m*M* sodium phosphate buffer pH 8 (left); water adjusted to pH 12 with NaOH (NaOH stripped) (middle) or solublized in 0.5% Triton X-100 in 56 m*M* sodium borate pH 8 (right). After centrifugation, aliquots of pellet (P) and supernatant (S) fractions derived from 10 μl of ghosts were electrophoresed and the gels stained with Coomassie Blue. TD, tracking dye. Bands are identified in the text. (From Steck, T. L., *J. Cell Biol.,* 62, 1, 1974. With permission.)

Today, our view of membrane structure is a cross between the fluid mosaic concept of Singer and Nicolson,[6] in which mobility is restricted to the plane of the membrane, and the structurally rigid view of the membrane espoused by workers in the late 1920s and 1930s where fluidity was not considered.[7,8] The composite view of membrane structure came into focus with the discovery of erythrocyte spectrin[9-12] and the subsequent detailed analysis of the proteins of the red cell membrane.[13-15] The human erythrocyte membrane is one of the best characterized cell membranes, owing to the ease with which it can be isolated and to its relative stability and simplicity of composition. These attributes support detailed biophysical studies, which require biochemically well-defined and stable systems with which to work.

The proteins of the erythrocyte membrane have been extensively characterized in recent years.[13,16-24] They fall into two classes: peripheral and integral.[14,16] The distinction between these classes is most clearly illustrated by gel electrophoretic patterns[13] of white ghosts[25] after various treatments. The normal ghost pattern is shown in Figure 1 (control, P = pellet, S = supernatant). The bands are numbered according to Fairbanks and co-workers.[24] Bands 1 and 2 are called spectrin,[9-12] band 2.1 is known as ankyrin,[26,27] bands 4.1 to 4.2 are discussed below, and band 5 is erythrocyte actin.[28,29] Band 6 is actually the cytosolic enzyme G3PD (glyceraldehyde 3-P dehydrogenase) which is found associated with isolated ghost preparations.[30] Band 7 is unidentified. After NaOH exposure, almost all of the Coomassie Blue staining bands are eluted into the supernatant fraction (Figure 1). These are the erythrocyte peripheral proteins. The major Coomassie Blue staining protein which remains associated with the membranous pellet is band

3. The minor bands 4.5 and 7 also seem to be integral. Sialoglycoproteins are similarly integral, but they do not stain with Coomassie Blue and are not observed in Figure 1.

As NaOH strips away peripheral proteins from ghosts, so too does Triton X-100 "strip away" the lipid bilayer and the integral proteins from their association with the underlying peripheral proteins. The detergent solubilizes the lipid bilayer, releasing integral proteins into the supernatant fraction (Figure 1). The structural component remaining is a very large mass of proteins which can be pelleted in a high-speed centrifuge. The proteins composing the pellet (P) are spectrin, actin, a small fraction of band 3, and some 2.1 and 4.1 to 4.2. The structure of the Triton "shell" of peripheral proteins has been visualized under the EM by Yu and co-workers.[31] This study and more recent evidence show that the peripheral proteins exist as a network.[17-21,32,33] The arrangement and mode of association of the integral membrane components and the underlying network are important further considerations.

B. THE MAJOR INTEGRAL PROTEINS

Glycoproteins are the predominant type of erythrocytic integral membrane protein. They may be divided into two classes on the basis of the sialic acid content of the carbohydrate moiety. One class has little or no sialic acid and is weakly stained with periodic acid Schiff (PAS) stain. It contains proteins which are stained by Coomassie Blue, predominantly band 3. The second class of integral protein contains most of the red cell sialic acid, stains with PAS but not with Coomassie Blue, is released upon addition of Triton X-100, and contains several proteins collectively known as the glycophorins.[13,22,23] Although the sialoglycoproteins were originally believed to be a single protein, glycophorin,[34-38] it has become clear in recent years that these proteins are composed of a major and several different minor polypeptides.[39-47]

Removal of sialic acid residues from glycophorin by treatment with trypsin promotes the binding of an anti-band 3 antibody to the membrane,[48] suggesting that an intimate connection exists between glycophorin and band 3. Furthermore, addition of an antibody against glyco-phorin slows the rotational diffusion rate of band 3.[49] Yet, for those humans who lack glycophorin (En[a-] variants), it seems not to be essential to health or to the function of band 3.[50-52] The rabbit also lacks glycophorin,[53,54] yet rabbit band 3 is functional.[55] Still, there are some subtle differences which may be ascribed to the absence of glycophorin. Gahmberg and co-workers,[56] using C12 to C15 spin-labeled stearic acid probes, showed that En(a-) cell mem-branes are more internally fluid. In contrast, C5 probes showed more stability nearer the lipid bilayer surface. Protein motion was also decreased in En(a-) cell membranes. These changes alone could have indirect modulatory consequences for band 3, but none have been directly demonstrated to date.

C. THE MAJOR PERIPHERAL PROTEINS

The various peripheral proteins found in the Triton shell (Figure 1) have been isolated in pure form and extensively studied.[16-24] Spectrin is a very large, single polypeptide which has been visualized under the EM as a flexible filament with a length of 100 nm.[57] It is composed of two parallel polypeptides of 260 kDa (alpha-spectrin) and 225 kDa (beta-spectrin). Spectrin heterodimers self-associate to form tetramers of 200 nm in length. Each alpha-spectrin is thought to be linked to a beta-spectrin such that there are no homodimeric contacts.[18] The tetrameric form of spectrin is considered to be the predominant state of association, but higher oligmeric states may exist.

Erythrocyte actin was discovered by Ohnishi.[28] It is similar to other actins except for the length of the actin polymers formed. Erythrocyte actin exists as short filamentous oligomers containing 12 to 17 actin subunits.[58,59] The limitation on filament size may be due to the presence of other actin-binding proteins such as band 4.9 and tropomyosin.[18,60,61]

Spectrin binds F-actin through a lateral association which is promoted by band 4.1.[18] There is evidence that spectrin, F-actin, and band 4.1 are associated into a ternary complex at the tails of the spectrin tetramer.[62,63] Spectrin also binds ankyrin (one per dimer).[26] Very recently Gardner and Bennett[64] discovered a new protein which they call *adducin* which (1) binds tightly to *in vitro* spectrin-actin complexes but not tightly to either protein alone; (2) promotes the assembly of additional spectrin molecules onto actin filaments; and (3) is inhibited in these actions by micromolar quantities of calmodulin plus calcium.

D. MODE OF ASSOCIATIONS

Erythrocyte spectrin and actin are not abruptly apposed to the lipid bilayer. Instead, a few copies of certain peripheral connecting proteins exist, the function of which is to help organize the cytoskeleton and attach the structure to the bilayer. One such protein is band 4.1, which binds to spectrin and is involved in attaching the cytoskeleton to the membrane. It consists of two polypeptides of molecular weights differing by 2 kDa (78 kDa vs. 80 kDa). It has an apparent charge asymmetry with an acidic domain of about 48 kDa and a basic domain of 30 kDa. The latter contains the spectrin binding site.[65] It may be noted that if the basic domain binds spectrin, the acidic domain could be available for binding to a positive center on the membrane. On this basis, glycophorin would be an unlikely site for 4.1 binding as it presents a highly negatively charged cytoplasmic extension.

A second connecting peripheral protein is ankyrin, which is one of the largest of cytoskeletal proteins (band 2.1 in Figure 1, mol wt = 215 kDa).[18] There are only 100,000 copies of this protein present per cell, which is equivalent to about 10% of the number of copies of band 3, yet ankyrin serves to link spectrin to the membrane by binding to band 3. The spectrin binding site of ankyrin is a 72-kDa chymotryptic domain of the protein. The band 3 binding site is in the 90-kDa domain. It is interesting that the tubulin binding domain of ankyrin is also the band 3 binding domain.[18]

One clear indication of the importance of the ankyrin-band 3 interaction in membrane structure has been revealed in studies on the biosynthesis of band 3 and the cytoskeleton. The mature mammalian erythrocyte membrane lacks all protein synthetic mechanisms and is not active in the *de novo* biosynthesis of fatty acids. The earliest nucleated stages of erythroid cells which perform the various syntheses are found in bone marrow. Before reaching the distinctive erythroblast stages, the pluripotent stem cell becomes committed to the erythroid cell lineage and then proceeds through two replicative progenitor stages (burst forming unit-erythroid, BFU-E and colony forming unit-erythroid, CFU-E).[66] The final differentiation of these erythroid progenitors involves modification of the plasma membrane structure, including biogenesis of the cytoskeleton.

The biosynthesis of band 3 has been studied by Lodish and Braell[67-69] and by Sabban and co-workers.[70,71] In the cell-free expression systems,[67-69] the expression of erythroid spleen cell mRNA from anemic mice could be observed. After synthesis, band 3 was found to be inserted into the microsomal membranes in its mature configuration. The N-terminal end was exposed to the cytoplasm while the C-terminal portion spanned the bilayer. In the reticulocyte lysate system[68] it took about 60 to 65 min for completion of the band 3 polypeptide. This corresponds to a rate of elongation of about 14 residues per minute. Once the so-called read-off period had ended, no additional band 3 was synthesized. Microsomal membranes could be added to this system as late as 35 to 40 min after the start of synthesis and still allow normal insertion of the subsequently completed polypeptide.[68] This and other evidence suggested that the insertion of band 3 occurs after 55 to 60% of the distance from the amino terminus has been synthesized. The insertion of band 3 is prevented only when microsomes are added after the protein is half complete, favoring an internal location for the signal sequence for band 3.

Woods and co-workers[72] followed the kinetics of synthesis and assembly of the cytoskeleton in cell lines which did and which did not synthesize band 3 protein. They used avian erythroblastosis virus (AEV) and S13-transformed erythroid progenitor cell as a model system. They found that AEV-transformed cells and S13-transformed cells express cytoskeletal proteins without expressing band 3. In kinetic studies it was shown that the cytoskeletal component proteins are inefficiently assembled into the final cross-linked product, with turnover of the feasible product. The kinetics of alpha- and beta-spectrin, ankyrin, and protein 4.1 were followed in pulse-chase studies. The transient nature of the assembly process was evident in this cell line which was shown not to synthesize band 3. This was compared with similar kinetic studies of mitotic primitive erythroblasts from 3- to 4-day-old chick embryos. Erythroblasts at this stage have a doubling time similar to that of AEV-transformed cells. The assembled pools of cytoskeletal components were stable, with no evidence of turnover. Since the AEV and S13-transformed erythroblasts do not express band 3, the authors suggested that band 3 synthesis confers long-term stability on the assembled erythroid cytoskeleton at the final stages of differentiation.

In summary, we have a picture of the red cell membrane where a few major integral proteins serve to anchor a peripheral network of proteins to the lipid bilayer. Band 3 is one of these anchoring sites, and it should be considered a multifunctional porter with at least two functions in the red cell. These two functions should be reflected in its structure. One, the porter function, will be discussed later; the other is a connecting function offering stabilizing links to the cytoskeleton. A problem seen in later discussion is that the number of ankyrin molecules is too small to bind directly to all of the band 3 molecules. Also, in later reading it will be noted that band 3 offers sites for the association of cytosolic enzymes and hemoglobin. Could there be isoforms of band 3 present for each purpose? Does some type of post-translational modification direct the various cytosolic interactions? Considering the diversity of associations, one might expect a porter extension of great proportion. The various interactions could be satisfied by a series of independent sites along this extension. The porter extension could interconvert between several conformations, depending on which site was occupied. These transitions could, in turn, modulate cytosolic interactions in a dynamic fashion, with conformational signaling to the porter active sites. Further exploration of these possibilities is facilitated by the study of the disposition and structure of band 3 porter in the membrane.

III. THE DISPOSITION OF BAND 3

A. HOW IS THE BAND 3 MONOMER PLACED WITHIN THE MEMBRANE?

The fact that band 3 porter serves a structural purpose in addition to its porter function leads to the anticipation of structural asymmetry and functional specialization at the two membrane surfaces. The biosynthetic studies referred to above showed that the actual insertion of the porter occurs only after about one half of its mass is formed;[67-71] this supports asymmetric membrane placement. The usual approach to establishing such structural asymmetry of the mature product is to add selectively reagents, proteases, or other agents to one or the other side of the membrane. Selective reactivity of protein parts after satisfactory demonstration of probe sidedness allows assignment of the reacted portion of the protein to a given side of the membrane.[13] Several investigations have used this approach[73-86] since the pioneering work of Berg.[73] Using proteolytic and other methods, Drickamer[86] showed that the N-terminal end of band 3 is cytoplasmic and is blocked by acetylation of a terminal methionine. The C-terminal portion is membrane bound and contains exofacially placed carbohydrates.[86] This disposition is unique, since other membrane proteins use an N-terminal signal sequence, which results in an exofacial N-terminal end after processing.[87] That the cytosolic N-terminus of band 3 contains about one half of the mass of the protein and is water soluble had been demonstrated in earlier dissection studies by Steck and co-workers.[84,85] The actual disposition (internal or external) of the very C-terminal end of the protein was not known until very recently when Lieberman and Reithmeier[88] showed that it too is cytoplasmically disposed. In this summary there is a general picture of the synthesis of band 3 in which intramonomeric signal sequences are formed that help insert most of the C-terminal half of the protein into the membrane, with the very C-terminus and the N-terminal, water-soluble half extended into the cytoplasmic space.[67-71] A more detailed picture of the

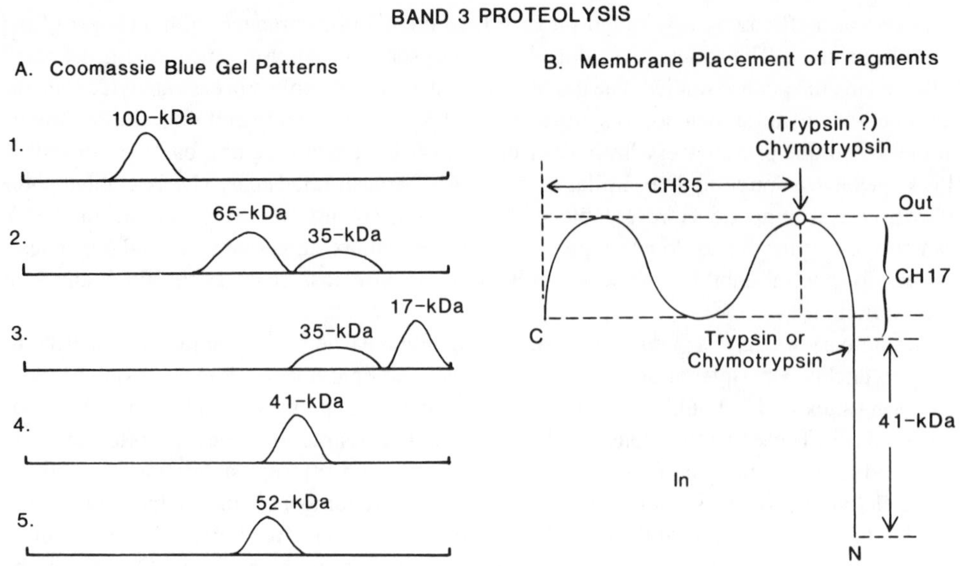

BAND 3 PROTEOLYSIS

FIGURE 2. Schematic drawing of Coomassie Blue stained gels (A, 1 through 5) of electrophoretic patterns of band 3 fragments from controlled proteolysis experiments. (B) Membrane placement of fragments.

structural asymmetry of the mature product is gained by constructing a general proteolytic map to define the two major domains of the protein (integral, C terminal and water-soluble, N-terminal) and their subdomains. These definitions will be referred to throughout the remainder of the book.

Band 3 may be cleaved at the exofacial surface under certain conditions (Figure 2).[79] Untreated, NaOH-stripped membranes present a single Coomassie Blue-staining peak at 90 to 100 kDa (Figure 2A, gel pattern No. 1). Addition of chymotrypsin to human red blood cells at physiological chloride, cleaves band 3 at a single exofacial site to generate 65-kDa and 35-kDa fragments (Figure 2A, gel pattern No. 2). However, the ability to cleave band 3 with chymotrypsin seems to be species dependent.[79] Neither bovine, horse, nor sheep band 3 can be cleaved under conditions which cleave human band 3 exofacially.[79] There are similar species differences and additional puzzling differences in effects of trypsin on the exofacial aspect of band 3. Trypsin is commonly believed to be unable to cleave band 3 at the exofacial surface. However, this is not a generally valid statement, for there are notable exceptions. It is true that human red cells and resealed ghosts are insensitive to trypsin at the exofacial surface when the reaction is carried out at physiological salt.[79] However, bovine band 3 is sensitive to trypsin under those conditions[89] while it is insensitive to chymotrypsin.[79] Surprisingly, when the ionic strength (i.e., chloride concentration) is lowered on both sides of the intact human red cell membrane through the use of valinomycin while physiological osmotic pressure is maintained, trypsin is able to cleave human band 3 to yield the two products seen, with chymotrypsin addition at physiological chloride (Figure 2A, gel pattern No. 2).[90,91] Jennings and co-workers[91] suggested that the ionic strength dependence for exofacial trypsin sensitivity was due to *minor* configurational changes in an otherwise firmly held protein, but this explanation needs to be more thoroughly examined. The reason is that Steck and co-workers[77,92,93] have shown that band 3 in Mg^{2+}-sealed right-side-out vesicles (ROVs) is insensitive to trypsin at low ionic strength. How is it that band 3 is insensitive to trypsin at the exofacial surface of ROVs at low ionic strength,[77,92] while in intact cells[90,91] lowering the ionic strength promotes exofacial trypsin cleavage? Owing to the insensitivity of band 3 in ROVs at low ionic strength, some other mechanism must account for the sensitivity of band 3 to trypsin when the ionic strength is lowered on both sides of the membrane in intact red cells. The reason for these differences remains unknown and needs further exploration.

Band 3 may be cleaved at internal sites by either trypsin or chymotrypsin. When trypsin is added to inside-out vesicles (IOVs) or to unsealed ghosts, two fragments are formed under certain conditions.[85] One is water soluble and is released into the supernatant. Its molecular weight is approximately 41 kDa (Figure 2A, gel pattern No. 4). More vigorous proteolysis can cleave this cytoplasmic fragment into two fragments of 22 and 16 kDa (not shown here). The second fragment generated by cytoplasmic trypsin digestion is an integral 52-kDa fragment (Figure 2A, gel pattern No. 5). Finally, the 35-kDa integral fragment and a new integral 17-kDa fragment may be generated by addition of chymotrypsin to unsealed ghosts (Figure 2A, gel pattern No. 3). Chymotrypsin bilateral digestion cuts the protein at the same extracellular location and also at an intracellular location, causing the release of the water-soluble, cytoplasmic fragment. The only difference between the cytoplasmic tryptic and chymotryptic sites of the 17-kDa fragment is that the chymotryptic fragment contains an N-terminal lysine, while the tryptic polypeptide lacks this residue.[94] Figure 2B shows a highly schematic representation of the dissection processes just described.

B. WHAT IS THE STATE OF ASSOCIATION OF BAND 3 AND WHAT FACTORS INFLUENCE ASSOCIATION STATE?

Another aspect of band 3 disposition concerns whether band 3 is a free-floating monomer in the membrane or whether it associates to stable oligomeric forms. There are several approaches which have been used to assess the state of association and the in-plane mobility of band 3 (which may be related to association state). A static method is the use of EM observations on isolated membranes and IOVs derived from membranes stripped of the cytoskeleton.[95-103] Chemical and photochemical cross-linking studies of unsealed ghosts and intact cells have been extensively utilized.[104-120]

Spectroscopic methods have been employed to assess the association state and the mobility of band 3.[49,121-130] The role of association state in porter function has been studied with the radiation inactivation methodology.[131,132] Finally, there is an increasing number of studies on the state of association of isolated band 3 in detergent solutions[133-151] and on planar lipid bilayers.[152] Although no one method may be considered definitive, together the methods point to the existence of oligomeric states of association *in situ*. Newer evidence suggests that band 3 ligation by substrate analogues and inhibitors may influence either the state of association or the quaternary structure of a preexisting oligomer.[120,139]

Steck[104] originally showed that band 3 may exist as a dimer in the membrane by using mild air oxidation to cross-link band 3 sulfhydryls of two cytoplasmic extensions. This finding has been confirmed in several papers, with some showing the presence of higher association states in membrane preparations.[106,108-110] These findings pose at least three important questions. One is whether or not the observed cross-linked products formed from a preexisting stable oligomer in the isolated membrane. The second is whether or not oligomeric associations exist *in situ*. The third is a more complex question. Most of the cross-linking reactions just cited took place at the cytoplasmic extension or at unknown sites. Is the integral domain associated to the same degree as the cytosolic extension?

To address the first problem concerning preexistence of stable complexes, Clarke[133] and Yu and Steck[134] studied subunit assembly and cross-linking after solubilization of unsealed ghosts in Triton X-100. They found that the dimer of band 3 was the predominant stable form. Others have studied associations of band 3 in different detergents and have found evidence for mixtures of dimers and tetramers[135,138,139] or mixtures of monomers, dimers, and tetramers.[136,137] As we will see, there is evidence that the monomeric form of the porter may be one which is denatured,[141] although not irreversibly.[153] In addition, evidence exists that one population of covalently labeled band 3 does not exchange labeled monomers with a second unlabeled population, suggesting that the oligomers present form stable complexes.[150]

What are the association states of the water-soluble extension and the integral domain (Figure

2) when they are separated from each other? Yu and Steck[134] and others[110,146-149] have clearly established that the cytoplasmic extension forms a stable noncovalent dimer. The state of association of the integral domain of band 3 in detergents has been studied and shows a more complex pattern. Bovine integral domain tends to aggregate to higher than dimeric states of association.[139,141] In contrast, human integral domain forms a singular dimeric state.[151] The differences could be due to diversity of conditions,[139] but it is interesting to note that pretreatment of bovine band 3 with the anion transport inhibitor DIDS (4,4′-diisothiocyanostilbene-2,2′-disulfonate) causes the aggregate to dissociate, yielding a pure dimeric form.[139] It would seem that the integral domain and the cytoplasmic extension can each independently form at least a stable dimer. The dimers seen in various detergent solutions support Steck's cross-linking results in unsealed ghosts,[104] but they do not preclude the existence of higher oligomeric states in the membrane *in situ*.

The question of the association state of band 3 in isolated membranes is most directly studied in EM experiments.[95-103] Freeze-fracture studies of red cell membranes define four membrane surfaces. The natural surfaces are called extracellular (ES) and protoplasmic (PS). Freeze-fracture cleavage generates two new surfaces which are the fracture face of the protoplasmic leaflet of the membrane (PF) and the fracture face of the extracellular leaflet (EF). IMPs (intramembranous particles) are seen on the two fracture faces and are called IMP_p for those on PF and IMP_e for those on EF.[100] In the fractured membrane, band 3 is associated largely with the inner leaflet (IMP_p). The extracellular surface lacks discernible substructure, but discrete populations of ES particles become visible following extracellular proteolysis with chymotrypsin. The topography of the ES particles corresponds to IMP_p. It may be that chymotrypsin unmasks the outer surface poles of ES particles, perhaps by cleavage of proteolytically sensitive sialoglycoproteins which are believed to be associated with band 3 in the membrane.[96] Although band 3 and glycophorin could be associated within the membrane, Gahmberg and co-workers[101] have shown that the presence of IMPs does not depend on glycophorin since En(a-) cells, which lack glycophorin, still show IMPs.

The most dramatic and revealing effect of controlled proteolysis on the IMP was demonstrated by Weinstein and co-workers[96] when they studied the effect of trypsin on the P surface of IOVs, which are devoid of spectrin and actin. There is a granulofibrillar structure (gf) and a population of particles with an average diameter of about 90 Å. Digestion of this inner surface with trypsin or chymotrypsin is known to cause the release of the 41-kDa water-soluble domain of band 3 into the supernatant (Figure 2). In the Weinstein experiments, proteolysis caused the removal of the gf component without affecting the 90-Å PS particles. Weinstein and co-workers[98] suggested that the gf component of the inner surface contains at least two 41-kDa cytoplasmic extensions of the band 3 dimer.

Since the IMP contains band 3, it was of interest to compare the number of IMPs with the number of band 3 molecules determined by other methods. One way to find the number of band 3 molecules in the membrane is to correlate the binding of a specific inhibitor of anion transport with the fraction of transport inhibition. If the stoichiometry is known, then the number of active band 3 molecules can be estimated by measuring the number of bound inhibitors necessary to fully inhibit transport. The most widely used inhibitor for this purpose has been DIDS, which binds to the band 3 monomer with a 1:1 stoichiometry.[154,155] Weinstein and co-workers[98] compared EM data from several laboratories and arrived at a number of 3.6 to 4.5×10^5 IMP_p per cell. Fairbanks and co-workers[24] originally estimated band 3 to be about 1.2×10^6 per cell, based on staining intensity. The DIDS inhibition studies have yielded values of between 0.8 and 1.2×10^6 (see next chapter). Thus, the numbers of IMPs are about one third as great as the numbers of band 3 monomers. There is evidence that the size of the IMP is heterogeneous.[102] This could mean that some IMPs may contain dimers of band 3, while others may contain tetramers. Weinstein and co-workers[103] have presented evidence favoring a tetrameric state of band 3 association within the IMP[98,103] which would be roughly consistent with the 1:3 stoichiometry of IMP to band 3 monomer.

The dynamic aspects of band 3 within the membrane have been studied with spectroscopic methods, and some light thereby has been shed on the various associations of the protein. Transient absorption anisotropic measurements on ghosts with eosin maleimide-labeled band 3 have been made by Cherry and co-workers.[122] The anisotropic decay measurements showed the existence of two populations of band 3 molecules, one with a very slow rate. Nigg and Cherry[123] found, through cross-linking studies, that the rapidly rotating form is at least a dimer, since cross-linking band 3 to dimers had no effect on the rotational correlation time. Later, the same authors[124] showed that salt stripping or removal of the N-terminal 42-kDa cytoplasmic domain by trypsin digestion did not change the intrinsic rotational correlation times, but increased dramatically the proportion of rapid over slowly rotating forms. The effect of trypsin is related to cleavage of the cytoplasmic domain and the associated elimination of interactions of band 3 with the cytoskeleton. It was suggested that the interaction with the cytoskeleton apparently inhibits the rotation of band 3, possibly by favoring the formation of tetramers. Yet, it will be recalled that there are too few ankyrin molecules to directly accomplish such a task. Bennett[18] has given arguments suggesting that one ankyrin molecule could immobilize two band 3 dimers as a tetramer. This would explain the effect of trypsin on the rotational mobility. The slowly rotating component could be assigned to band 3 monomers in an immobilized tetramer, while the rapid component could be the free dimer. That there is a fast component present would be consistent with the EM evidence seen previously, suggesting heterogeneous association states of band 3 in isolated membranes. However, none of these results speaks directly to the *in situ* condition.

If the association state of band 3 to tetramers is tenuous, then many factors which affect the state of the lipid or the state of the cytoskeleton could change the state of association between dimers and tetramers or even change the folded structure of the monomer. These changes in state may have subtle functional consequences. There have been several studies quantitating the general effects of lipids on the structure and reactivity of band 3.[156-170] One integral component which has been shown to influence the state of association of band 3 is cholesterol.[125] Increasing the cholesterol content promotes band 3 association to higher oligomers, while decreasing cholesterol promotes dissociation.[156] Band 3 shows a very strong interaction with cholesterol,[157,158] which may be due to a specific cholesterol-binding site on band 3.[159] These cholesterol-induced changes in band 3 association may be correlated with (1) an effect of cholesterol content on the conformation of band 3 (determined using fluorescence energy transfer methods);[160] and (2) a decrease in the rate of anion transport with increasing cholesterol.[161] Recent studies have investigated effects of fatty-acid acyl chain length, degree of unsaturation, and head-group composition as well as cholesterol.[168-170] All can have effects on the structure and, very probably, the transport activity of band 3.[170]

Integral and peripherally attached proteins may influence the association state of band 3. There is some evidence that band 3 interacts with glycophorin A.[49] However, the rotation of band 3 in En(a-) erythrocytes, which lack glycophorin A, is not significantly different from normal.[126] In addition, lateral mobility of band 3 in the membrane seems to be strongly influenced by interactions with the cytoskeleton.[127] Tsuji and Ohnishi[128] have shown that addition of exogenous ankyrin to unsealed ghost preparations slows band 3 lateral mobility.

If the evidence in nonionic detergent solution is combined with the EM and spectroscopic evidence for unsealed ghosts, it may be concluded that porter dimers are stable forms, while porter tetrameric states are more tenuous and depend on various conditions. Is the porter tetramer essential to the anion transport function? Very probably not. Resealed ghosts are able to conduct anion exchange,[171] and even removal of the cytoplasmic extension by trypsin does not stop transport;[172,173] yet trypsin apparently dissociates band 3 tetramers to dimers.[124] On the other hand, it is very likely that porter states of association beyond the dimer level can have a significant modulatory effect on porter function as suggested by the effects of cholesterol already described. Indeed, there is a growing body of evidence which suggests that changes in state and function of band 3 which occur upon osmotic hemolysis might be expected to disrupt or alter band 3-cytosolic contacts. Although these changes have not been directly correlated with states of band 3 association, such experiments may be possible in the future due to some new discoveries of cross-linking band 3 in intact red cells.

Rao[174] showed one of the first indications that changes in band 3 structure could occur upon hemolysis. She found that sulfhydryl reactivity is altered with hemolysis. More recently, Beth and co-workers,[129,130] using a specific spin label which binds to band 3, have shown that there is a significant increase in rotational mobility of band 3 with hemolysis. Salhany and co-workers[175] have shown that hemolysis and resealing partially deinhibits covalent PLP (pyridoxal 5′-phosphate) inhibition of anion transport and that this is related to exposure of a lysine residue on the CH17 integral subdomain of band 3. CH17 is the part of the integral domain connected to the cytoplasmic extension where cytoskeletal and cytosolic proteins are attached. A new band 3 mutant recently described by Kay and co-workers[176] supports the CH17 connection by showing altered anion transport and altered ankyrin binding consequent to an insertion mutation within the CH17 subdomain. Very recently Ojcius and co-workers[177,178] have shown that the stoichiometry of pCMBS (*p*-chloromercuribenzene sulfonate) inhibition of water and urea transport is consistent with a band 3 tetrameric functional unit, but that the ability of pCMBS to inhibit transport is virtually completely lost in white resealed ghosts.[177] The pCMBS inhibitory site involved is thought to be on CH17 of band 3. It is clear from all of this evidence that although the protein still possesses anion-exchange activity in resealed ghosts, function must be studied over broader conditional ranges in order to detect possible changes in mechanism or strengths of interactions. The newer results point to the significance of band 3-cytosolic interactions in determining structure and function of band 3. These results continue to raise the major issue as to just what is the state of association of band 3 *in situ*. First, there is the possibility of integral interactions between the monomers of the stable dimer. Then there is the possibility of modulatory interactions, through changes in either association state and/or the quaternary structure of preexisting tetramer.

Although there has been much functional evidence to suggest the existence of the tetramer *in situ*, almost all of the structural work has been performed with unsealed ghosts. Most of the cross-linking reagents added to ghosts have been directed at the cytosolic extension. Membrane-permeable reagents on intact red cells have been directed at unknown sites making an interpretation difficult. The association state of the integral domain in intact red cells was studied by Staros,[117] who synthesized a membrane-impermeant reagent known as BS³ (bis[sulfosuccinimidyl] suberate). Work with this reagent has shown that band 3 is predominantly cross-linkable into dimers in intact red cells.[117-119] Jennings and Nicknish[119] did observe some oligomeric product which would be consistent with a tetramer. However, this form was only observed in ghosts which were not subsequently treated with proteolytic enzymes, and the fraction present was small. One of the problems in working with BS³ is that complete product formation is not necessarily obtained because *N*-hydroxysuccinimide reactions in aqueous solution consist of two competing reactions. One reaction involves reactivity with primary amines, while the other involves hydrolysis of the ester. Hydrolysis decreases the efficiency of the cross-linking reaction.

Salhany and Sloan[120] have used the Staros reagent BS³ to cross-link band 3 half saturated with the substrate and affinity probe PLP. They found that PLP caused the conversion of the cross-linking pattern from a predominantly dimer-cross-linkable (DC) product, in the absence of PLP, to an exclusively oligomeric product of a higher molecular weight than dimer with PLP covalently bound (Figure 3).[120] The authors were able to detect a small fraction of oligomeric product in the control in agreement with Jennings and Nicknish.[119] These findings suggest that PLP reaction with certain lysines must change the arrangement of the remaining lysines so that at least two types of cross-links can form. One needs to be intradimeric. The other cross-link needs to form between the cross-linked dimer and the second entity to make the cross-linked oligomer, tentatively identified as a tetramer.

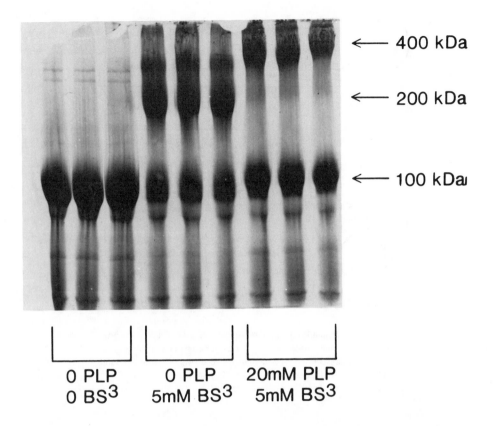

FIGURE 3. Coomassie Blue staining pattern of a 6% acrylamide SDS gel of alkali-stripped human erythro-cyte membranes. Band 3 was reacted and fixed in the presence or absence of pyridoxal 5'-phosphate (PLP) within intact red cells. The free PLP was washed away and the cells were reacted with bis(sulfosuccinimidyl)suberate (BS³). Three conditions are shown in triplicate lanes. (From Salhany, J. M and Sloan, R. L., *Biochem. Biophys. Res. Commum.*, 156, 1215, 1988. With permission.)

In the next chapter of the book, the significance of these findings as they relate to the mechanism of inhibition of anion transport by PLP will be discussed. For now, simply stated, there is evidence for intermonomeric cooperativity in PLP binding to the band 3 dimer.[179] The conformational change responsible is either a change in dimer quaternary structure for two dimers within a tetramer, or there is a tetrameric functional unit *in situ*. Association of dimers to tetramers could also be responsible (see below). Newer evidence from our lab suggests that the cross-linked product cannot be a trimer of band 3. In any case, a change in quaternary structure is proposed to be responsible for the new BS³ cross-linking pattern. The scheme is illustrated in Figure 4.

Since PLP is an extremely slowly transported anion, it is natural to wonder if the tetramer cross-linkable state (TC state) is one liganded state on the transport pathway, perhaps an outward-facing or intermediate-liganded quaternary structure. Jennings and Nicknish[119] studied the BS³ reaction in the absence and presence of DNDS (4,4'-dinitrostilbene-2,2'-disulfonate). However, unlike the results with PLP, the researchers could not find evidence for the TC state. One major difference in the experimental approach was that Jennings and Nicknish[119] treated their unsealed ghosts with trypsin in order to analyze the data more easily, while Salhany and Sloan did not. Jennings and Nicknish[119] found that the only cross-linked product was a 104-kDa fragment which they assumed was a cross-linked fragment consisting of two 52-kDa integral domains of a band 3 dimer. Salhany and Sloan[281] have recently retested the effect of DNDS on the BS³ cross-linking pattern but without including a trypsin post-treatment step. They found

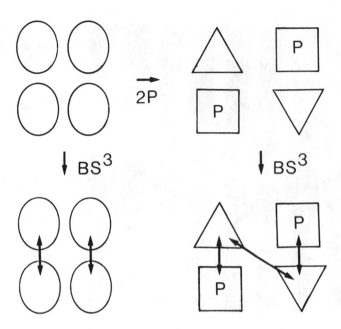

FIGURE 4. A schematic representation of the events associated with partial PLP labeling of band 3 followed by BS[3] cross-linking of band 3 protomers. Each symbol represents a band 3 monomer. The arrows represent intermonomeric BS[3] cross-links. See text for details. (From Salhany, J. M. and Sloan, R. L., *Biochem. Biophys. Res. Commun.*, 156, 1215, 1988. With permission.)

that DNDS, like PLP, can exclusively populate the TC state of a band 3 in intact red cells. In an extremely important experiment, they also found that pretreatment with DNDS followed by extensive washing, restores the original cross-linking pattern, strongly suggesting that the transition between the DC state and the TC state is a reversible change in quaternary structure mediated by transport-site ligands. These findings will be reported shortly. Since the TC state was found to exist to a small degree in the presence of rapidly diffusible anions, and since slowly permeable anions or impermeant anions greatly populate this state, the change in cross-linking pattern is probably not due to local ligand-induced changes in the amino acids of each monomer. The pattern change probably reflects a change in the quaternary structure of the porter. The functional significance of this allosteric conformational change will be discussed in the next chapter, and then in Chapter 4, and based on the available evidence, will show how the existence of two quaternary states can be used for cytosolic modulation.

To summarize this section, the dimeric form of band 3 is seen as one of the more stable states of association both in solution and in the membrane. Higher association states are also present and may even predominate *in situ*. The ability to populate and cross-link these states is influenced by integral membrane components, by cytoskeletal interactions, and significantly by ligands of the transport domain. We suggest that ligand binding to band 3 changes the global conformation within a preexisting tetramer between two reversibly interconvertible quaternary structures. However, other mechanisms have not been totally ruled out as of this writing. The role of the tetramer and of changes in quaternary structure in anion transport is less clear at the moment, but it would be consistent with the quaternary-based transport models introduced in Chapter 1. Quaternary structural changes may also be of major consequence to interactions of the cytosolic extension of band 3, since covalent DIDS binding to the transport site has been shown to alter hemoglobin binding to the band 3 cytosolic extension.[180]

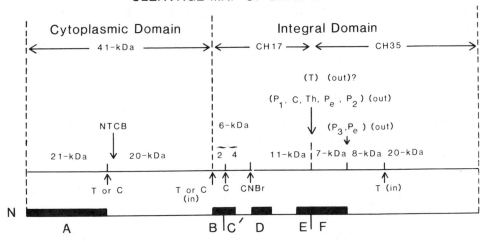

CLEAVAGE MAP OF BAND 3

FIGURE 5. Chemical and proteolytic map of the band 3 monomer. The symbols are T = trypsin; NTCB = (2-nitro 5-thiocyanobenzoic acid); C = chymotrypsin; P = papain; Pe = pepsin; Th = thermolysin; and CNBr = cyanogen bromide. Lettered segments on the bottom represent fragments for which the amino acid sequence has been directly determined.

IV. THE STRUCTURE OF THE BAND 3 MONOMER

A. INTRODUCTION

The findings just discussed seem to fit a modulation theory if the changes in quaternary structure which have been identified are functionally significant. But whether the quaternary structural changes modulate transport sites within a common channel formed by the oligomer or whether each monomer contains a separate channel with channel-channel interactions being modulated by the change in quaternary structure needs to be known. To carry the discussion further, we need to study the structure of the monomer. Ultimately, it will be important to search for data which may indicate how the folded structure of the monomer depends on the quaternary structure and/or the presence of the cytosolic extension.

B. SUMMARY OF PRINCIPAL CLEAVAGE SITES ON BAND 3

Figure 2 showed that chymotrypsin and trypsin digestion can define three major proteolytic fragments of the band 3 monomer, two of which are integral (CH17 and CH35) and one of which is cytosolic and water soluble (41-kDa tryptic fragment). Other enzymes and chemical cleavage methods can further degrade these major domains into smaller subdomains.

1. Cytoplasmic Domain

Digestion of unsealed ghosts or IOVs with 5 μg/ml of trypsin cleaves all copies of band 3 to yield the cytoplasmic extension.[84,85] This internal trypsin cleavage site is shown schematically in Figure 5, as the second T site from the left. The product of this digestion is a 41-kDa cytoplasmic fragment. Trypsin digestion produces three kinds of water-soluble fragments from IOVs, depending on conditions. They are the 41-kDa piece and two smaller pieces of 21 kDa and 20 kDa, produced by an additional cleavage at the first T site from the left.[84,85]

Mild papain (P) digestion of IOVs also releases water-soluble fragments.[84] Major bands of 40 kDa and 31 kDa are observed. These products are not shown in Figure 5.

Chymotrypsin (C), like trypsin, cleaves band 3 at the membrane cytosolic interface to yield a 41-kDa water-soluble fragment (second C site from the left in Figure 5). It also cleaves at a subsite approximately 21 kDa from the N-terminus (first C site from the left).[181] Chymotrypsin attacks this subsite less vigorously than trypsin. Makino and co-workers[89] showed that chymotrypsin digestion of isolated bovine band 3 in the nonionic detergent $C_{12}E_9$ results in extensive proteolysis of the integral domain and produces a 38-kDa water-soluble, cytoplasmic piece. This domain is resistant to further degradation but becomes degradable when it is dissociated into monomers by dimethylmaleic anhydride.[89]

Hydroxylamine hydrolyzes asparagine-glycine bonds and generates an N-terminal 11-kDa fragment and a 33-kDa piece (not shown).[182] N-bromosuccinamide hydrolyzes at tryptophan residues and cleaves the cytoplasmic domain at four locations, releasing a 12-kDa N-terminal fragment, a 30-kDa piece, and some smaller fragments (not shown).[182] Nitro-5-thiocyanobenzoic acid (NTCB) cleaves the cytoplasmic domain at a sensitive cysteine residue yielding 23-kDa and 17-kDa fragments (Figure 5).[84,183,184] Excess cyanide ions cleave the peptide bond at cysteine residues in a similar manner[185] and essentially duplicate NTCB cleavage of the cytoplasmic domain when 2 mM NaCN is used, if band 3 is first cross-linked via *o*-phenanthroline plus copper sulfate.[84]

2. CH17 Integral Subdomain

The CH17 subdomain is generated by mild extracellular chymotrypsin digestion and intracellular digestion with trypsin or chymotrypsin.[84,173] The generation of CH17 by bilateral chymotrypsin digestion in unsealed ghosts can be accomplished by 100 μg/ml of the enzyme.[84] However, higher concentrations (1.5 mg/ml) for longer times (1.5 h at 37°C) cause generation of a smaller, 15-kDa fragment by removal of a 2-kDa peptide from the N-terminal end.[186,187] This is thought to occur at the third chymotryptic site from the left in Figure 5.

The CH17 segment of band 3 may be subdivided into two fragments based on the principal cyanogen bromide cleavage site which yields two fragments (Figure 5). One is an 11-kDa C-terminal piece, and the other is a 6-kDa piece (shown as 2-kDa and 4-kDa pieces in Figure 5).[94,182,183,188] The 11-kDa fragment can be further cleaved into two fragments of 7 kDa (C-terminal) and 4 kDa (N-terminal) by excess cyanogen bromide or hydroxylamine (not shown).[81] There is also an N-bromosuccinamide cleavage site in the 4-kDa C-terminal fragment (not shown) of the 11-kDa source fragment.[189]

3. CH35 Integral Subdomain

The CH35 integral fragment of band 3 may be generated by digestion of intact erythrocytes with chymotrypsin,[84] as already discussed. Thermolysin[190,191] and low concentrations of pronase[74,80] also generate the 35-kDa C-terminal fragment. At higher concentrations, extracellular papain cleaves at three principal sites.[192,193] The first two are in the vicinity of the principal chymotrypsin site. The third is located about 7 kDa further toward the C-terminus (Figure 5). The result is a papain-generated 28-kDa piece and a 7-kDa N-terminal piece of CH35 which Jennings calls P7.[192,193]

Tanner and co-workers[194,195] have studied the effects of pepsin cleavage of leaky ghosts. One pepsin cleavage site is the same as the principal chymotrypsin cleavage site which yields CH35. The second pepsin cleavage site in Figure 5 is placed in the vicinity of the third papain site (P_3).

It has been generally thought that the only internal trypsin sites are the ones which yield the 41-kDa fragment and which further split that fragment into 21-kDa and 20-kDa parts. However, Jennings and co-workers[91] have recently found an *internal* trypsin cleavage site in the the CH35 subdomain. Here, band 3 is cleaved to form a C-terminal 20-kDa fragment (Figure 5). What is very unusual about this cleavage product is that it is not generated in significant amount until the ionic strength is lowered.[91] Jennings and co-workers[91] suggest that this is due to local ionic strength effects at the inner surface of band 3. However, the ion being changed is a ligand of band 3. Could the difference in reactivity be due to differences in band 3 conformation due to ligation? This seems probable. DIDS binding to its site at the outer surface prevents trypsin digestion at the internal C-terminal site even at low ionic strength.[91] This seems to be a clear example of a

ACIDIC N-TERMINAL 23 AMINO ACIDS
OF HUMAN ERYTHROCYTE BAND 3.

1   8   10
MET-GLU-GLU-LEU-GLN-ASP-ASP- TYR-GLU -ASP-ASP

20   21
MET-GLU-GLU-ASN-LEU-GLU-GLN-GLU-GLU-TYR-GLU-ASP

FIGURE 6. Amino acid sequence of the first 23 N-terminal amino acids of human erythrocyte band 3.

transmembrane allosteric effect where DIDS binding to the transport domain at the outer surface changes an enzyme reactivity on the liganded porter at the inner surface. It is one of many such changes which have been identified (e.g., difference in hemoglobin binding with DIDS ligation[180]).

C. SEGMENTS OF HUMAN BAND 3 WHOSE PRIMARY STRUCTURE HAS BEEN DIRECTLY DETERMINED

Figure 5 also shows the segments of human erythrocyte band 3 (A through F) where the primary amino acid sequence has been directly determined.[86,94,181,187,192,195-197] Segment A of Figure 5 has been completely sequenced by Kaul and co-workers.[181] The N-terminal portion of this segment of band 3 is involved in the binding of the glycolytic enzymes (Chapter 4). In keeping with this function, it is highly acidic, containing five aspartic acids and nine glutamic acids (Figure 6). The N-terminal alpha-amino group is blocked by acetylation.[86,181] The last 23 residues of the N-terminus (Figure 6) form two 11-amino acid sequences which are nearly perfect repeats.[181] This suggests gene duplication and could explain the elongated N-terminus of a band 3 mutant discovered by Mueller and Morrison.[198] A final feature noted by Kaul and co-workers[181] is the bipolar nature of the 21-kDa fragment where, in contrast to the acidic N-terminal third, the C-terminal two thirds of the fragment has a predominantly basic charge character.

The sequence of the 2-kDa B segment of Figure 5 for human band 3 has been determined.[94,196,197] One notable feature of this region is that the N-terminal amino acid differs according to whether trypsin or chymotrypsin is used to cleave the 41-kDa water-soluble fragment. Trypsin cleavage of human erythrocyte band 3 causes the release of the N-terminal fragment with a C-terminal lysine, while chymotrypsin does not cleave that lysine residue.[94]

Segments C′ (N-terminus of 4 kDa) and D (N-terminus of 11 kDa) of Figure 5 have also been sequenced.[94,187] The latter segment was originally thought to contain the lysine residue which covalently binds DIDS.[187,199] However, that part of band 3 does not contain lysines,[94] and the discrepancy remains unresolved.

The two segments E (C-terminus of 11 kDa) and F (Jenning's P7) of Figure 5 generated by papain and chymotrypsin digestion have also been sequenced.[192,193] The cleavage of the second papain site in Figure 5 produces major changes in the binding of both competitive[193] and noncompetitive[200] inhibitors, without affecting substrate binding to the transport site.[193] The amino acid sequence from the pepsin cleavage studies[195] overlaps the CH35 N-terminus and Jenning's P7 fragment.

D. DEDUCTION OF THE AMINO ACID SEQUENCE OF BAND 3 FROM THE NUCLEOTIDE SEQUENCE OF A COMPLEMENTARY DNA CLONE

The isolation and sequence determination of the fragments of band 3 just described required much effort. Direct sequence determination of the entire protein, including several hydrophobic segments, has proved intractable. These technical problems have been circumvented by the application of modern techniques for the cloning and sequencing of cDNA encoding the full length of murine[201] and human nonerythroid[202] messenger RNA. A problem in applying these techniques to the solution of the structure of band 3 was that mature mammalian erythrocytes lack the protein synthetic mechanism, and it is not possible to obtain significant amounts of mRNA encoding the band 3 polypeptide. Braell and Lodish[67,68] solved this problem by utilizing anemic mouse spleen as a source for band 3 mRNA, since this tissue contains a significant population of erythroid precursor cells. Murine band 3 mRNA was shown to be present by means of specific immunoprecipitation of the polypeptide from in vitro translation. Proteolytic gel patterns indicate similarity of murine and human band 3.

With this system established, Kopito and Lodish[201] constructed a cDNA library in the expression vector lambda-gt11. They isolated clones encoding murine band 3 by antibody screening and determined the complete nucleotide and corresponding amino acid sequence for murine band 3. Demuth and his co-workers[202] have identified polypeptides immunologically related to erythrocyte band 3 in several nonerythroid cells and have determined the primary structure of this human protein. These two sequences are listed in Tables 1 (murine) and 2 (human nonerythroid).

Brock and Tanner[203] have recently determined the sequences of two fragments of human erythrocyte band 3 generated by pepsin at intracellular proteolytic sites and compared this sequence with the murine sequence. These fragments are, using the murine numbering system, 416 to 434 and 795 to 813 (Table 1). It was noted that eight differences exist between the N-terminal sequence of human (416 to 434) and the murine protein; five are contiguous and their compositions in this region are nearly the same. The sequence of human erythrocyte band 3 between 795 to 813 is conserved.

A more complete comparison of sequence homology was possible with the determination of the primary structure of a human nonerythroid band 3 (Table 2).[202] The human protein was called pHKB3 (Table 2) in that paper, while the mouse protein was called MEB3 (Table 1). One primary difference between the two proteins (pHKB3 and MEB3) is that pHKB3 has a 29-amino acid insertion at position 582 in the pHKB3 sequence. This is the Z region of the hydropathy plot in Figure 7 (see below for further discussion of this figure). The introduction of this insertion allows optimal alignment of the two band 3. Excluding this segment, the two integral domains have a sequence homology of 71%, which corresponds to the level of homology seen when the published, directly determined sequences of fragments of the membrane-bound domain are compared.[202]

Certain lysine residues thought to be intimately involved in anion transport are among those amino acids which are conserved when the sequences of the two species are compared. At least one of these reacts with the anion transport inhibitor DIDS.[155] The conserved lysines are 449, 558, and 561 within the MEB3 sequence (Table 1).[201] In addition to these lysines, Brock and co-workers[194] identified lysines 608, 610, and 618 at the inner membrane surface of human erythrocyte band 3, one of which seemed important to anion transport. Lysines 608 and 610 are conserved in pHKB3.

The cytoplasmic domain of pHKB3[202] was compared to mouse MEB3[201] and human band 3 [181] by Demuth and co-workers.[202] There is a substantial divergence of cytoplasmic domain of nonerythroid pHKB3 from the erythroid versions. This divergence strongly contrasts with the high degree of homology seen for the integral domain. The authors point to three regions of the cytoplasmic domain where the sequence homology is high. There are 20 amino acids from position 157 to 177 in pHKB3 where there is a 75% sequence homology to both human band 3 and MEB3. This cytoplasmic region contains a subdomain where amino acids 167 to 177 show 90% homology with MEB3; it may be the ankyrin binding site.[202] There is a region between amino acids 193 and 198 significantly enriched in proline residues which has been proposed[149]

TABLE 1
Amino Acid Sequence of Murine Band 3

```
LEU-GLU-ILE-PRO-ASP-ARG-ASP-SER-GLU-GLU-GLU-LEU-GLU-ASN-ILE-
                                                            25
ILE-GLY-GLN-ILE-ALA-TYR-ARG-ASP-LEU-THR-ILE-PRO-VAL-THR-GLU-
                                                            40
MET-GLN-ASP-PRO-GLU-ALA-LEU-PRO-THR-GLU-GLN-THR-ALA-THR-ASP-
                                                            55
TYR-VAL-PRO-SER-SER-THR-SER-THR-PRO-HIS-PRO-SER-SER-GLY-GLN-
                                                            70
VAL-TYR-VAL-GLU-LEU-GLN-GLU-LEU-MET-MET-ASP-GLN-ARG-ASN-GLN-
                                                            85
GLU-LEU-GLN-TRP-VAL-GLU-ALA-ALA-HIS-TRP-ILE-GLY-LEU-GLU-GLU-
                                                            100
ASN-LEU-ARG-GLU-ASP-GLY-VAL-TRP-GLY-ARG-PRO-HIS-LEU-SER-TYR-
                                                            115
LEU-THR-PHE-TRP-SER-LEU-LEU-GLU-LEU-GLN-LYS-VAL-PHE-SER-LYS-
                                                            130
GLY-THR-PHE-LEU-LEU-GLY-LEU-ALA-GLU-THR-SER-LEU-ALA-GLY-VAL-
                                                            145
ALA-ASN-HIS-LEU-LEU-ASP-CYS-PHE-ILE-TYR-GLU-ASP-GLN-ILE-ARG-
                                                            160
PRO-GLN-ASP-ARG-GLU-GLU-LEU-LEU-ARG-ALA-LEU-LEU-LEU-LYS-ARG-
                                                            175
SER-HIS-ALA-GLU-ASP-LEU-GLY-ASN-LEU-GLU-GLY-VAL-LYS-PRO-ALA-
                                                            190
VAL-LEU-THR-ARG-SER-GLY-GLY-ALA-SER-GLU-PRO-LEU-LEU-PRO-HIS-
                                                            205
GLN-PRO-SER-LEU-GLU-THR-GLN-LEU-TYR-CYS-GLY-GLN-ALA-GLU-GLY-
                                                            220
GLY-SER-GLU-GLY-PRO-SER-THR-SER-GLY-THR-LEU-LYS-ILE-PRO-PRO-
                                                            235
ASP-SER-GLU-THR-THR-LEU-VAL-LEU-VAL-GLY-ARG-ALA-ASN-PHE-LEU-
                                                            250
GLU-LYS-PRO-VAL-LEU-GLY-PHE-VAL-ARG-LEU-LYS-GLU-ALA-VAL-PRO-
                                                            265
LEU-GLU-ASP-LEU-VAL-LEU-PRO-GLU-PRO-VAL-GLY-PHE-LEU-LEU-VAL-
                                                            280
LEU-LEU-GLY-PRO-GLU-ALA-PRO-HIS-VAL-ASP-TYR-THR-GLN-LEU-GLY-
                                                            295
ARG-ALA-ALA-ALA-THR-LEU-MET-THR-GLU-ARG-VAL-PHE-ARG-ILE-THR-
                                                            310
ALA-SER-MET-ALA-HIS-ASN-ARG-GLU-GLU-LEU-LEU-ARG-SER-LEU-GLU-
                                                            325
SER-PHE-LEU-ASP-CYS-SER-LEU-VAL-LEU-PRO-PRO-THR-ASP-ALA-PRO-
                                                            340
SER-GLU-LYS-ALA-LEU-LEU-ASN-LEU-VAL-PRO-VAL-GLN-LYS-GLU-LEU-
                                                            355
LEU-ARG-ARG-ARG-TYR-LEU-PRO-SER-PRO-ALA-LYS-PRO-ASP-PRO-ASN-
                                                            370
LEU-TYR-ASN-THR-LEU-ASP-LEU-ASN-GLY-GLY-LYS-GLY-GLY-PRO-GLY-
                                                            385
ASP-GLU-ASP-ASP-PRO-LEU-ARG-ARG-THR-GLY-ARG-ILE-PHE-GLY-GLY-
                                                            400
LEU-ILE-ARG-ASP-ILE-ARG-ARG-ARG-TYR-PRO-TYR-TYR-LEU-SER-ASP-
                                                            415
ILE-THR-ASP-ALA-LEU-SER-PRO-GLN-VAL-LEU-ALA-ALA-VAL-ILE-PHE-
                                                            430
ILE-TYR-PHE-ALA-ALA-LEU-SER-PRO-ALA-VAL-THR-PHE-GLY-GLY-LEU-
                                                            445
```

TABLE 1 (continued)
Amino Acid Sequence of Murine Band 3

```
LEU-GLY-GLU-LYS-THR-ARG-ASN-LEU-MET-GLY-VAL-SER-GLU-LEU-LEU-
                                                            460
ILE-SER-THR-ALA-VAL-GLN-SER-ILE-LEU-PHE-ALA-LEU-LEU-GLY-ALA-
                                                            475
GLN-PRO-LEU-LEU-VAL-LEU-GLY-PHE-SER-GLY-PRO-LEU-LEU-VAL-PHE-
                                                            490
GLU-GLU-ALA-PHE-PHE-SER-PHE-CYS-GLU-SER-ASN-ASN-LEU-GLU-TYR-
                                                            505
ILE-VAL-GLY-ARG-ALA-TRP-ILE-GLY-PHE-TRP-LEU-ILE-LEU-LEU-VAL-
                                                            520
MET-LEU-VAL-VAL-ALA-PHE-GLU-GLY-SER-PHE-LEU-VAL-GLN-TYR-ILE-
                                                            535
SER-ARG-TYR-THR-GLN-GLU-ILE-PHE-SER-PHE-LEU-ILE-SER-LEU-ILE-
                                                            550
PHE-ILE-TYR-GLU-THR-PHE-SER-LYS-LEU-ILE-LYS-ILE-PHE-GLN-ASP-
                                                            565
TYR-PRO-LEU-GLN-GLN-THR-TYR-ALA-PRO-VAL-VAL-MET-LYS-PRO-LYS-
                                                            580
PRO-GLN-GLY-PRO-VAL-PRO-ASN-THR-ALA-LEU-PHE-SER-LEU-VAL-LEU-
                                                            595
MET-ALA-GLY-THR-PHE-LEU-LEU-ALA-MET-THR-LEU-ARG-LYS-PHE-LYS-
                                                            610
ASN-SER-THR-TYR-PHE-PRO-GLY-LYS-LEU-ARG-ARG-VAL-ILE-GLY-ASP-
                                                            625
PHE-GLY-VAL-PRO-ILE-SER-ILE-LEU-ILE-MET-VAL-LEU-VAL-ASP-SER-
                                                            640
PHE-ILE-LYS-GLY-THR-TYR-THR-GLN-LYS-LEU-SER-VAL-PRO-ASP-GLY-
                                                            655
LEU-LYS-VAL-SER-ASN-SER-SER-ALA-ARG-GLY-TRP-VAL-ILE-HIS-PRO-
                                                            670
LEU-GLY-LEU-TYR-ARG-LEU-PHE-PRO-THR-TRP-MET-MET-PHE-ALA-SER-
                                                            685
VAL-LEU-PRO-ALA-LEU-LEU-VAL-PHE-ILE-LEU-ILE-PHE-LEU-GLU-SER-
                                                            700
GLN-ILE-THR-THR-LEU-ILE-VAL-SER-LYS-PRO-GLU-ARG-LYS-MET-ILE-
                                                            715
LYS-GLY-SER-GLY-PHE-HIS-LEU-ASP-LEU-LEU-LEU-VAL-VAL-GLY-MET-
                                                            730
GLY-GLY-VAL-ALA-ALA-LEU-PHE-GLY-MET-PRO-TRP-LEU-SER-ALA-THR-
                                                            745
THR-VAL-ARG-SER-VAL-THR-HIS-ALA-ASN-ALA-LEU-THR-VAL-MET-GLY-
                                                            760
LYS-ALA-SER-GLY-PRO-GLY-ALA-ALA-ALA-GLN-ILE-GLN-GLU-VAL-LYS-
                                                            775
GLU-GLN-ARG-ILE-SER-GLY-LEU-LEU-VAL-SER-VAL-LEU-VAL-GLY-LEU-
                                                            790
SER-ILE-LEU-MET-GLU-PRO-ILE-LEU-SER-ARG-ILE-PRO-LEU-ALA-VAL-
                                                            805
LEU-PHE-GLY-ILE-PHE-LEU-TYR-MET-GLY-VAL-THR-SER-LEU-SER-GLY-
                                                            820
ILE-GLN-LEU-PHE-ASP-ARG-ILE-LEU-LEU-LEU-PHE-LYS-PRO-PRO-LYS-
                                                            835
TYR-HIS-PRO-ASP-VAL-PRO-PHE-VAL-LYS-ARG-VAL-LYS-THR-TRP-ARG-
                                                            850
MET-HIS-LEU-PHE-THR-GLY-ILE-GLN-ILE-ILE-CYS-LEU-ALA-VAL-LEU-
                                                            865
TRP-VAL-VAL-LYS-SER-THR-PRO-ALA-SER-LEU-ALA-LEU-PRO-PHE-VAL-
                                                            880
```

TABLE 1 (continued)
Amino Acid Sequence of Murine Band 3

LEU-ILE-LEU-THR-VAL-PRO-LEU-ARG-ARG-LEU-ILE-LEU-PRO-LEU-ILE-
895
PHE-ARG-GLU-LEU-GLU-LEU-GLN-CYS-LEU-ASP-GLY-ASP-ASP-ALA-LYS-
910
VAL-THR-PHE-ASP-GLU-GLU-ASN-GLY-LEU-ASP-GLU-TYR-ASP-GLU-VAL-
925
PRO-MET-PRO-VAL

TABLE 2
Amino Acid Sequence of Human Nonerythroid Band 3

GLU-LEU-ARG-ARG-THR-LEU-ALA-HIS-GLY-ALA-VAL-LEU-LEU-ASP-LEU-
15
ASP-GLN-GLN-THR-LEU-PRO-GLY-VAL-ALA-GLN-VAL-VAL-GLU-GLN-MET-
30
VAL-ILE-SER-ASP-GLN-ILE-LYS-ALA-GLU-ASP-ARG-ALA-ASN-VAL-LEU-
45
ARG-ALA-LEU-LEU-LEU-LYS-HIS-SER-HIS-PRO-SER-ASP-GLU-LYS-ASP-
60
PHE-SER-PHE-PRO-ARG-ASN-ILE-SER-ALA-GLY-SER-LEU-GLY-SER-CYS-
75
TRP-GLY-ILE-THR-MET-VAL-ARG-GLY-LEU-ARG-VAL-THR-PRO-THR-SER-
90
PRO-SER-LEU-SER-TRP-GLU-VAL-PHE-LEU-ARG-THR-ARG-LEU-GLU-VAL-
105
GLU-ARG-GLU-ARG-ASP-VAL-PRO-PRO-PRO-ALA-PRO-PRO-ALA-GLY-ILE-
120
THR-ARG-SER-LYS-SER-LYS-HIS-GLU-LEU-LYS-LEU-LEU-GLU-LYS-ILE-
135
PRO-GLU-ASN-ALA-GLU-ALA-THR-VAL-VAL-LEU-VAL-GLY-CYS-VAL-GLU-
150
PHE-LEU-SER-ARG-PRO-THR-MET-ALA-PHE-VAL-ARG-LEU-ARG-GLU-ALA-
165
VAL-GLU-LEU-ASP-ALA-VAL-LEU-GLU-VAL-PRO-VAL-PRO-VAL-ARG-PHE-
180
LEU-PHE-LEU-LEU-LEU-GLY-PRO-SER-SER-ALA-ASN-MET-ASP-TYR-HIS-
195
GLU-ILE-GLY-ARG-SER-ILE-SER-THR-LEU-MET-SER-ASP-LYS-GLN-PHE-
210
HIS-GLU-ALA-ALA-TYR-LEU-ALA-ASP-GLU-ARG-GLU-ASP-LEU-LEU-THR-
225
ALA-ILE-ASN-ALA-PHE-LEU-ASP-CYS-SER-VAL-VAL-LEU-PRO-PRO-SER-
240
GLU-VAL-GLN-GLY-GLU-GLU-LEU-LEU-ARG-SER-VAL-ALA-HIS-PHE-GLN-
255
ARG-GLN-MET-LEU-LYS-LYS-ARG-GLU-GLU-GLN-GLY-ARG-LEU-LEU-PRO-
270
THR-GLY-ALA-GLY-LEU-GLU-PRO-LYS-SER-ALA-GLN-ASP-LYS-ALA-LEU-
285
LEU-GLN-MET-VAL-GLU-ARG-GLN-GLY-GLN-LEU-LYS-MET-ILE-PRO-SER-
300
ALA-ASP-GLY-ALA-ALA-PHE-GLY-GLY-LEU-ILE-ARG-ASP-VAL-ARG-ARG-
315
ARG-TYR-PRO-HIS-TYR-LEU-SER-ASP-PHE-ARG-ASP-ALA-LEU-ASP-PRO-
330
GLN-CYS-LEU-ALA-ALA-VAL-ILE-PHE-ILE-TYR-PHE-ALA-ALA-LEU-SER-
345

TABLE 2 (continued)
Amino Acid Sequence of Human Nonerythroid Band 3

PRO-ALA-ILE-THR-PHE-GLY-GLY-LEU-LEU-GLY-GLU-LYS-THR-GLN-ASP-
360
LEU-ILE-GLY-VAL-SER-GLU-LEU-ILE-MET-SER-THR-ALA-LEU-GLN-GLY-
375
VAL-VAL-PHE-CYS-LEU-LEU-GLY-ALA-GLN-PRO-LEU-LEU-VAL-ILE-GLY-
390
PHE-SER-GLY-PRO-LEU-LEU-VAL-PHE-GLU-GLU-ALA-PHE-PHE-SER-PHE-
405
CYS-SER-SER-ASN-HIS-LEU-GLU-TYR-LEU-VAL-GLY-ARG-VAL-TRP-ILE-
420
GLY-PHE-TRP-LEU-VAL-PHE-LEU-ALA-LEU-LEU-MET-VAL-ALA-LEU-GLY-
435
GLY-SER-PHE-LEU-VAL-ARG-PHE-VAL-SER-ARG-PHE-THR-ARG-GLU-ILE-
450
PHE-ALA-PHE-LEU-ILE-SER-LEU-ILE-PHE-ILE-TYR-GLU-THR-PHE-TYR-
465
LYS-LEU-VAL-LYS-ILE-PHE-GLN-GLU-HIS-PRO-LEU-HIS-GLY-CYS-SER-
480
ALA-SER-ASN-SER-SER-GLU-VAL-ASP-GLY-GLY-GLU-ASN-MET-THR-TRP-
495
ALA-GLY-ALA-ARG-PRO-THR-LEU-GLY-PRO-GLY-ASN-ARG-SER-LEU-ALA-
510
GLY-GLN-SER-GLY-GLN-GLY-LYS-PRO-ARG-GLY-GLN-PRO-ASN-THR-ALA-
525
PRO-LEU-SER-LEU-VAL-LEU-MET-ALA-GLY-THR-PHE-PHE-ILE-ALA-PHE-
540
PHE-LEU-ARG-LYS-PHE-LYS-ASN-SER-ARG-PHE-PHE-PRO-GLY-ARG-ILE-
555
ARG-ARG-VAL-ILE-GLY-ASP-PHE-GLY-VAL-PRO-ILE-ALA-ILE-LEU-ILE-
570
MET-VAL-LEU-VAL-ASP-TYR-SER-ILE-GLU-ASP-THR-TYR-THR-GLN-LYS-
585
LEU-SER-VAL-PRO-SER-GLY-PHE-SER-VAL-THR-ALA-PRO-GLU-LYS-ARG-
600
GLY-TRP-VAL-ILE-ASN-PRO-LEU-GLY-GLU-LYS-SER-PRO-PHE-PRO-VAL-
615
TRP-MET-MET-VAL-ALA-SER-LEU-LEU-PRO-ALA-ILE-LEU-VAL-PHE-ILE-
630
LEU-ILE-PHE-MET-GLU-THR-GLN-ILE-THR-THR-LEU-ILE-ILE-SER-LYS-
645
LYS-GLU-ARG-MET-LEU-GLN-LYS-GLY-SER-GLY-PHE-HIS-LEU-ASP-LEU-
660
LEU-LEU-ILE-VAL-ALA-MET-GLY-GLY-ILE-CYS-ALA-LEU-PHE-GLY-LEU-
675
PRO-TRP-LEU-ALA-ALA-ALA-THR-VAL-ARG-SER-VAL-THR-HIS-ALA-ASN-
690
ALA-LEU-THR-VAL-MET-SER-LYS-ALA-VAL-ALA-PRO-GLY-ASP-LYS-PRO-
705
LYS-ILE-GLN-GLU-VAL-LYS-GLU-GLN-ARG-VAL-THR-GLY-LEU-LEU-VAL-
720
ALA-LEU-LEU-VAL-GLY-LEU-SER-ILE-VAL-ILE-GLY-ASP-LEU-LEU-ARG-
735
GLN-ILE-PRO-LEU-ALA-VAL-LEU-PHE-GLY-ILE-PHE-LEU-TYR-MET-GLY-
750
VAL-THR-SER-LEU-ASN-GLY-ILE-GLN-PHE-TYR-GLU-ARG-LEU-HIS-LEU-
765
LEU-LEU-MET-PRO-PRO-LYS-HIS-HIS-PRO-ASP-VAL-THR-TYR-VAL-LYS-
780

TABLE 2 (continued)
Amino Acid Sequence of Human Nonerythroid Band 3

```
LYS-VAL-ARG-THR-LEU-ARG-MET-HIS-LEU-PHE-THR-ALA-LEU-GLN-LEU-
                                                            795
LEU-CYS-LEU-ALA-LEU-LEU-TRP-ALA-VAL-MET-SER-THR-ALA-ALA-SER-
                                                            810
LEU-ALA-PHE-PRO-PHE-ILE-LEU-ILE-LEU-THR-VAL-PRO-LEU-ARG-MET-
                                                            825
VAL-VAL-LEU-THR-ARG-ILE-PHE-THR-ASP-ARG-GLU-MET-LYS-CYS-LEU-
                                                            840
ASP-ALA-ASN-GLU-ALA-GLU-PRO-VAL-PHE-ASP-GLU-ARG-GLU-GLY-VAL-
                                                            855
ASP-GLU-TYR-ASN-GLU-MET-PRO-MET-PRO-VAL
```

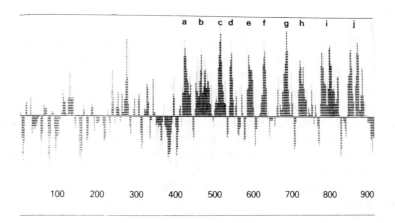

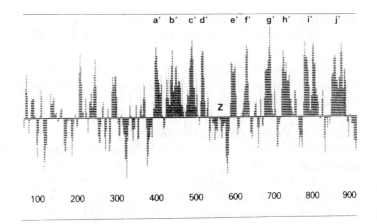

FIGURE 7. Hydropathy plot of murine band 3 (top) and human nonerythroid band 3 (bottom). See Tables 1 and 2 for the complete amino acid sequences. (From Demuth, D. R., Showe, L. C., Ballantine, M., Palumbo, A., Fraser, P. J., Cioe, L., Rovera, G., and Curtis, P. J., *EMBO J.*, 5, 1205, 1986. With permission.)

to be a "hinge" region of the cytoplasmic domain. Two additional regions of homology were identified by Demuth and co-workers.[202] They are residues 398 to 423 (80% homology) and residues 232 to 336 (50% homology).

Several other regions of the primary structure of the cytoplasmic domain have been characterized.[149] For example, all of the tryptophans of the cytoplasmic domain are located between residues 89 and 119 of the murine sequence. Also, the extremely acidic nature of the N-terminus seen in human band 3[181] is not a common feature of avian (chicken) and rodent band 3, which have significantly fewer acidic N-terminal residues. This difference leads to reduction or elimination of cytoplasmic protein binding (see Chapter 4).

E. HYDROPATHY PLOTS OF BAND 3

Having determined the primary structure of murine band 3, Kopito and Lodish[201] calculated the hydrophobicity index using the algorithm of Kyte and Doolittle.[204] The hydrophobicities were averaged over 11 successive spans of amino acids and the results are shown in Figure 7 (top plot). There are two notable features about this structure. First, the protein can be divided roughly into two major domains. The N-terminal half (amino acids 1 to 400) is predominantly hydrophilic, in agreement with experiment. Secondly, an integral domain is defined which is rather large compared to other integral membrane transport proteins (52 kDa). This domain contains about 450 amino acids and is predominantly amphipathic. Clusters of hydrophobic residues (corresponding to peaks a to j) are placed between polar, predominantly basic residues. Finally, the 32 C-terminal residues are rather acidic (11 glu or asp residues). Kopito and Lodish[201] suggested that this may constitute a third domain of the protein and that it should be water soluble and not buried within the lipid bilayer.

These structural interpretations for murine band 3 have been fully confirmed and extended to human nonerythroid band 3 in the study by Demuth and his co-workers.[202] Figure 7 shows comparative hydrophobicity plots for murine band 3 (top) and for pHKB3 (bottom). The plots were aligned from the C terminus, and the amino acids are numbered according to Kopito and Lodish.[201] The hydrophobicity patterns for these two proteins are quite similar, save for the conspicuous and extremely hydrophilic Z insert sequence in pHKB3 mentioned above. Both proteins contain ten hydrophobic regions (a to j in MEB3 and a' to j' in pHKB33). The high degree of conservation between the two structures in the membrane-spanning domain is consistent with the high level of sequence homology present within this domain (71%).

V. THE FOLDED STRUCTURE OF THE WATER-SOLUBLE CYTOPLASMIC DOMAIN OF BAND 3 (CDB3)

The primary function of the water-soluble, N-terminal cytoplasmic domain of band 3 (CDB3) is to provide an anchoring site for cytoskeletal proteins and also to bind glycolytic enzymes and hemoglobin in human band 3.

A. HYDRODYNAMIC PROPERTIES OF CDB3

Low and co-workers[147,148] have investigated the hydrodynamic properties of CDB3 while Makino and co-workers[146] performed similar studies on bovine CDB3. Gel filtration studies were used to determine Stokes' radius, while sedimentation velocity studies were performed to determine the molecular weight. The data from these studies is given in Table 3. Bovine and human CDB3 have similar hydrodynamic properties. Low and co-workers[147] found that the molecular weight of CDB3 was not significantly dependent on pH. In addition, there was no protein concentration dependence over the ranges studied. They concluded that the isolated cytoplasmic domain retains the dimeric form under all solution conditions examined.

Changes in CDB3 morphology can be deduced by measuring changes in Stokes' radius as a function of pH (Figure 8).[147] The value of the Stokes' radius increases from 55 at pH 6 to 66 at pH 10. A spherical protein with a mass of 95 kDa and a partial specific volume of 0.74 cm^3/g[148] should have a radius of about 30 Å. Values of 55 to 66 strongly suggest that CDB3 is highly asymmetric. Based on the CDB3 frictional ratio of 1.6, Low[149] calculates an axial ratio of 10 and after other assumptions, concludes that the CDB3 dimer should be about 25 Å in diameter and 250 Å long. These estimates of the CDB3 dimensions are consistent with the EM studies of Weinstein and co-workers[96,98-100] discussed above.

TABLE 3
Physical-Chemical Characteristics of CDB3

	Stokes' radius (Å)	Sedimentation coefficient (s)	Polypeptide mol wt (× 10⁻³)	No. subunits	Frictional ratio	Ref.
Human CDB3	53	4.1	40.0	2	1.6	148
Bovine CDB3	52	4.7	50.0	2	1.55	146

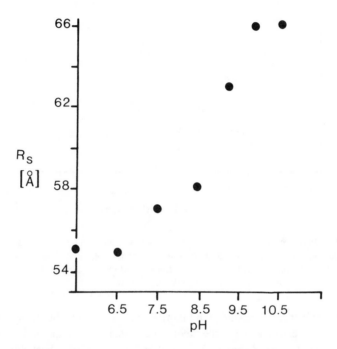

FIGURE 8. The Stokes' radius (R_s) of the isolated cytoplasmic domain of band 3 as a function of pH. (From Low, P. S., Westfall, M. A., Allen, D. P., and Appell, K. C., *J. Biol. Chem.*, 259, 13070, 1984. With permission.)

B. CIRCULAR DICHROISM STUDIES OF CDB3

The optical activity of proteins in solution and in membranes has been used to determine protein structural properties,[205] in particular the circular dichroism (CD) spectrum of the protein. CD is the difference in sample absorbance of left and right circularly polarized light.[205] One of the more useful applications of this form of spectroscopy is the estimation of the degree of alpha-helical content assumed by a polypeptide, since the optical activity depends profoundly upon conformation of the peptide. The alpha-helix is characterized by two negative dichroic bands at 222 and 209 nm as well as a positive dichroic band at 191 nm.[205] There is a characteristic "notch" in the negative CD at 215 nm. By way of contrast, the CD for a disordered chain shows a small negative band at 238 nm, a weak positive CD maximum at 217 nm, and a strong negative band at 198 nm.

Appell and Low[148] published a CD spectrum for human CDB3 and calculated the amount of alpha-helical content using the ellipticity at 208 nm according to the method of Greenfield and Fasman.[206] They obtained a value of about 37%. A similar value was obtained by Moriyama and co-workers for bovine CDB3 using the same approach.[146] More recently Oikawa and co-workers[207] have performed similar measurements and found a significantly smaller alpha-

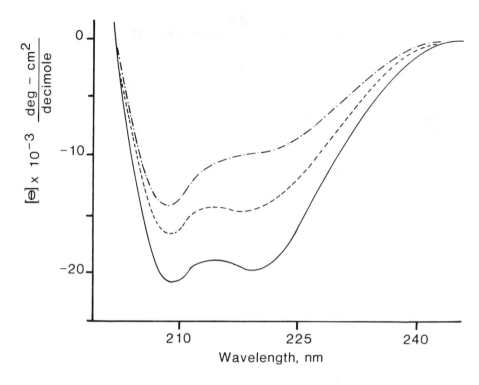

FIGURE 9. Far ultraviolet circular dichroism spectra of purified band 3 in $C_{12}E_8$ (- - -), of the cytoplasmic domain of band 3 in 150 mM NaCl and 20 mM sodium phosphate (–●–) and of the membrane associated domain in the above detergent (—). All samples were at pH 8. (From Oikawa, K., Lieberman, D. M., and Reithmeier, R. A. F., *Biochemistry*, 24, 2843, 1985. With permission.)

helical content. Their spectra are shown in Figure 9. Also shown are the CD spectra of purified band 3 in a nonionic detergent and of the membrane-associated domain in the same detergent. The researchers found a helical content for CDB3 of 27% and a beta-sheet content of 48%. By comparison, the membrane-bound domain had a much higher alpha-helix content, and the sum of the helical content of the two domains equaled that of the whole molecule. The lower helical content of CDB3 compared to the other studies may be attributed to differences in CD collection conditions and to differences in the way the helical value was calculated. Oikawa and co-workers[207] used the method of Chen and co-workers,[208] employing the entire CD spectrum, while Appell and Low[148] made single wavelength calculations. Kaul and co-workers[181] made Chou-Fasman type calculations of the amount of alpha-helical content based on their direct determination of the primary structure of the first 201 N-terminal amino acids. They obtained a value of about 40% alpha-helical content. They suggest that serine-182 to proline-188 constitutes a beta-turn region of the peptide, which would seem to agree with the findings of Kopito and co-workers.[209] Finally, Oikawa and co-workers[207] found that the cytoplasmic domain was readily denatured by guanidine HCl, while the purified membrane-bound domain was resistant.

C. FLUORESCENCE SPECTROSCOPY OF CDB3

Low and co-workers[147,148,210] and Bjerrum and associates[211] have presented fluorescence spectroscopic evidence for the existence of multiple conformations of CDB3. Figure 10, from Low,[147,149] shows the effects of pH on the conformational equilibrium of CDB3 with and without denaturation by heat or by 8 M urea. The fluorescence arises from the cluster of tryptophan residues located in the 21-kDa N-terminal portion of CDB3. Two apparent pK values are seen: one at pH 7.2 and the other at pH 9.2. These titration curves were interpreted in terms of three

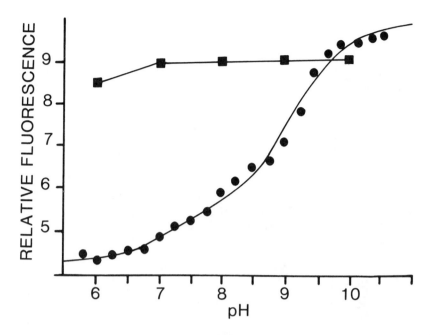

FIGURE 10. The pH and temperature dependence of the conformational equilibrium of the cytoplasmic domain of band 3 monitored by intrinsic fluorescence as a function of pH (●). The relative fluorescence of heat-denatured or 8-*M* urea-denatured fragment is also plotted as a function of pH (■). (From Low, P. S., Westfall, M. A., Allen, D. P., and Appell, K. C., *J. Biol. Chem.*, 259, 13070, 1984. With permission.)

native and reversibly interconvertible conformations of CDB3. The curves are believed to be the conformations responsible for the variation in Stokes' radius. These structural transitions can also be detected in ghost preparations using calorimetry.[210]

The changes in hydrodynamic properties with pH suggested that CDB3 is in a more extended structure at high pH.[147] The changes do not appear to involve alterations in the degree of self-association of the fragments. Fluorescence kinetic studies show that the equilibria are rapidly attained and involve a change in tertiary structure.[147] Low and co-workers[147] presented fluorescence energy transfer data to support the hypothesis that the tertiary conformational changes involved a pivoting of the two subdomains of CDB3 around the proline "hinge" between them. The authors showed this by labeling the –SH groups of the 20-kDa C-terminal (with respect to the hinge) subdomain with the sulfhydryl fluorescent reagent 1,5-IAEDANS (*N*-[iodoacetylaminoethyl]-5-naphthylamine-1-sulfonate). They then measured fluorescence energy transfer efficiency between that moiety and the band 3 tryptophan residues which are conveniently clustered within the N-terminal 21-kDa subdomain. Figure 11 shows a comparison of fluorescence energy transfer efficiencies between the two fluorophores at pHs 6.5 and 10.[147] The efficiency of energy transfer estimated from the ratio of donor quantum yield in the presence and absence of acceptor was 0.34 at pH 6.5 and 0.22 at pH 10. The decrease in energy transfer efficiency at higher pH occurred in the face of a twofold increase in donor quantum yield. This fact strongly supports the hypothesis that the donor and acceptor are closer to each other at pH 6.5 than at pH 10.

The authors raised several points of caution about the interpretation of their results. One of the most interesting was the demonstration that modification of the –SH groups of CDB3 completely changed the character of the pH-dependent transition seen in Figure 10. Instead of multiple titrations, only a single titration could be seen after modification of the –SH groups of the fragment. The single pK observed was now at pH 8.7, while the total fluorescence change was comparable to the combined transitions shown in Figure 10. The authors concluded that –SH modification causes superposition of the two structural transitions into a single conformational event.[147] The number of significant states has been reduced by –SH modification.

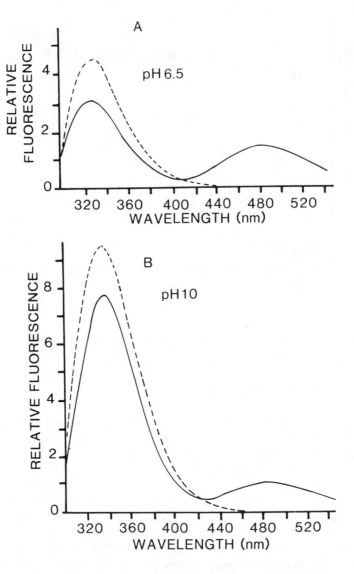

FIGURE 11.   Comparison of the efficiency of fluorescence energy transfer from the cytoplasmic domain tryptophans to covalently attached IAEDANS at pH 6.5 (A) and pH 10 (B). Dashed lines (- - -) and solid lines (—) represent the emission spectra (lambda$_{ex}$, 290 nm) of the unlabeled and IAEDANS-labeled cytoplasmic domains, respectively. All four spectra were conducted at identical domain concentrations and spectrophotometer settings, and therefore, they can be directly compared. (From Low, P. S., Westfall, M. A., Allen, D. P., and Appell, K. C., *J. Biol. Chem.,* 259, 13070, 1984. With permission.)

D. STATE OF SULFHYDRYL GROUPS ON CDB3

The possibility that sulfhydryl reactive reagents perturb the conformation of CDB3[147] raises the question of the number and disposition of –SH groups in CDB3. Rao and Reithmier[110,212] first showed that the sulfhydryl groups are clustered in the C-terminal 20-kDa subdomain and that human CDB3 contains about two reactive sulfhydryl groups. One is located (in the linear amino acid sequence) very close to the site of trypsin digestion that yields the 20-kDa piece, while the second group is located 15-kDa N-terminal to that site.[110] However, despite the fact that the two sulfhydryl groups are well separated in the linear sequence, each of the cystines participates in interdomain[110] and intradomain[151] disulfide bond formation. These findings strongly suggest that the two sulfhydryl groups are spatially close within the CDB3 dimer and may form a cluster within a pocket at the interface between the two CDB3 monomers.

Salhany and Cassoly[213] have recently probed the structure of the CDB3 dimer by studying the stopped-flow kinetics of *p*-chloromercuribenzoate (PMB) binding to CDB3 sulfhydryls. This method has been extensively used by Gibson and Antonini and their co-workers[214] in the hemoglobin research field to detect conformational differences between oxy- and deoxyhemoglobin. The time-course data of Figure 12 for PMB reaction with isolated CDB3 show the presence of two equally weighted exponentials. The concentration dependence of the rate constants for both phases showed saturation behavior (Figure 13). Salhany and Cassoly[213] proposed a model where PMB reacts with the sulfhydryl cluster on the C-terminal 20-kDa half of CDB3 through a mechanism like that shown in Figure 14. This mechanism implies that PMB approaches a saturable sulfhydryl pocket and then chemically reacts with the –SH groups. The PMB reaction will be used in Chapter 4 to show how hemoglobin can alter the conformation of CDB3.

E. A STRUCTURAL MODEL FOR CDB3

The possibility of a conformational hinge and of rapid, pH-induced tertiary conformational changes led Low and his co-workers[147] to propose the model for CDB3 shown in Figure 15. The very N-terminal acidic portion is shown as an elongated, highly charged structure which binds enzymes, hemoglobin, and hemichromes. The locations of the tryptophan cluster, an IgG binding site, and the ankyrin binding site are shown, relative to the regulated hinge. The –SH group cluster is shown in the 20-kDa subdomain. It seems clear that the highly elongated nature of CDB3 has the purpose of multisite interactions with cytosolic components. However, are these interactions static or do they occur in a dynamic concert depending on conditions in the cytosol? Can ligand binding alter conformation of CDB3 which is then transmitted to the integral domain? Several papers have been cited which suggest that some form of connection is needed to explain changes in the structure of the integral domain which occur upon hemolysis (Section III. B).

VI. STRUCTURAL STUDIES OF THE 52-KDA INTEGRAL DOMAIN OF BAND 3

A. INTRODUCTION

Figure 7 showed that the integral domain of band 3 has more hydrophobic and amphipathic character than the water-soluble cytoplasmic half of the protein. The integral domain is thought to function in anion exchange since it contains numerous inhibitor binding sites. The fundamental question is how the structure of the domain explains the anion-exchange kinetics. How many physiological anion binding sites are there on one band 3 monomer? How far apart are they? Does the monomer form a channel or do oligomeric states contribute to channel formation? Unfortunately, we do not know the crystal structure of band 3, so all detailed structural interpretations to date must be considered speculative. In fact, many rather detailed structural and kinetic models have been presented, yet there are almost no detailed studies of anion transport inhibition from the inner surface of the membrane. Furthermore, there are no direct measurements of the binding stoichiometry of either chloride, bicarbonate, or sulfate to isolated band 3. All of these functional problems will be discussed in detail later. They are mentioned here to emphasize the fact that we are at a primitive state of knowledge concerning the structure/function of band 3.

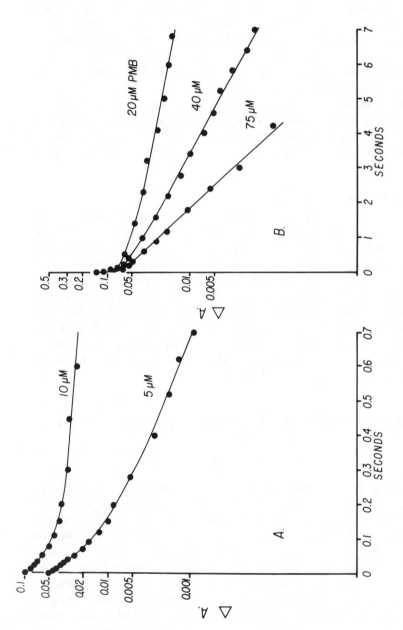

FIGURE 12. Time courses of PMB binding to the sulfhydryl groups on CDB3. The final protein concentration was 5 μ*M* in CDB3 monomer. The final PMB concentrations for each curve are shown in the figure. The samples were in 5 m*M* phosphate buffer, pH 6. The temperature was 25°C. The reaction was followed at 255 nm in a 2-cm cell. A shows data at low PMB for the initial time periods. The lines drawn in both A and B are based on computer fits to an equation representing the weighted sum of two exponentials:

$$\Delta A = \Delta A_f \exp(-k_f t) + \Delta A_s \exp(-k_s t)$$

where ΔA is the observed absorbance change and the ks are apparent rate constants with f and s meaning fast and slow, respectively. (From Salhany, J. M. and Cassoly, R., *J. Biol. Chem.*, 264, 1399, 1989. With permission.)

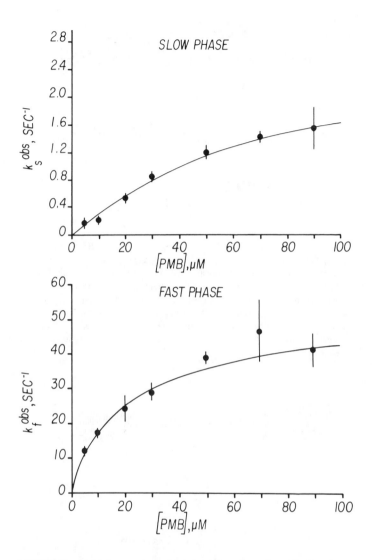

FIGURE 13. Plot of computer-extracted rate constants from kinetic progress curves at various PMB concentrations. The kinetic constants from double exponential fits like those shown in Figure 12 were plotted vs. their respective PMB concentrations. The data were fit to Equation 2 of Figure 14. The lines drawn come from the fits and the constants are fast phase: $k_{+2} = 50$ sec^{-1}; $K_{-1} = 20$ μM and slow phase: $k_{+2} = 3.1$ sec^{-1}; $K_{-1} = 80$ μM. (From Salhany, J. M. and Cassoly, R., *J. Biol. Chem.,* 264, 1399, 1989. With permission.)

B. PHYSICAL-CHEMICAL PROPERTIES OF THE INTEGRAL 52-KDA DOMAIN

There are several methods available for isolating intact band 3[134,142-145] and its various proteolytic fragments[141,142,151] in nonionic detergents. Reithmeier[151] and later Makino and Nakashima[141] studied the detergent binding properties and state of association of the 52-kDa domain of human and bovine band 3. These authors showed that this domain comprises the bulk of nonionic detergent binding sites. They also determined the hydrodynamic and molecular parameters of the 52-kDa domain. After removal of the cytoplasmic domain with trypsin and solubilization in Triton X-100, Reithmeier[151] characterized the purified protein using gel filtration and sucrose density gradient centrifugation. The values of the various physical parameters for both human and bovine fragments are given in Table 4. In Triton X-100, the integral domain of human band 3 exists as a dimer.[151] This contrasts with the various oligomeric

$$1.\ P + S \xrightleftharpoons[k_{-1}]{k_{+1}} (PS)^* \xrightarrow{k_{+2}} (PS)$$

$$2.\ k_{obs} = (k_{+2}(P_0)/K_{-1} + (P_0))$$

$$where\ K_{-1} = k_{-1}/k_{+1}$$

FIGURE 14.   Mechanism of PMB binding to a single CDB3 sulfhydryl group. This mechanism proposes a reversible preequilibrium of PMB with the protein followed by a chemical reaction step (Equation 1) where P = PMB; S = sulfhydryl groups; (PS)* is the initial complex; and (PS) the final covalent complex. The scheme can be described by the second equation with the terms defined as shown and with P_0 being the total concentration of PMB after mixing. Equation 2 was used to fit the data shown in Figure 13. (From Salhany, J. M. and Cassoly, R., *J. Biol. Chem.* 264, 1399, 1989. With permission.)

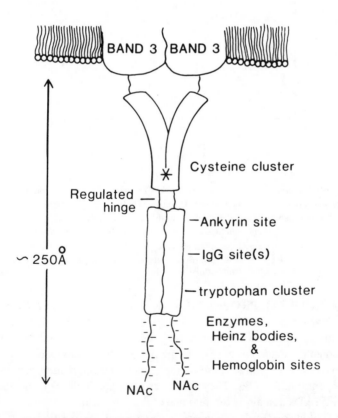

FIGURE 15.   Sketch of the major structural features of CDB3.(From Low, P. S., Westfall, M. A., Allen, D. P., and Appell, K. C., *J. Biol. Chem.*, 259, 13070, 1984. With permission.)

TABLE 4
Physical-Chemical Properties of Band 3 and the Integral Domain of
Band 3 for Human and Bovine

	Human band 3	Human 52-kDa	Bovine band 3	Bovine 52-kDa
Detergent	Triton	Triton	$C_{12}E_9$	$C_{12}E_9$
Sed. coeff. (S)	6.9	5.7	—	—
Partial sp vol (ml/mg)	0.81	0.84	—	—
Stokes' radius (Å)	80	73	80	90
Subunits	2	2	2, 4	Oligomers

states observed in the nonionic detergent $C_{12}E_9$ with bovine band 3.[141] Chymotrypsin digestion at the outer surface (which does not affect anion transport when performed with low concentrations) does not cause CH17 and CH35 to dissociate when isolated in Triton X-100.[151]

C. DISPOSITION OF SULFHYDRYL GROUPS ON THE INTEGRAL DOMAIN OF BAND 3

The modification of band 3 sulfhydryl groups by either organic mercurials[215] or N-ethylmaleimide (NEM)[174] does not affect the rate of anion exchange. The amino acid sequence shown in Table 1 indicates that mouse erythrocyte band 3 has six sulfhydryl groups. They are located at positions 152, 215, 330, 498, 861, and 903.[201] The amino acid composition of human erythrocyte band 3 also suggests the presence of six sulfhydryl groups.[85] However, the recently determined primary structure of human nonerythroid band 3 (Table 2) shows nine sulfhydryl groups.[202] According to the numbering system of Table 2, they are located at residues 75, 148, 233, 332, 379, 406, 479, 797, and 839. Mouse 903, 861, and 498 correspond to human nonerythroid 839, 797, and 406. Human nonerythroid band 3 has two more integral sulfhydryl groups at 379 and 332 which are not found in the mouse or apparently in human erythroid sequences. The latter two contain alanine at 471. Residue 424 in mouse is a valine, while no information is available about human erythroid band 3 at that position (see Addendum).

The number of sulfhydryl groups present in a given protein sequence is not, of course, always equal to the number of chemically reactive sulfhydryls observed experimentally. Rao[174] studied sulfhydryl reactivity using membrane permeant and impermeant maleamides. She found five reactive sulfhydryl groups, all of which were accessible only to the membrane-permeant reagent NEM. Two of the sulfhydryl groups are on CDB3, and three reactive groups are present in the integral domain, two of which are localized to CH35. Extensive proteolytic digestion experiments have further localized these two groups to an 8 to 9-kDa fragment of CH35 (groups 861 and 903 of the murine sequence).[216,217]

Although the entire sequence of human erythrocyte band 3 is not known as of this writing, (see Addendum), there is reason to believe that there is a sixth sulfhydryl group present in the integral domain which is not reactive toward NEM. This sixth, or so-called cryptic, sulfhydryl group is on the integral domain of human erythrocyte band 3, located in the CH17 subdomain.[216,217] This group is not reactive toward NEM in intact cells, but does apparently react with pCMBS.[218-220] The exact residue containing this sulfhydryl group is not known for the human erythrocyte version of band 3. In mouse, cys 498 is a likely candidate. However, human nonerythroid band 3 has a cystine at a position only ten residues from lysine 561 of the murine numbering system. This proximity could account for the fact that pCMBS binding alters both the extent and the rate of reversible stilbene disulfonate binding. Finally, Toon and co-workers[220] also presented evidence that DTNB (5,5'-dithiobis-[2-nitrobenzoate]) binding reduces the rate of reversible stilbene-disulfonate binding. However, DTNB reacts covalently with a sulfhydryl on NEM pretreated membranes at a seventh and distinct cryptic sulfhydryl which reacts with neither NEM or pCMBS.[220] This site does not seem to affect any transport process. There is a second low affinity DTNB site which is a reversible binding, nonsulfhydryl-containing domain and which inhibits anion transport when occupied.[220,221] This second site also inhibits water transport and has been used to show that band 3 is involved in that process as well. If the integral domain of human erythrocyte band 3 is comparable to that of human nonerythroid band 3, then there are at least three additional integral sulfhydryls which could account for the new DTNB covalent site.[220]

D. DIRECT EVIDENCE ON THE NUMBER OF MEMBRANE CROSSINGS
1. General Considerations

One of the initial indications of the number of membrane crossings came from work with the enzyme pepsin.[222,223] Bilateral digestion of ghosts with pepsin digests all exposed portions of band 3 and produces five different 4-kDa membrane-bound fragments.[223] A helical segment of this size would be expected to cross the membrane one time. In Figure 9 the removal of the cytosolic extension greatly increased the degree of alpha-helical content as revealed in the CD spectrum. This result, in combination with the pepsin digestion studies (where all peripheral extensions of band 3 would be cut), supports the view that there may be at least five integral alpha-helices within the 52-kDa domain.[223]

Enzymatic digestion has been used to define the orientation of the N-terminal and the C-terminal ends of the 52-kDa fragment. It is well established that the N-terminus of band 3 enters the cytoplasm, since the water-soluble 41-kDa fragment is only released when trypsin or chymotrypsin is added at the cytoplasmic face. Lieberman and co-workers[88,224] have recently employed carboxypeptidase Y to digest band 3 and have shown that amino acids were released from the C-terminus and from the 52-kDa domain of band 3 isolated in nonionic detergents. In ghosts, digestion only occurred when cytoskeletal proteins were stripped by alkali or high salt, and the band 3 of intact red cells was not affected at all. The researchers concluded that the C-terminus of band 3 is located at the cytoplasmic side of the membrane.[224] In a more recent study,[88] polyclonal antibodies were raised against a synthetic peptide corresponding to the 12 amino acids of the C-terminal sequence of murine band 3. Carboxypeptidase Y digestion of mouse membranes eliminated antibody binding, which occurs in ghosts and permeabilized cells, but not in intact erythrocytes. The authors concluded that since both amino and carboxyl termini are cytoplasmic, band 3 should cross the membrane an even number of times, with either 8, 10, or 12 transmembrane segments.[88]

2. Number of CH17 Crossings

The apparent molecular weight of CH17 has been reported to be as low as 14.5 kDa[94] and as high as 20 kDa,[191] depending on the type of gel electrophoretic system used. A fragment that size could conceivably have five transmembrane helical crossings. Williams and co-workers[191] performed mapping studies by labeling band 3 with lactoperoxidase iodination. This was followed by digestion of the protein with thermolysin and trypsin. Thermolysin cleaves at four extracellular sites including one very near the major extracellular chymotryptic site (Figure 5). On the basis of these studies, they proposed a model with three membrane crossings between the cytoplasmic N-terminus and the principal thermolysin cleavage site.[191] These crossings include one intracellular and two extracellular loops. Other workers have proposed a similar number of crossings.[192,217,225]

Jennings and Nicknish[188] investigated the topology of CH17 with chemical labeling and proteolytic cleavage methods. They studied two well-defined CNBr-generated peptides from CH17. One is an N-terminal 6-kDa fragment and the other is a C-terminal 11-kDa piece (Figure 5). They studied labeling of three exofacial lysine residues on CH17, one located on the 6-kDa fragment and the other two on the 11-kDa piece. The 11-kDa fragment contains the covalent

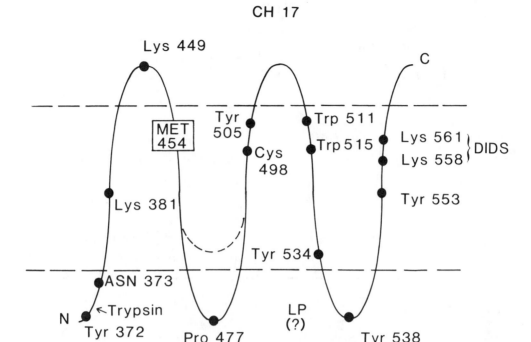

FIGURE 16. Schematic of the CH17 integral subdomain of murine band 3. LP = lactoperoxidase labeling sites.

extracellular DIDS labeling site in its C-terminus near the extracellular chymotryptic site. They discovered that the lysine residue in the 6-kDa fragment can be labeled from the extracellular surface of the membrane.[188] Thus, it appears that CH17 must span the bilayer more than once.

Figure 16 summarizes the major conclusions concerning the number of times CH17 may cross the bilayer. The sequence numbers of the residues are those of the murine sequence (Table 1). The N-terminal trypsin cleavage site is at Tyr 372, yielding an N-terminal asparagine (373) for the resulting integral domain of murine band 3. The next experimentally established site is Lys 449, which is the exofacial site of reductive methylation on the 6-kDa CNBr fragment.[188] The 6-kDa fragment is defined from Asn 373 to Met 454, while the 11-kDa fragment runs from Met 454 to the principal extracellular chymotryptic site at Tyr 572 (not shown). One of the main questions to consider is the number of times the 11-kDa CNBr fragment partially or fully crosses the bilayer before reaching the outer surface. Jay and Cantley[226] do not favor a structure in which a complete crossing occurs for the N-terminal segment of the 11-kDa CNBr piece leading to Cys 498. They suggest that the proline at 477 may cause the peptide to turn out toward the extracellular surface. In addition, this part of the segment seems too small to form a transmembrane alpha-helix.

The results of Williams and co-workers[191] seem clearly to identify an intracellular lactoperoxidase iodination site on what would be the Jennings and Nicknish 11-kDa CNBr fragment of CH17. According to the murine sequence, Tyr 534 or 538 would be likely sites for intracellular iodination. The region between Tyr 505 and the extracellular C-terminal chymotryptic site is large enough to cross the membrane and has charged groups that would exist within the bilayer if the secondary structure were alpha-helical. Furthermore, the only two tryptophans of CH17 are at 511 and 515. Kleinfeld and co-workers,[227] using fluorescence methods, showed that the tryptophans of the integral domain are located on the extracellular half of the helices.

Pradhan and Lala[228] have very recently studied photochemical labeling of the hydrophobic core of band 3 using tritiated 2-diazofluorene. The label was equally distributed between CH17

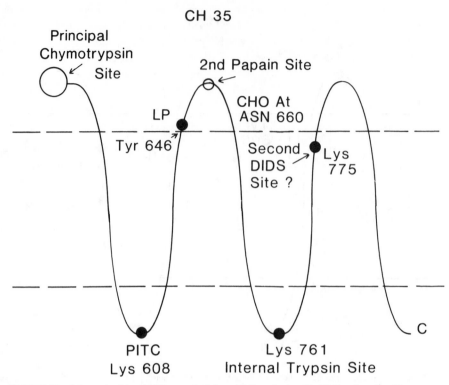

FIGURE 17.   Schematic of the CH35 integral subdomain of murine band 3. PITC = phenylisothiocyanate; LP = lactoperoxidase labeling site; and CHO = glycosylation site.

and CH35. In a recent personal communication, Lala states that all three fragments which can result from extensive CNBr cleavage are labeled by the reagent. This further suggests that CH17 has at least three integral or transmembrane segments.

3. Number of CH35 Crossings

On the basis of size alone, CH35 could be expected, theoretically, to form about ten transmembranal helices, giving a total of 15 transmembrane crossings for the entire 52-kDa fragment. As we saw earlier (Figure 5), there are three extracellular papain cleavage sites. Two are very near the principal chymotrypsin site and one is C-terminal to that site. In Figure 17, the third papain cleavage site of Figure 5 (P$_3$ of that figure) is designated as the second principal cleavage site. The two principal extracellular papain cleavage sites (P$_1$ or P$_2$ and P$_3$, Figure 5) generate a 7- to 8-kDa integral fragment which Jennings and co-workers call P7, and also a 28-kDa C-terminal fragment.[192,193] The 65-residue P7 segment probably crosses the membrane twice (Figure 17). Brock and co-workers[194] sequenced a 72-amino acid fragment which roughly corresponds to P7. P7 contains an exofacial lactoperoxidase iodination site (Tyr 646 in the murine sequence). In addition, lysine 608 can be labeled by phenylisothiocyanate (PITC) at the inner surface, which would favor two crossings.[194]

The structural outline of the remainder of the 28-kDa fragment is incomplete. However, some recent papers have been published which identify an internal trypsin cleavage site[91] and which show that the C-terminus is cytoplasmic.[88,224] Jennings and co-workers[91] demonstrated the presence of an internal trypsin cleavage site at lysine 761 of the murine sequence. It lies between the extracellular papain cleavage site (which generates P7 and the 28-kDa fragments) and the cytoplasmically placed C-terminus (Figure 17). The stretch of peptide between the extracellular papain site and the internal trypsin site must cross the membrane at least once, but owing to its size, probably crosses three times. Finally, there is a second DIDS-reactive lysine residue which is involved in cross-linking CH17 to CH35 at alkaline pH.[154] Jennings and co-workers[91] showed that it lies between 70 and 168 residues from the C-terminus and could therefore be lysine 775, 832, 835, 844, or 847, of the murine sequence (Table 1).

In summary, the experimental evidence would support at least three and possibly five transmembrane crossings for CH35, approximately one half the number expected theoretically for a fragment this size.

E. SOME SPECULATIONS ON THE ARRANGEMENT OF THE BAND 3 SEGMENTS OF THE INTEGRAL DOMAIN

Hydropathy plots of murine and human nonerythroid band 3 show that there is a striking degree of conservation within the integral domain in that both encompass ten amphipathic regions (Figure 7). This structural similarity between the two species does not seem coincidental. Regions like the ten amphipathic segments of the integral domain shown in Figure 7, containing at least 23 amino acids with hydropathy averages greater than 1.5, are often tightly associated with the lipid. The high helical content of the core structure of band 3 as shown in CD measurements strongly suggests that these regions are alpha-helices. Kopito and Lodish[201,229] analyzed the sequence further and concluded that the ten amphipathic regions could form 12 transmembrane helices with virtually all potentially membrane-spanning helices showing amphipathic character. Kopito and Lodish[229] suggested further that these helices could cluster to form at least one or possibly two hydrophilic regions in which the charged residues involved in the anion-exchange process are allowed to pair and form a stable structure.

The algorithm used by Kopito and Lodish to determine the helices obviously influences the conclusions. However, Lodish[230] has recently questioned the use of that algorithm. He now favors a model with eight membrane-spanning helices forming an outer ring in contact with lipid. The remainder of the C-terminus would consist of shorter alpha-helices (about ten residues long) forming an inner ring of helices in contact with the outer ring, but not in contact with the lipid bilayer. The inner helices would form the anion passageway and undergo the conformational change that causes alternation of the anion site from inward- to outward-facing forms. This proposal may be more consistent with a realistic packing of the helices. It is also consistent with the newer results from Jennings and co-workers[91] indicating the presence of an internal trypsin cleavage site at lysine 761 of the murine sequence discussed earlier. In the last analysis, it must be concluded that the structure of the integral domain of the monomer is unknown. There is no direct evidence as to whether or not it forms a channel. It could form at least one channel, it is large enough to form two channels,[229] but it may form none. Amino acids involved at the transport sites may be contributing to a common channel formed by the band 3 dimer.

The possible arrangement of the integral CH17 and CH35 subdomains with respect to the binding site of the transport inhibitor DIDS was elucidated in a revealing study published by Jennings and Passow.[154] They discovered that the two chymotryptic integral domains could be cross-linked by DIDS to form the 100-kDa band 3, when the pH was raised to alkaline levels (pH 9 or greater). Was the cross-linked product formed by inter- or by intramolecular DIDS cross-linking? This point was tested by treating the cells with DIDS at alkaline pH without chymotrypsin pretreatment. The authors did not observe formation of covalent dimers, despite the fact that the two integral fragments were cross-linked. Formation of intramolecular cross-links by DIDS, combined with its ability to inhibit linearly anion transport, has suggested that each monomer contains one transport site or class of sites and that both chymotryptic subdomains are intimate with that site.

Several studies have addressed the question of the spatial arrangement of the CH17 and CH35 subdomains within the dimer.[118,119] Staros and Kakkad[118] have provided evidence through cross-linking that the CH17 fragment of one monomer is in close contact with the CH35 fragment of the other monomer. The results of their study would be consistent with a model of the anion-

A. Subdomains Form Common Channel

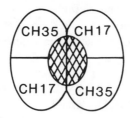

B. Subdomains Form Separate Channels

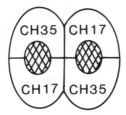

FIGURE 18.   Possible structural arrangement of the integral subdomains within a band 3 dimer forming a common channel between monomers or with separate channels on each monomer.

exchange channel in which subunits form a head-to-head dimer with a twofold axis of symmetry perpendicular to the plane of the membrane. They further pointed out that their cross-linking data were not consistent with a tetrameric model in which four subunits are related by a fourfold axis of symmetry. Jennings and Nicknish[119] presented cross-linking studies which confirmed those just described. They also showed that the intermolecular cross-linking site for BS[3] is near the exofacial chymotryptic cleavage site, an indication that this region of the 52-kDa domain is at the dimer subunit interface. However, the discovery of the BS[3] cross-linked tetramer by Salhany and Sloan[120] shows that more than one intermonomeric cross-link can form, depending on quaternary structure. In the TC-state, one cross-links intermonomerically to form the dimer, and one cross-links two dimers to form a tetramer.

Figure 18 shows two possible structures of the band 3 dimer that would be consistent with the cross-linking results. The tetramer would form by cross-linking two of these dimers. In each case CH17 of one monomer is arranged to be near CH35 of the other. In the first model, the four subdomains of the dimer contribute to a common channel. The second model shows a single channel per monomer. Very recently, Beth and co-workers[231] have found that the minimum distance between each monomeric stilbene site is 16 Å. This distance could favor a two-channel dimer (Figure 18B) and shows that these sites are too far apart for steric interactions between stilbene molecules. These distance measurements are consistent with previous fluorescence measurements.[121,150]

VII. EFFECT OF QUATERNARY STRUCTURE ON THE FOLDED STRUCTURE AND INHIBITOR-BINDING CAPACITY OF THE INTEGRAL DOMAIN OF THE MONOMER

The strength of the association between CH17 and CH35 in nonionic detergents was emphasized in studies by Makino and Nakashima[141] of the CD spectrum of bovine 52-kDa

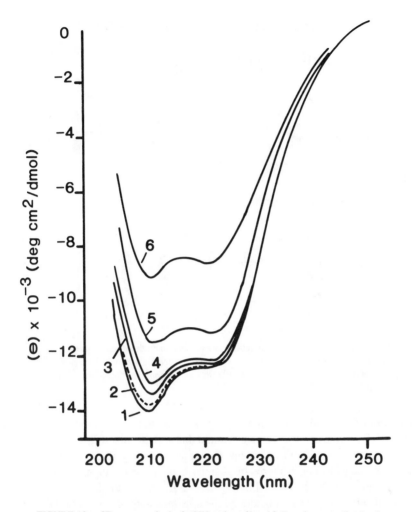

FIGURE 19. CD spectrum in the far UV region of band 3. Proteins were dissolved in a 50 mM NaCl, 10 mM Tris-HCl, 2 mM NaN$_3$, pH 8 buffer containing C$_{12}$E$_9$ or 0.25% deoxycholate. Curve 1, band 3 dimer in 0.25% deoxycholate; curve 2, band 3 tetramer in 0.25% deoxycholate; curve 3, fragmented band 3 in 0.1% detergent; curve 4, band 3 in 0.1% detergent; curve 5, DMMA (2,3-dimethylmaleic anhydride)-treated fragmented band 3 in 0.1% detergent; and curve 6, DMMA-treated band 3 in 0.1% detergent. The spectra were recorded at room temperature. Fragmented band 3 was generated by extracellular chymotrypsin digestion. (From Makino, S. and Nakashima, H., *J. Biochem. (Tokyo)*, 92, 1069, 1982. With permission.)

domain in C$_{12}$E$_9$. Native and chymotrypsin-digested band 3 had a similar CD spectrum, indicating that cleavage did not change the structure significantly. However, DMMA (2,3-dimethylmaleic anhydride) caused a significant decrease in the negative CD intensity (Figure 19).[141] DMMA is known to cause band 3 to dissociate partially into monomers.[135,141] The authors[141] suggest that the helical structure of the segments is disrupted by a DMMA-induced monomerization. Normally, the two fragments of the integral domain mutually interact such that the dimeric state is important to the formation of the folded structure of the monomer. The fact that tetramers and dimers have the same CD suggests that higher-order states of association do not alter the folded structure of each monomer.

The dependence of the folded structure of the band 3 transport site on the dimeric state[141] would explain the findings of Boodhoo and Reithmeier[153] showing that isolated monomers do not bind stilbene disulfonates. As pointed out above, stilbene disulfonates are potent anion-

Monomerization of the Band 3 Dimer

A. Separate Channels Collapse

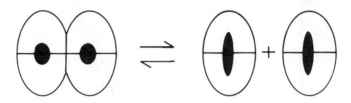

B. Common Channel

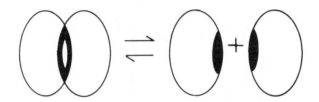

FIGURE 20.   Schematic of the effect of monomerization on the structure of band 3 channels for two separate channels per monomer (A) and for a model where each monomer has tightly packed monomeric helices with transport sites contributing to a common channel (B).

transport inhibitors which bind to band 3 with a 1:1 stoichiometry per monomer and linearly inhibit transport.[155] Boodhoo and Reithmeier[153] found that stilbene disulfonate does not bind to the isolated monomer. Reassociation of the same monomers restores stilbene binding to normal.

If stilbene-disulfonate binding is altered by changes in the folded structure of the monomer, does the reverse hold true? Does stilbene binding detectably change the folded structure of the monomer? Ligand and inhibitor binding altered the apparent state of association of band 3 as seen earlier, or it may change the quaternary structure of a preexisting tetrameric state as reflected in BS[3] cross-linking patterns.[120] Werner and Reithmeier[140] purified and characterized human band 3 in the nonionic detergent octyl glucoside. Sedimentation experiments showed that band 3 existed in a high oligomeric state of heterogeneous composition. CD measurements did not show major changes in structure with stilbene-disulfonate binding. The solubilized protein could bind stilbene disulfonates reversibly, and the dissociation constant was comparable to the stilbene transport inhibition constant. Oikawa and co-workers[207] investigated the effects of several other factors on the stability of band 3 folded structure. The ellipticity of band 3 at 222 nm was insensitive to pH between pHs 4 and 10.5. DIDS binding to isolated band 3 also did not significantly affect the CD spectrum, nor did DIDS binding alter guanidine HCl-induced denaturation. However, DIDS binding had a significant stabilizing effect on heat denaturation of band 3.[207] Is this effect perhaps more directly correlated with changes at the interfacial energies between monomers?

Taken together these findings suggest that any changes in association to higher than dimeric states do not seem to significantly alter the folded structure of the monomer, nor does inhibitor binding. Inhibitor binding does seem to directly alter either the quaternary structure or the state of association, or at the very least the BS[3] cross-linking pattern, to yield tetramers.[120] However, once the monomers are separated from each other, the active site seems to fall apart and it can no longer bind stilbene disulfonates. Figure 20 shows two models for the effect of monomerization on the active site. If each monomer forms a separate channel in the dimer, monomerization

TABLE 5
Carbohydrate Composition of Band 3 Oligosaccharide Fraction
(Molar Ratio to Mannose = 3)

	F	M	G	N-Glu	N-Gal
Unfractionated	2.1	3.0	6.6	8.5	0.3
N = I	1.6	3.0	8.5	10.5	0.2
N = II	0.6	3.0	2.8	5.6	0.0

Note: F = fructose, M = mannose, G = galactose, N-Glu = *N*-acetyl glucosamine, and N-Gal = *N*-acetylgalactosamine.

could cause the collapse of each channel. This would explain the CD change and the inability of monomers to bind stilbenes. Alternatively, if each monomer has a tightly packed integral domain and contributes sites to a common channel, one might expect diminished inhibitor binding, but not necessarily a change in the folded structure with monomerization. On the basis of these considerations a model would be favored with two separate channels (one on each monomer),[121,150,231] the structural integrity of which depends on the quaternary structure of the dimer.

Does the attachment of the cytoplasmic domain affect the structure of the integral domain? As seen in Section III.B, the structure of the integral domain can be altered by changes in cytosolic interactions. However, there are few quantitative correlations with changes in quaternary structure or states of association. There is one quantitative study showing that DIDS binding to the transport site alters hemoglobin binding to CDB3.[180] Chapter 4 will discuss newer data suggesting that CDB3 effects can alter the DIDS binding site and anion transport.

VIII. MISCELLANEOUS ASPECTS OF BAND 3 STRUCTURE

A. BAND 3 HETEROGENEITY AND GENETIC VARIANTS

It is quite common to observe more than one type of given protein within a cell. Band 3 migrates on SDS gels as a broad band, and this led to some early speculation that there may be various isoforms of band 3. Although there are minor protein components which migrate on the gel in the position of band 3,[83,232] they are unrelated to the anion-transport function. Over 90% of the integral protein in the band 3 region is homogeneous with respect to two-dimensional gel electrophoresis, DIDS binding and cross-linking, and to extracellular proteolysis.[84,104,154,233]

1. Carbohydrate Heterogeneity

The broad banding seen in the band 3 region on SDS gels is largely related to heterogeneity in the carbohydrate content of the various copies of band 3,[86,196,197,234-238] as illustrated in the paper by Tsuji and co-workers.[236] The distribution of band 3 forms can be narrowed considerably by treating intact cells with endo-beta-galactosidase from *Escherichia freundii*.[239] In this procedure, band 3 was first purified by gel chromatography in SDS, and the carbohydrate was released by hydrazinolysis. The released oligosaccharides were N-acetylated and chromatographed on DEAE-cellulose columns. Most of the band 3 was free of sialic acid, and when the neutral fraction was subjected to gel chromatography on Sephadex G-50, two broad peaks could be seen which indicated size heterogeneity in the oligosaccharides. The results confirm those of Drickamer.[86] The molecular-weight ranges of the two peaks (N-I and N-II) were 3000 to 8000 and 1500 to 2500, respectively. The two fractions were further characterized as to carbohydrate composition. The compositions of the two peaks and of the unfractionated material are presented in Table 5. Galactose, mannose, *N*-acetylglucosamine, and fructose are seen in all fractions. There was a small amount of *N*-acetylgalactosamine in the high molecular-weight fraction

(N-I). The higher molecular-weight fraction also had higher galactose and *N*-acetylglucosamine content than the lower one. Subfractions of N-I were also analyzed. The structures of the oligosaccharides from N-I were reported in the same paper[236] and the structure of the lower molecular-weight fraction in a second paper.[237] Fukuda and co-workers determined the entire structure for the oligosaccharide chain in both adult and fetal forms of band 3.[240,241]

When band 3 is cleaved at the extracellular chymotryptic site, the resulting CH65 fragment usually migrates as a sharp band indicating protein homogeneity. The CH35 integral domain still migrates as a diffuse band, suggesting that the carbohydrate is attached to this subdomain. Pretreatment of cells with endo-beta-galactosidase followed by chymotrypsin has no effect on the sharpness of CH65, but radically sharpens the CH35 band.[192] The carbohydrate attachment site is a single asparagine on CH35. The location of the glycosylation site has been mapped to 280 residues from the C-terminus of band 3.[242] Papain digestion of chymotrypsin-treated cells produces a C-terminal 28-kDa fragment which contains the glycosylation site.[192] Of the two possible attachment sites in the murine sequence one can be ruled out, and a residue immediately C-terminal to the second principal papain cleavage site can be postulated (Figure 17).

2. Phosphorylation

Although carbohydrate heterogeneity is well defined, this cannot explain all examples of band 3 heterogeneity. Ideguchi and co-workers[243] found an example of band 3 heterogeneity which is probably not due to the carbohydrate component since it was observed in the chymotryptic CH65 fragment. Isoelectric focusing revealed three major bands. This result confirms the earlier work of Ross and McConnell,[244] who suggested that different degrees of phosphorylation could account for the heterogeneity. This idea and the finding that the heterogeneity occurs in CH65 agree with Drickamer's[183] demonstration that phosphorylation of band 3 occurs mainly on the N-terminal cytoplasmic domain. Waxman[245] showed that phosphorylation occurs exclusively within the N-terminus of the cytoplasmic domain. A major site of phosphorylation *in vitro* is tyrosine 8 (Figure 6).[246]

Considerable attention has been paid to the role of membrane protein phosphorylation in regulation of function. A general discussion of the regulatory mechanisms which control protein kinase function can be found in the review by Flockhart and Corbin.[247] Tao and his co-workers have extensively studied protein kinases from human erythrocytes.[248-251] They demonstrated that one fraction of protein kinase activity is membrane bound and that it can phosphorylate band 3. Several investigators have shown that the human erythrocyte contains a tyrosine kinase which phosphorylates tyrosine 8 of the cytoplasmic domain of band 3.[246,252-254] Lu and Tao[255] showed that a red cell casein kinase they had studied earlier could also phosphorylate protein tyrosine. The molecular properties of the tyrosine kinase and the casein kinase are similar. Thus, although casein kinase primarily phosphorylates serine or threonine residues, it can phosphorylate tyrosine and may be involved in that function in the red cell.[255] Bursaux and co-workers[256] have studied band 3 phosphorylation in buffers containing vanadate (a phosphatase inhibitor) and Mg^{2+} and Mn^{2+} to differentiate the effects of casein kinases (Mg^{2+} dependent) and tyrosine kinases (Mn^{2+} dependent). They showed that band 3 was phosphorylated to the same extent in the presence of the two types of cation, but that in the presence of Mg^{2+}, tyrosine and serine as well as threonine are equally phosphorylated, while phosphotyrosine represents 80% of the total when Mn^{2+} is the activator. Hillsgrove and co-workers[257] have demonstrated that the avian erythrocyte contains a tightly bound tyrosine-specific protein kinase identical to or closely related to pp60[c-src]. This enzyme is a normal cellular tyrosine kinase of unknown function which is closely related to the transforming protein of Rous sarcoma virus (RSV; 4,5) pp60[c-src].

The exact function of band 3 phosphorylation is unclear. Chapter 4 will show glycolytic enzymes and ankyrin bind to this domain in human red cells. G3PD significantly inhibits band 3 phosphorylation,[254] and tyrosine phosphorylation of band 3 inhibits binding of that enzyme and hemoglobin.[258] However, band 3 phosphorylation does not alter ankyrin binding.[259]

Phosphorylation of band 3 seems to affect the rate of anion exchange,[260] and a phosphotyrosyl phosphatase has been isolated.[261] Clearly, the cytoplasmic fragment of band 3 may be a regulatory location where phosphorylation-dephosphorylation cycles operate, promoting and inhibiting cytosolic protein binding and anion transport.

Pontremoli and co-workers[262] have studied the role of calpain in band 3 phosphorylation in normal red cells and cells from hypertensive subjects. Phosphorylation of band 3 is selectively increased upon activation of calpain. Calpain activity may modulate band 3 structure-function through phosphorylation. There is increased phosphorylation of band 3 in hypertensives, which may be related to an uncontrolled intracellular calpain-mediated proteolytic system.

3. Methylation

Reversible methyl esterification of glutamate residues on membrane proteins is important in the chemotactic mechanism of enteric bacteria.[263,264] There are specific enzymes which catalyze the transfer of methyl groups from S-adenosylmethionine to substrate proteins.[265] Protein methylation occurs in mammalian cells, but the exact physiological function is obscure.[265] The cytosol of the human erythrocyte also contains enzyme activity which catalyzes the addition of methyl groups from S-adenosylmethionine.[266] Galletti and co-workers[267] first showed that methyl groups can be introduced into red cell membrane proteins including band 3. Terwilliger and Clarke[268] have extensively studied erythrocyte membrane protein methylation. They found that the aspartate residues on the inner surface of band 3 are methylated. One methylation site is the hinge region between the membrane and the cytosolic domains (Figure 2). Recent evidence suggests that carboxymethylation of band 3 does not affect the rate of anion (phosphate) exchange.[269] At present, band 3 methylation has not been correlated with any specific physiological or pathophysiological function.

4. Genetic Variants

The apparent homogeneity of the protein portion of band 3 does not preclude the existence of genetic variants. As noted in Chapter 1, there is physiological evidence that band 3 anion exchange may be totally inhibited with only a minor (14%) reduction in CO_2 output at the lung in the resting, anesthetized animal. Grossly abnormal physiology may not be a useful marker for genetic variation in band 3 if the mutations do not lead to major functional abnormalities. Nevertheless, careful screening of blood has led to the discovery of interesting variants of band 3.

Mueller and Morrison[198] have identified a variant band 3 in which CH65 migrates as a doublet. The variant has a higher molecular weight by about 3 kDa on SDS gels in the Laemmli buffer system. The integral domain of this mutant seems structurally normal, as is the rate of anion transport. However, the cytoplasmic domain, which binds glycolytic enzymes and hemoglobin, is elongated at the amino-terminal 23-kDa portion. Investigation of over 400 randomly selected blood bank donors showed that between 5 and 6% of the population has this variant. Most individuals were heterozygotes. There was no obvious clinical abnormality associated with this elongation, but many questions may be asked. For example, is glycolytic enzyme and hemoglobin binding to this variant normal? Is the variant phosphorylated to the same degree and at the same sites? Do ankyrin and band 3 tyrosine kinase bind in the same manner?

A second variant of band 3 has recently been discovered by Hsu and Morrison.[270] This is an interesting mutant for unlike the one just discussed, the abnormality seems to involve part of the anion-transport site. The erythrocyte donor was a double heterozygote in that he possessed normal band 3 plus the band 3 variant with the elongated cytoplasmic domain as well as a second variation at the DIDS binding site. The variant reacts more readily with stilbene disulfonates than normal. Also, intramolecular cross-linking by DIDS is less efficient in the variant than in normal band 3. The authors surmised that the DIDS binding site is more exposed in the variant.

However, it is not clear whether the mutation actually occurs at an amino acid directly involved in anion transport since there is no apparent abnormality in the rate of anion transport. More sensitive kinetic methods may be needed to detect any subtle changes in transport. Perhaps the nonphysiological size of the stilbene disulfonate molecule makes it much more sensitive to conformational differences not directly related to anion transport.

Kay and co-workers[176] have recently described an interesting mutant form of band 3. Several functional abnormalities were discovered, including alterations in (1) anion transport, (2) band 3 rotational diffusion, and (3) the number of high-affinity ankyrin binding sites. Two-dimensional gel electrophoresis revealed a 2- to 4-kDa insertion in the CH17 subdomain of the transport site. This subdomain is connected to the cytoplasmic domain of band 3 which binds ankyrin, the glycolytic enzymes, and hemoglobin. It has taken on renewed and increasing importance in transport inhibition studies.

5. "Physical-Chemical" Heterogeneity

There is a new report by Swanson and co-workers[271] which is distinct from the kind of chemical heterogeneity just discussed. It may be called "physical-chemical" heterogeneity since the heterogeneity was discovered through examination of different physical-chemical properties within a single band 3 population. They discovered that two populations of band 3 exist which differ in phase partition between a detergent and aqueous phase. Partitioning into Triton X-1114 was used in combination with countercurrent distribution to examine the phase properties. This was followed by electrophoresis and immunoblotting to identify the products of each phase. The authors found that 65% of the band 3 population was localized into the detergent phase, while 35% was isolated in the aqueous phase. This bipartite phasing was not due to either glycosylation or phosphorylation. While the integral domain solely partitions into the detergent phase, isolated CH65 was found to have biphasic partitioning, but now 70% of the material was found in the aqueous phase and only 30% in the detergent phase. Since CH65 is dominated by the water-soluble CDB3 domain, the change in proportion is not surprising, but mechanistic basis for the heterogeneity is unknown. It is probably not due to differences in protein sequence based on current genetic information. Rather, it seems likely that the difference is due to conformational or charge differences between two physically and chemically distinct states within the population. It is interesting that covalent DIDS binding did not change the partitioning patterns according to the authors.

B. BAND 3 AND ENDOGENOUS PROTEOLYSIS

If contaminating leukocytes are removed from blood, the only well-established proteolytic activity remaining is a calcium-activated protease of the erythrocyte membrane.[272-276] This protease is primarily found in the cytoplasm and requires nonphysiological calcium concentrations to be activated. Proof that there exists a membrane-bound protease which can degrade band 3 is at best inconclusive. There is evidence for proteolytic digestion of Triton X-100 extracted band 3 under certain conditions.[277] Morrison and co-workers[278] have carefully studied band 3 catabolism in human erythrocytes, and their paper may be consulted for further details.

In summary, band 3 from most donors seems to be a homogeneous polypeptide. The predominant heterogeneity arises from posttranslational modifications. Certain mutant forms have been discovered in less than 5% of the population.

IX. CONCLUSIONS

Several themes have emerged from this survey of the structure and disposition of band 3 within the erythrocyte membrane. Among the most potentially significant is the fact that the dimeric state of association seems to have a major impact on the state of the folded structure of the monomer. Monomerization produces major changes in the CD spectrum, and it virtually eliminates stilbene-disulfonate binding. If the monomeric helices were tightly packed and if inhibitors like stilbene disulfonates required a dimeric niche to bind, then dissociation to monomers might be expected to cause a diminution in stilbene binding, but without affecting the folded structure of the tightly packed monomer. On the other hand, if each monomer formed a separate channel which binds stilbenes and if the folded structure was dependent on the quaternary structure of the dimer, then monomerization would be expected to cause a collapse in the channel structure, and a collapsed channel would block stilbene binding. These arguments obviously do not constitute a proof for any one structure, but they offer a plausible basis for explaining allosteric communication between two classes of functional sites within a dimeric unit. Furthermore, since new measurements show distance between the stilbene sites on each monomer to be >16 Å, the sites would seem to be too far apart for steric explanations of cooperativity.[231] The fact that the folded structure does change implies that there must be strong energies of interactions between the monomers of a dimer. Such interactions could be expected to translate into functional interactions if each monomer were, in the dimeric state, capable of independently exchanging anions (using sites on both CH17 and CH35 subdomains of one monomer). The intermonomeric allosteric interactions would be superimposed for modulation. This is a very common theme in the biochemistry of allosteric enzymes. That the same theme may hold for porter activity was originally suggested by Jardetzky over 20 years ago.[279] Singer[280] specifically suggested that each monomer of an oligomeric porter could contain an active site with allosteric interactions between sites. The structural description given here for the band 3 porter seems to have many of these features, making classic homotropic protein allosterism a very plausible consideration. The fact that transport site ligands can reversibly convert the protein between two quaternary structures (the DC-state and the TC-state) shows that changes in the global structure of this porter can no longer be ignored in the interpretation of functionality. It may be at the very heart of function.

The asymmetric disposition of the porter with fully one half of its mass extended over 250 Å into the cytosolic space (as a dimer) clearly has a structural purpose for the cell. It is also a convenient arrangement for heterotropic, allosteric, modulatory interactions with cytosolic ligands. It does not appear that there is a singular purpose for the cytosolic extension. Indeed, the number of copies of cytoskeletal connecting proteins is far less than stoichiometric. Such nonstoichiometric associations seem poised for regulation by any number of cytosolic effects, including oxygen-linked hemoglobin binding and phosphorylation. Pathological interactions may also disrupt tenuous interactions with the cytoskeleton; this in turn could have functional consequences. In Chapter 4, there is evidence of a rapid exchange of ankyrin-free for ankyrin-bound band 3. Modulation of the state of association of band 3 through interactions with the cytoskeleton could affect the interaction energies between monomers which, we will show, modulate the anion-exchange activity. Why is band 3 asymmetrically placed and multifunctional? The evidence will show that it is because band 3 porter is a center for control. As such, allosteric modulation would be expected. If the results of the last 100 years of study with soluble proteins is any indication of how proteins use conformational changes for control, protein oligomers and multisite allosterism must be involved.

REFERENCES

1. **Klingenberg, M.,** Membrane protein oligomeric structure and transport function, *Nature (London)*, 290, 449, 1981.
2. **Overton, E.,** Über die allgemeinen osmotischen Eigenschaften der Zelle, ihre vermutlichen Ursachen und ihre Bedeutung für die Physiologie, *Vierteljahrsschr. Naturforsch. Ges. Zuerich*, 88, 1899.
3. **Gorter, E. G. and Grendel, F.,** Bimolecular layers of lipids on the chromocytes of blood, *Proc. K. Ned. Akad. Wet. (Amsterdam)*, 29, 314, 1926.

4. **Danielli, J. F. and Harvey, E. N.,** The tension at the surface of mackerel egg oil, with remarks on the nature of the cell surface, *J. Cell. Comp. Physiol.,* 5, 483, 1935.
5. **Danielli, J. F. and Davson, H.,** A contribution to the theory of permeability of thin films, *J. Cell. Comp. Physiol.,* 5, 495, 1935.
6. **Singer, S. J. and Nicolson, G. L.,** The fluid mosaic model of the structure of cell membranes, *Science,* 175, 720, 1972.
7. **Seifriz, W.,** The physical properties of erythrocytes, *Protoplasma,* 1, 345, 1926.
8. **Norris, C. H.,** The tension at the surface and other physical properties of the nucleated erythrocyte, *J. Cell. Comp. Physiol.,* 14, 117, 1939.
9. **Marchesi, V. T. and Steers, E., Jr.,** Selective solubilization of a protein component of the red cell membrane, *Science,* 159, 203, 1968.
10. **Marchesi, S. L., Steers, E., Marchesi, V. T., and Tillack, T. W.,** Physical and chemical properties of a protein isolated from red cell membranes, *Biochemistry,* 9, 50, 1970.
11. **Tillack, T. W., Marchesi, S. L., Marchesi, V. T., and Steers, E., Jr.,** A comparative study of spectrin: a protein isolated from red blood cell membranes, *Biochim. Biophys. Acta,* 200, 125, 1970.
12. **Clarke, M.,** Isolation and characterization of a water-soluble protein from bovine erythrocyte membranes, *Biochem. Biophys. Res. Commun.,* 45, 1063, 1971.
13. **Steck, T. L.,** The organization of proteins in the human red blood cell membrane, *J. Cell Biol.,* 62, 1, 1974.
14. **Singer, S. J.,** The molecular organization of membranes, *Annu. Rev. Biochem.,* 43, 805, 1974.
15. **Elgsaeter, A. and Branton, D.,** Intramembrane particle aggregation in erythrocyte ghosts, *J. Cell Biol.,* 63, 1018, 1974.
16. **Guidotti, G.,** Membrane proteins. Structure, arrangement and disposition in the membrane, in *Physiology of Membrane Disorders,* Andreoli, T. E., Hoffman, J. F., Fanestil, D. D., and Schultz, S. G., Eds., Plenum Press, New York, 1986, 45.
17. **Chasis, J. A. and Shohet, S. B.,** Red cell biochemical anatomy and membrane properties, *Annu. Rev. Physiol.,* 49, 237, 1987.
18. **Bennett, V.,** The membrane skeleton of human erythrocytes and its implications for more complex cells, *Annu. Rev. Biochem.,* 54, 273, 1985.
19. **Gratzer, W. B.,** The red cell membrane and its cytoskeleton, *Biochem. J.,* 198, 1, 1981.
20. **Branton, D., Cohen, C. M., and Tyler, J.,** Interaction of cytoskeletal proteins on the human erythrocyte membrane, *Cell,* 24, 24, 1981.
21. **Lux, S. E.,** Spectrin-actin membrane skeleton of normal and abnormal red blood cells, *Semin. Hematol.,* 16, 21, 1979.
22. **Marchesi, V. T.,** The red cell membrane skeleton: recent progress, *Blood,* 61, 1, 1983.
23. **Marchesi, V. T. and Furthmayr, H.** The red cell membrane, *Annu. Rev. Biochem.,* 45, 667, 1976.
24. **Fairbanks, G., Steck, T. L., and Wallach, D. F. H.,** Electrophoretic analysis of the major polypeptides of the human erythrocyte membrane, *Biochemistry,* 10, 2606, 1971.
25. **Wood, P. G. and Passow, H.,** Techniques for the modification of the intracellular composition of red blood cells, *Tech. Cell. Physiol.,* P112, 1, 1981.
26. **Bennett, V.,** Immunoreactive forms of human erythrocyte ankyrin are present in diverse cells and tissues, *Nature (London),* 281, 597, 1979.
27. **Tyler, J. M., Hargreaves, W. R., and Branton, D.,** Purification of two spectrin-binding proteins: biochemical and electron microscopic evidence for site-specific reassociation between spectrin and bands 2.1 and 4.1, *Proc. Natl. Acad. Sci. U.S.A.,* 76, 5192, 1979.
28. **Ohnishi, T.,** Extraction of actin- and myosin-like proteins from erythrocyte membrane, *J. Biochem. (Tokyo),* 52, 307, 1962.
29. **Tilney, L. G. and Detmers, P.,** Actin in erythrocyte ghosts and its association with spectrin. Evidence for a nonfilamentous form of these two molecules *in situ, J. Cell Biol.,* 66, 508, 1975.
30. **Tanner, M. J. A. and Gray, W. R.,** The isolation and functional identification of a protein from the human erythrocyte "ghost", *Biochem. J.,* 125, 1109, 1971.
31. **Yu, J., Fischman, D. A., and Steck, T. L.,** Selective solubilization of proteins and phospholipids from red blood cell membranes by nonionic detergents, *J. Supramol. Struct.,* 1, 233, 1973.
32. **Hainfeld, J. F. and Steck, T. L.,** The sub-membrane reticulum of the human erythrocyte: a scanning electron microscope study, *J. Supramol. Struct.,* 6, 301, 1977.
33. **Liu, S. C., Derick, L. H., and Palek, J.,** Separation of the lipid bilayer from the membrane skeleton during echinocytic transformation of red cell (RBC) ghosts, *J. Cell Biol.,* 105, 291a, 1987.
34. **Winzler, R. J.,** A glycoprotein in human erythrocyte membranes, in *Red Cell Membrane Structure and Function,* Jamieson, G. A. and Greenwalt, T. J., Eds., J. B. Lippincott, Philadelphia, 1969, 157.
35. **Marchesi, V. T. and Andrews, E. P.,** Glycoproteins: isolation from cell membranes with lithium diiodosalicylate, *Science,* 174, 1247, 1971.

36. **Marchesi, V. T., Tillack, T. W., Jackson, R. L., Segrest, J. P., and Scott, R. E.,** Chemical characterization and surface orientation of the major glycoprotein of the human erythrocyte membrane, *Proc. Natl. Acad. Sci. U.S.A.,* 69, 1445, 1972.

37. **Segrest, J. P., Jackson, R. L., Andrews, E. P., and Marchesi, V. T.,** Human erythrocyte membrane glycoprotein: reevaluation of the molecular weight as determined by SDS polyacrylamide gel electrophoresis, *Biochem. Biophys. Res. Commun.,* 44, 390, 1971.

38. **Segrest, J. P., Kahane, I., Jackson, R. L., and Marchesi, V. T.,** Major glycoprotein of the human erythrocyte membrane: evidence for an amphipathic molecular structure, *Arch. Biochem. Biophys.,* 155, 167, 1973.

39. **Owens, J. W., Mueller, T. J., and Morrison, M.,** A minor sialoglycoprotein of the human erythrocyte membrane, *Arch. Biochem. Biophys.,* 204, 247, 1980.

40. **Hamaguchi, H. and Cleve, H.,** Solubilization of human erythrocyte membrane glycoproteins and separation of the MN glycoprotein from a glycoprotein with I, S, and A activity, *Biochim. Biophys. Acta,* 278, 271, 1972.

41. **Tanner, M. J. A. and Boxer, D. H.,** Separation and some properties of the major proteins of the human erythrocyte membrane, *Biochem. J.,* 129, 333, 1972.

42. **Mueller, T. J. and Morrison, M.,** The transmembrane proteins in the plasma membrane of normal human erythrocytes, *J. Biol. Chem.,* 249, 7568, 1974.

43. **Dahr, W., Uhlenbruck, G., Janssen, E., and Schmalisch, R.,** Heterogeneity of human red cell membrane sialoglycoproteins, *Blut,* 32, 171, 1976.

44. **Mueller, T. J., Dow, A. W., and Morrison, M.,** Heterogeneity of the sialoglycoproteins of the normal human erythrocyte membrane, *Biochem. Biophys. Res. Commun.,* 72, 94, 1976.

45. **Gahmberg, C. G. and Andersson, L. C.,** Selective radioactive labeling of cell surface sialoglycoproteins by periodate-tritiated borohydride, *J. Biol. Chem.,* 252, 5888, 1977.

46. **Furthmayr, H.,** Structural comparison of glycophorins and immunochemical analysis of genetic variants, *Nature (London),* 271, 519, 1978.

47. **Furthmayr, H.,** Glycophorins A, B, and C: a family of sialoglycoproteins. Isolation and preliminary characterization of trypsin derived peptides, *J. Supramol. Struct.,* 9, 79, 1978.

48. **Kay, M. M. B.,** Aging of cell membrane molecules leads to appearance of an aging antigen and removal of senescent cells, *Gerontology,* 31, 215, 1985.

49. **Nigg, E. A., Bron, C., Girardet, M., and Cherry, R. J.,** Band 3-glycophorin A association in erythrocyte membranes demonstrated by combining protein diffusion measurements with antibody-induced cross-linking, *Biochemistry,* 19, 1887, 1980.

50. **Dahr, W., Uhlenbruck, G., Leikola, J., Pirkola, A., and Landfried, K.,** Studies on the membrane glycoprotein defect of En(a-) erythrocytes. I. Biochemical aspects, *J. Immunogenet.,* 3, 329, 1976.

51. **Gahmberg, C. G., Myllyla, G., Leikola, J., Pirkola, A., and Nordling, S.,** Absence of the major sialoglycoprotein in the membrane of human En(a-) erythrocytes and increased glycosylation of band 3, *J. Biol. Chem.,* 251, 6108, 1976.

52. **Tanner, M. J. A. and Anstee, D. J.,** The membrane change in En(a-) human erythrocytes. Absence of the major erythrocyte sialoglycoprotein, *Biochem. J.,* 153, 271, 1976.

53. **Lodish, H. F. and Small, B.,** Membrane proteins synthesized by rabbit reticulocytes, *J. Cell Biol.,* 65, 51, 1975.

54. **Light, N. D. and Tanner, M. J. A.,** Changes in surface-membrane components during the differentiation of rabbit erythroid cells, *Biochem. J.,* 164, 565, 1977.

55. **Rauenbuehler, P. B., Cordes, K. A., and Salhany, J. M.,** Identification of the hemoglobin binding sites on the inner surface of the erythrocyte membrane, *Biochim. Biophys. Acta,* 692, 361, 1982.

56. **Jansson, S.-E., Gripenberg, J., Hekali, R., and Gahmberg, C. G.,** Organization of membrane lipids and proteins in human En(a-) erythrocytes that lack the major sialoglycoprotein, glycophorin A. A spin-label study, *Biochem. J.,* 195, 123, 1981.

57. **Shotton, D. M., Burke, B. E., and Branton, D.,** The molecular structure of human erythrocyte spectrin. Biophysical and electron microscopic studies, *J. Mol. Biol.,* 131, 303, 1979.

58. **Brenner, S. L. and Korn, E. D.,** Spectrin/actin complex isolated from sheep erythrocytes accelerates actin polymerization by simple nucleation, *J. Biol. Chem.,* 255, 1670, 1980.

59. **Pinder, J. C. and Gratzer, W. B.,** Structural and dynamic states of actin in the erythrocyte, *J. Cell Biol.,* 96, 768, 1983.

60. **Fowler, V. M. and Bennett, V.,** Erythrocyte membrane tropomyosin. Purification and properties, *J. Biol. Chem.,* 259, 5978, 1984.

61. **Fowler, V. M. and Bennett, V.,** Tropomyosin: new component of the erythrocyte membrane skeleton, in *Erythrocyte Membranes 3: Recent Clinical and Experimental Advances,* Kruckeberg, W. C., Eaton, J. W., Aster, J, and Brewer, G. J., Eds., Alan R. Liss, New York, 1984, 57.

62. **Cohen, C. M. and Foley, S. F.,** Biochemical characterization of complex formation by human erythrocyte spectrin, protein 4.1 and actin, *Biochemistry,* 23, 6091, 1984.

63. **Ohanian, V., Wolfe, L. C., John, K. M., Pinder, J. C., Lux, S. E., and Gratzer, W. B.,** Analysis of the ternary interaction of the red cell membrane skeletal proteins spectrin, actin, and 4.1, *Biochemistry,* 23, 4416, 1984.

64. **Gardner, K. and Bennett, V.,** Modulation of spectrin-actin assembly by erythrocyte adducin, *Nature (London),* 328, 359, 1987.
65. **Leto, T. L. and Marchesi, V. T.,** A structural model of human erythrocyte protein 4.1, *J. Biol. Chem.,* 259, 4603, 1984.
66. **Metcalf, D. and Moore, M. A. S.,** in *Haemopoietic Cells, North Holland Research Monographs: Frontiers of Biology,* Vol. 24, North-Holland, Amsterdam, 1971.
67. **Braell, W. A. and Lodish, H. F.,** Biosynthesis of the erythrocyte anion transport protein, *J. Biol. Chem.,* 256, 11337, 1981.
68. **Braell, W. A. and Lodish, H. F.,** The erythrocyte anion transport protein is cotranslationally inserted into microsomes, *Cell,* 28, 23, 1982.
69. **Lodish, H. F. and Braell, W. A.,** Synthesis and maturation of the erythrocyte anion transport protein — an internal sequence for membrane insertion, *Biochem. Soc. Symp.,* 47, 193, 1982.
70. **Sabban, E. L., Marchesi, V., Adesnik, M., and Sabatini, D. D.,** Erythrocyte membrane protein band 3: its biosynthesis and incorporation into membranes, *J. Cell Biol.,* 91, 637, 1981.
71. **Sabban, E. L., Sabatini, D. D., Marchesi, V. T., and Adesnik, M.,** Biosynthesis of erythrocyte membrane protein band 3 in DMSO-induced Friend erythroleukemia cells, *J. Cell. Physiol.,* 104, 261, 1980.
72. **Woods, C. M., Boyer, B., Vogt, P. K, and Lazarides, E.,** Control of erythroid differentiation: asynchronous expression of the anion transporter and the peripheral components of the membrane skeleton in AEV- and S13-transformed cells, *J. Cell Biol.,* 103, 1789, 1986.
73. **Berg, H. C.,** Sulfanilic acid diazonium salt: label for the outside of the human erythrocyte membrane, *Biochim. Biophys. Acta,* 183, 65, 1969.
74. **Bender, W. W., Garan, H., and Berg, H. C.,** Proteins of the human erythrocyte membrane as modified by pronase, *J. Mol. Biol.,* 58, 783, 1971.
75. **Bretscher, M. S.,** Human erythrocyte membranes: specific labelling of surface proteins, *J. Mol. Biol.,* 58, 775, 1971.
76. **Phillips, D. R. and Morrison, M.,** Exterior proteins of the human erythrocyte membrane, *Biochem. Biophys. Res. Commun.,* 45, 1103, 1971.
77. **Steck, T. L., Fairbanks, G., and Wallach, D. F. H.,** Disposition of the major proteins in the isolated erythrocyte membrane. Proteolytic dissection, *Biochemistry,* 10, 2617, 1971.
78. **Hubbard, A. L. and Cohn, Z. A.,** The enzymatic iodination of the red cell membrane, *J. Cell Biol.,* 55, 390, 1972.
79. **Triplett, R. B. and Carraway, K. L.,** Proteolytic digestion of erythrocytes, resealed ghosts, and isolated membranes, *Biochemistry,* 11, 2897, 1972.
80. **Cabantchik, Z. I. and Rothstein, A.,** Membrane proteins related to anion permeability of human red blood cells. II. Effects of proteolytic enzymes on disulfonic stilbene sites of surface proteins, *J. Membr. Biol.,* 15, 227, 1974.
81. **Whiteley, N. M. and Berg, H. C.,** Amidination of the outer and inner surfaces of the human erythrocyte membrane, *J. Mol. Biol.,* 87, 541, 1974.
82. **Mueller, T. J. and Morrison, M.,** The transmembrane proteins in the plasma membrane of normal human erythrocytes. Evaluation employing lactoperoxidase and proteases, *Biochemistry,* 14, 5512, 1975.
83. **Reichstein, E. and Blostein, R.,** Arrangement of human erythrocyte membrane proteins, *J. Biol. Chem.,* 250, 6256, 1975.
84. **Steck, T. L., Ramos, B., and Strapazon, E.,** Proteolytic dissection of band 3, the predominant transmembrane polypeptide of the human erythrocyte membrane, *Biochemistry,* 15, 1154, 1976.
85. **Steck, T. L., Koziarz, J. J., Singh, M. K., Reddy, G., and Köhler, H.,** Preparation and analysis of seven major, topographically defined fragments of band 3, the predominant transmembrane polypeptide of human erythrocyte membranes, *Biochemistry,* 17, 1216, 1978.
86. **Drickamer, L. K.,** Orientation of the band 3 polypeptide from human erythrocyte membranes. Identification of NH_2-terminal sequence and site of carbohydrate attachment, *J. Biol. Chem.,* 253, 7242, 1978.
87. **Freifelder, D.,** *Molecular Biology,* 2nd ed., Jones and Bartlett, Boston, 1987.
88. **Lieberman, D. M. and Reithmeier, R. A. F.,** Localization of the carboxyl terminus of band 3 to the cytoplasmic side of the erythrocyte membrane using antibodies raised against a synthetic peptide, *J. Biol. Chem.,* 263, 10022, 1988.
89. **Makino, S., Moriyama, R., Kitahara, T., and Koga, S.,** Proteolytic digestion of band 3 from bovine erythrocyte membranes in membrane-bound and solubilized states, *J. Biochem. (Tokyo),* 95, 1019, 1984.
90. **Jenkins, R. E. and Tanner, M. J. A.,** Ionic-strength-dependent changes in the structure of the major protein of the human erythrocyte membrane, *Biochem. J.,* 161, 131, 1977.
91. **Jennings, M. L., Anderson, M. P., and Monaghan, R.,** Monoclonal antibodies against human erythrocyte band 3 protein. Localization of proteolytic cleavage sites and stilbenedisulfonate-binding lysine residues, *J. Biol. Chem.,* 261, 9002, 1986.

92. **Steck, T. L.,** The organization of proteins in human erythrocyte membranes, in *Membrane Research,* Fox, C. F., Ed., Academic Press, New York, 1972, 71.

93. **Steck, T. L.,** Preparation of impermeable inside-out and right-side-out vesicles from erythrocyte membranes, in *Methods in Membrane Biology,* Vol. 2, Korn, E. D., Ed., Plenum Press, New York, 1974, 245.

94. **Mawby, W. J. and Findlay, J. B. C.,** Characterization and partial sequence of diiodosulphophenyl isothiocyanate- binding peptide from human erythrocyte anion-transport protein, *Biochem. J.,* 205, 465, 1982.

95. **Yu, J. and Branton, D.,** Reconstitution of intramembrane particles in recombinants of erythrocyte protein band 3 and lipid: effects of spectrin-actin association, *Proc. Natl. Acad. Sci. U.S.A.,* 73, 3891, 1976.

96. **Weinstein, R. S., Khodadad, J. K., and Steck, T. L.,** Fine structure of the band 3 protein in human red cell membranes: freeze-fracture studies, *J. Supramol. Struct.,* 8, 325, 1978.

97. **Edwards, H. H., Mueller, T. J., and Morrison, M.,** Distribution of transmembrane polypeptides in freeze fracture, *Science,* 203, 1343, 1979.

98. **Weinstein, R. S., Khodadad, J. K., and Steck, T. L.,** The band 3 protein intramembrane particle of the human red blood cell, in *Membrane Transport in Erythrocytes,* Lassen, U. V., Ussing, H. H., and Wieth, J. O., Eds., Munksgaard, Copenhagen, 1980, 35.

99. **Khodadad, J. K. and Weinstein, R. S.,** The band 3-rich membrane of llama erythrocytes: studies on cell shape and the organization of membrane proteins, *J. Membr. Biol.,* 72, 161, 1983.

100. **Weinstein, R. S.,** Changes in plasma membrane structure associated with malignant transformation in human urinary bladder epithelium, *Cancer Res.,* 36, 2518, 1976.

101. **Gahmberg, C. G., Taurén, G., Virtanen, I., and Wartiovaara, J.,** Distribution of glycophorin on the surface of human erythrocyte membranes and its association with intramembrane particles: an immunochemical and freeze-fracture study of normal and En(a-) erythrocytes, *J. Supramol. Struct.,* 8, 337, 1978.

102. **Margaritis, L. H., Elgsaeter, A., and Branton, D.,** Rotary replication for freeze-etching, *J. Cell Biol.,* 72, 47, 1977.

103. **Weinstein, R. S., Khodadad, J. K., and Steck, T. L.,** Band 3 protein is a tetramer in the human red cell membrane, *J. Cell Biol.,* 87, 209a, 1980.

104. **Steck, T. L.,** Cross-linking the major proteins of the isolated erythrocyte membrane, *J. Mol. Biol.,* 66, 295, 1972.

105. **Salhany, J. M., Swanson, J. C., Cordes, K. A., Gaines, S. B., and Gaines, K. C.,** Evidence suggesting direct oxidation of human erythrocyte membrane sulfhydryls by copper, *Biochem. Biophys. Res. Commun.,* 82, 1294, 1978.

106. **Wang, K. and Richards, F. M.,** An approach to nearest neighbor analysis of membrane proteins. Applicaton to the human erythrocyte membrane of a method employing cleavable cross-linkages, *J. Biol. Chem.,* 249, 8005, 1974.

107. **Kiehm, D. J. and Ji, T. H.,** Photochemical cross-linking of cell membranes. A test for natural and random collisional cross-links by millisecond cross-linking, *J. Biol. Chem.,* 252, 8524, 1977.

108. **Haest, C. W. M., Kamp, D., Plasa, G., and Deuticke, B.,** Intra- and intermolecular cross-linking of membrane proteins in intact erythrocytes and ghosts by SH- oxidizing agents, *Biochim. Biophys. Acta,* 469, 226, 1977.

109. **Liu, S.-C., Fairbanks, G., and Palek, J.,** Spontaneous, reversible protein cross-linking in the human erythrocyte membrane. Temperature and pH dependence, *Biochemistry,* 16, 4066, 1977.

110. **Reithmeier, R. A. F. and Rao, A.,** Reactive sulfhydryl groups of the band 3 polypeptide from human erythrocyte membranes. Identification of the sulfhydryl groups involved in Cu²⁺-o-phenanthroline crosslinking, *J. Biol. Chem.,* 254, 6151, 1979.

111. **Wang, K. and Richards, F. M.,** Reaction of dimethyl-3,3'-dithiobispropionimidate with intact human erythrocytes. Cross-linking of membrane proteins and hemoglobin, *J. Biol. Chem.,* 250, 6622, 1975.

112. **Sato, S. and Nakao, M.,** Cross-linking of intact erythrocyte membrane with a newly synthesized cleavable bifunctional reagent, *J. Biochem. (Tokyo),* 90, 1177, 1981.

113. **Willingham, G. L. and Gaffney, B. J.,** Reactions of spin-label cross-linking reagents with red blood cell proteins, *Biochemistry,* 22, 892, 1983.

114. **Mikkelsen, R. B. and Wallach, D. F. H.,** Photoactivated cross-linking of proteins within the erythrocyte membrane core, *J. Biol. Chem.,* 251, 7413, 1976.

115. **Huang, C.-K. and Richards, F. M.,** Reaction of a lipid-soluble, unsymmetrical, cleavable, cross-linking reagent with muscle aldolase and erythrocyte membrane proteins, *J. Biol. Chem.,* 252, 5514, 1977.

116. **Sigrist, H., Allegrini, P. R., Kempf, C., Schnippering, C., and Zahler, P.,** 5-Isothiocyanato-1-naphthalene azide and *p*-azidophenylisothiocyanate. Synthesis and application in hydrophobic heterobifunctional photoactive cross-linking of membrane proteins, *Eur. J. Biochem.,* 125, 197, 1982.

117. **Staros, J. V.,** *N*-hydroxysulfosuccinimide active esters: bis(*N*-hydroxysuccinimide)esters of two dicarboxylic acids are hydrophilic, membrane-impermeant, protein cross-linkers, *Biochemistry,* 21, 3950, 1982.

118. **Staros, J. V. and Kakkad, B. P.,** Cross-linking and chymotryptic digestion of the extracytoplasmic domain of the anion exchange channel in intact human erythrocytes, *J. Membr. Biol.,* 74, 247, 1983.

119. **Jennings, M. L. and Nicknish, J. S.,** Localization of a site of intermolecular cross-linking in human red blood cell band 3 protein, *J. Biol. Chem.,* 260, 5472, 1985.

120. **Salhany, J. M. and Sloan, R. L.,** Partial covalent labeling with pyridoxal 5′-phosphate induces bis(sulfosuccinimidyl)-suberate crosslinking of band 3 protein tetramers in intact human red blood cells, *Biochem. Biophys. Res. Commun.,* 156, 1215, 1988.

121. **Macara, I. G. and Cantley, L. C.,** Interactions between transport inhibitors at the anion binding sites of the band 3 dimer, *Biochemistry,* 20, 5095, 1981.

122. **Cherry, R. J., Bürkli, A., Busslinger, M., Schneider, G., and Parish, G. R.,** Rotational diffusion of band 3 proteins in the human erythrocyte membrane, *Nature (London),* 263, 389, 1976.

123. **Nigg, E. A. and Cherry, R. J.,** Dimeric association of band 3 in the erythrocyte membrane demonstrated by protein diffusion measurements, *Nature (London),* 277, 493, 1979.

124. **Nigg, E. A. and Cherry, R. J.,** Anchorage of a band 3 population at the erythrocyte cytoplasmic membrane surface: protein rotational diffusion measurements, *Proc. Natl. Acad. Sci. U.S.A.,* 77, 4702, 1980.

125. **Cherry, R. J.,** Modulation of protein-protein interactions in membranes, *Biochem. Soc. Trans.,* 15, 91, 1987.

126. **Nigg, E. A., Gahmberg, C. G., and Cherry, R. J.,** Rotational diffusion of band 3 proteins in membranes from En(a-) and neuraminidase-treated normal human erythrocytes, *Biochim. Biophys. Acta,* 600, 636, 1980.

127. **Golan, D. E. and Veatch, W.,** Lateral mobility of band 3 in the human erythrocyte membrane studied by fluorescence photobleaching recovery: evidence for control by cytoskeletal interactions, *Proc. Natl. Acad. Sci. U.S.A.,* 77, 2537, 1980.

128. **Tsuji, A. and Ohnishi, S.,** Restriction of the lateral motion of band 3 in the erythrocyte membrane by the cytoskeletal network: dependence on spectrin association state, *Biochemistry,* 25, 6133, 1986.

129. **Beth, A. H., Conturo, T. E., Venkataramu, S. D., and Staros, J. V.,** Dynamics and interactions of the anion channel in intact human erythrocytes: an electron paramagnetic resonance spectroscopic study employing a new membrane-impermeant bifunctional spin-label, *Biochemistry,* 25, 3824, 1986.

130. **Beth, A. H., Conturo, T. E., Abumrad, N. A., and Staros, J. V.,** Studies of the dynamics and interactions of the anion channel in intact human erythrocytes by saturation transfer EPR spectroscopy, in *Membrane Proteins,* Goheen, S. C., Ed., Bio-Rad Publishers, Richmond, CA, 1987, 371.

131. **Cuppoletti, J., Goldinger, J., Kang, B., Jo, I., Berenski, C., and Jung, C. Y.,** Anion carrier in the human erythrocyte exists as a dimer, *J. Biol. Chem.,* 260, 15714, 1985.

132. **Verkman, A. S., Skorecki, K. L., Jung, C. Y., and Ausiello, D. A.,** Target molecular weights for red cell band 3 stilbene and mercurial binding sites, *Am. J. Physiol.,* 251, C541, 1986.

133. **Clarke, S.,** The size and detergent binding of membrane proteins, *J. Biol. Chem.,* 250, 5459, 1975.

134. **Yu, J. and Steck, T. L.,** Isolation and characterization of band 3, the predominant polypeptide of the human erythrocyte membrane, *J. Biol. Chem.,* 250, 9170, 1975.

135. **Nakashima, H. and Makino, S.,** State of association of band 3 protein from bovine erythrocyte membrane in nonionic detergent, *J. Biochem. (Tokyo),* 88, 933, 1980.

136. **Dorst, H.-J. and Schubert, D.,** Self-association of band 3 protein from human erythrocyte membranes in aqueous solutions, *HoppeSeyler's Z. Physiol. Chem.,* 360, 1605, 1979.

137. **Pappert, G. and Schubert, D.,** Self-association of band 3 protein from erythrocyte membranes in solutions of a nonionic detergent Ammonyx-LO, in *Protides of Biological Fluids,* Peeters, H., Ed., Pergamon Press, New York, 1982, 117.

138. **Nakashima, H., Nakagawa, Y., and Makino, S.,** Detection of the associated state of membrane proteins by polyacrylamide gradient gel electrophoresis with non-denaturing detergents. Application to band 3 protein from erythrocyte membranes, *Biochim. Biophys. Acta,* 643, 509, 1981.

139. **Tomida, M., Kondo, Y., Moriyama, R., Machida, H., and Makino, S.,** Effect of stilbenedisulfonate binding on the state of association of the membrane-spanning domain of band 3 from bovine erythrocyte membrane, *Biochim. Biophys. Acta,* 943, 493, 1988.

140. **Werner, P. K. and Reithmeier, R. A. F.,** Molecular characterization of the human erythrocyte anion transport protein in octyl glucoside, *Biochemistry,* 24, 6375, 1985.

141. **Makino, S. and Nakashima, H.,** Behavior of fragmented band 3 from chymotrypsin-treated bovine erythrocyte membrane in nonionic detergent solution, *J. Biochem. (Tokyo),* 92, 1069, 1982.

142. **Schubert, D. and Domning, B.,** A new method for the preparation of band 3, the main integral protein of the human erythrocyte membrane, *HoppeSeyler's Z. Physiol. Chem.,* 359, 507, 1978.

143. **Lukacovic, M. F., Feinstein, M. B., Sha'afi, R. I., and Perrie, S.,** Purification of stabilized band 3 protein of the human erythrocyte membrane and its reconstitution into liposomes, *Biochemistry,* 20, 3145, 1981.

144. **Pimplikar, S. W. and Reithmeier, R. A. F.,** Affinity chromatography of band 3, the anion transport protein of erythrocyte membranes, *J. Biol. Chem.,* 261, 9770, 1986.

145. **Moriyama, R., Nakashima, H., Makino, S., and Koga, S.,** A study on the separation of reconstituted proteoliposomes and unincorporated membrane proteins by use of hydrophobic affinity gels, with special reference to band 3 from bovine erythrocyte membranes, *Anal. Biochem.,* 139, 292, 1984.

146. **Moriyama, R., Kitahara, T., Sasaki, T., and Makino, S.,** Structural characterization of the cytoplasmic pole of band 3 from bovine erythrocyte membranes, *Arch. Biochem. Biophys.,* 243, 228, 1985.

147. **Low, P. S., Westfall, M. A., Allen, D. P., and Appell, K. C.,** Characterization of the reversible conformational equilibrium of the cytoplasmic domain of erythrocyte membrane band 3, *J. Biol. Chem.,* 259, 13070, 1984.

148. **Appell, K. C. and Low, P. S.,** Partial structural characterization of the cytoplasmic domain of the erythrocyte membrane protein, band 3, *J. Biol. Chem.,* 256, 11104, 1981.

149. **Low, P. S.,** Structure and function of the cytoplasmic domain of band 3: center of erythrocyte membrane-peripheral protein interactions, *Biochim. Biophys. Acta,* 864, 145, 1986.

150. **Macara, I. G. and Cantley, L. C.,** The structure and function of band 3. *Cell Membranes: Methods and Reviews,* Elson, E., Frazier, W., and Glasser, L., Eds., Plenum Press, New York, 1983, 41.

151. **Reithmeier, R. A. F.,** Fragmentation of the band 3 polypeptide from human erythrocyte membranes. Size and detergent binding of the membrane-associated domain, *J. Biol. Chem.,* 254, 3054, 1979.

152. **Benz, R., Tosteson, M. T., and Schubert, D.,** Formation and properties of tetramers of band 3 protein from human erythrocyte membranes in planar lipid bilayers, *Biochim. Biophys. Acta,* 775, 347, 1984.

153. **Boodhoo, A. and Reithmeier, R. A. F.,** Characterization of matrix-bound band 3, the anion transport protein from human erythrocyte membranes, *J. Biol. Chem.,* 259, 785, 1984.

154. **Jennings, M. L. and Passow, H.,** Anion transport across the erythrocyte membrane, in situ proteolysis of band 3 protein and cross-linking of proteolytic fragments by 4,4′-diisothiocyano dihydrostilbene-2,2′-disulfonate, *Biochim. Biophys. Acta,* 554, 498, 1979.

155. **Passow, H.,** Molecular aspects of band 3 protein-mediated anion transport across the red blood cell membrane, *Rev. Physiol. Biochem. Pharmacol.,* 103, 61, 1986.

156. **Mühlebach, T. and Cherry, R. J.,** Influence of cholesterol on the rotation and self association of band 3 in the human erythrocyte membrane, *Biochemistry,* 21, 4225, 1982.

157. **Klappauf, E. and Schubert, D.,** Interactions of band 3 protein from human erythrocyte membranes with cholesterol and cholesterol analogues, *HoppeSeyler's Z. Physiol. Chem.,* 360, 1225, 1979.

158. **Seigneuret, M., Favre, E., Marrot, G., and Devaux, P. F.,** Strong interactions between a spin-labeled cholesterol analog and erythrocyte proteins in the human erythrocyte membrane, *Biochim. Biophys. Acta,* 813, 174, 1985.

159. **Schubert, D. and Boss, K.,** Band 3 protein—cholesterol interactions in erythrocyte membranes, *FEBS Lett.,* 150, 4, 1982.

160. **Klugerman, A. H., Gaarn, A., and Parkes, J. G.,** Effect of cholesterol upon the conformation of band 3 and its transmembrane fragment, *Can. J. Biochem. Cell Biol.,* 62, 1033, 1984.

161. **Grunze, M., Forst, B., and Deuticke, B.,** Dual effect of membrane cholesterol on simple and mediated transport processes in human erythrocytes, *Biochim. Biophys. Acta,* 600, 860, 1980.

162. **Gregg, V. A. and Reithmeier, R. A. F.,** Effect of cholesterol on phosphate uptake by human red blood cells, *FEBS Lett.,* 157, 159, 1983.

163. **Jackson, P. and Morgan, D. B.,** The relation between the membrane cholesterol content and anion exchange in the erythrocytes of patients with cholestasis, *Biochim. Biophys. Acta* 693, 99, 1982.

164. **Cabantchik, Z. I., Baruch, D., Keren-Zur, Y., Zangvill, M., and Ginsburg, H.,** The modulatory effect of membrane viscosity on structural and functional properties of the anion exchange protein of human erythrocytes, *Membr. Biochem.,* 6, 197, 1986.

165. **Deuticke, B. and Haest, C. W. M.,** Lipid modulation of transport proteins in vertebrate cell membranes, *Annu. Rev. Physiol.,* 49, 221, 1987.

166. **Wilbers, K. H., Haest, C. W. M., Von Benthem, M., and Deuticke, B.,** Influence of enzymatic phospholipid cleavage on the permeability of the erythrocyte membrane. II. Protein-mediated transfer of monosaccharides and anions, *Biochim. Biophys. Acta,* 554, 400, 1979.

167. **Sandermann, H., Jr.,** Regulation of membrane enzymes by lipids, *Biochim. Biophys. Acta,* 515, 209, 1978.

168. **Gruber, H. J. and Low, P. S.,** Interaction of amphiphiles with integral membrane proteins. I. Structural destabilization of the anion transport protein of the erythrocyte membrane by fatty acids, fatty alcohols, and fatty amines, *Biochim. Biophys. Acta,* 944, 414, 1988.

169. **Gruber, H. J.,** Interaction of amphiphiles with integral membrane proteins. II. A simple, minimal model for the nonspecific interaction of amphiphiles with the anion exchanger of the erythrocyte membrane, *Biochim. Biophys. Acta,* 944, 425, 1988.

170. **Maneri, L. R. and Low, P. S.,** Structural stability of the erythrocyte anion transporter, band 3, in different lipid environments. A differential scanning calorimetric study, *J. Biol. Chem.,* 263, 16170, 1988.

171. **Funder, J. and Wieth, J. O.,** Chloride transport in human erythrocytes and ghosts: a quantitative comparison, *J. Physiol. (London),* 262, 679, 1976.

172. **Lepke, S. and Passow, H.,** Effects of incorporated trypsin on anion exchange and membrane proteins in human red blood cell ghosts, *Biochim. Biophys. Acta,* 455, 353, 1976.

173. **Grinstein, S., Ship, S., and Rothstein, A.,** Anion transport in relation to proteolytic dissection of band 3 protein, *Biochim. Biophys. Acta,* 507, 294, 1978.

174. **Rao, A.,** Disposition of the band 3 polypeptide in the human erythrocyte membrane. The reactive sulfhydryl groups, *J. Biol. Chem.,* 254, 3503, 1979.

175. **Salhany, J. M., Rauenbuehler, P. B., and Sloan, R. L.,** Alterations in pyridoxal 5′-phosphate inhibition of human erythrocyte anion transport associated with osmotic hemolysis and resealing, *J. Biol. Chem.,* 262, 15974, 1987.

176. **Kay, M. M. B., Bosman, G. J. C. G. M., and Lawrence, C.,** Functional topography of band 3: specific structural alteration linked to functional aberrations in human erythrocytes, *Proc. Natl. Acad. Sci. U.S.A.,* 85, 492, 1988.

177. **Ojcius, D. M., Toon, M. R., and Solomon, A. K.,** Is an intact cytoskeleton required for red cell urea and water transport?, *Biochim. Biophys. Acta,* 944, 19, 1988.

178. **Ojcius, D. M. and Solomon, A. K.,** Sites of *p*-chloromercuri-benzenesulfonate inhibition of red cell urea and water transport, *Biochim. Biophys. Acta,* 942, 73, 1988.

179. **Salhany, J. M., Rauenbuehler, P. B., and Sloan, R. L.,** Characterization of pyridoxal 5′-phosphate affinity labeling of band 3 protein. Evidence for allosterically interacting transport inhibitory subdomains, *J. Biol. Chem.,* 262, 15965, 1987.

180. **Salhany, J. M., Cordes, K. A., and Gaines, E. D.,** Light-scattering measurements of hemoglobin binding to the erythrocyte membrane. Evidence for transmembrane effects related to a disulfonic stilbene binding to band 3, *Biochemistry,* 19, 1447, 1980.

181. **Kaul, R. K., Murthy, S. N. P., Reddy, A. G., Steck. T. L., and Kohler, H.,** Amino acid sequence of the N^{α}-terminal 201 residues of human erythrocyte membrane band 3, *J. Biol. Chem.,* 258, 7981, 1983.

182. **Drickamer, L. K.,** Fragmentation of the 95,000-Dalton transmembrane polypeptide in human erythrocyte membranes. Arrangement of the fragments in the lipid bilayer, *J. Biol. Chem.,* 251, 5115, 1976.

183. **Drickamer, L. K.,** Fragmentation of the band 3 polypeptide from human erythrocyte membranes. Identification of regions likely to interact with the lipid bilayer, *J. Biol. Chem..,* 252, 6909, 1977.

184. **Fukuda, M., Eshdat, Y., Tarone, G., and Marchesi, V. T.,** Isolation and characterization of peptides derived from the cytoplasmic segment of band 3, the predominant intrinsic membrane protein of the human erythrocyte, *J. Biol. Chem.,* 253, 2419, 1978.

185. **Catsimpoolas, N. and Wood, J. L.,** Specific cleavage of cystine peptides by cyanide, *J. Biol. Chem.,* 241, 1790, 1966.

186. **Ramjeesingh, M., Grinstein, S., and Rothstein, A.,** Intrinsic segments of band 3 that are associated with anion transport across the red blood cell membranes, *J. Membr. Biol.,* 57, 95, 1980.

187. **Ramjeesingh, M., Gaarn, A., and Rothstein, A.,** The location of a disulfonic stilbene binding site in band 3, the anion transport protein of the red blood cell membrane, *Biochim. Biophys. Acta,* 599, 127, 1980.

188. **Jennings, M. L. and Nicknish, J. S.,** Erythrocyte band 3 protein: evidence for multiple membrane-crossing segments in the 17000-dalton chymotryptic fragment, *Biochemistry,* 23, 6432, 1984.

189. **Knauf, P. A.,** Anion transport in erythrocytes, in *Physiology of Membrane Disorders,* Andreoli, T. E., Hoffman, J. F., Fanestil, D. D., and Schultz, S. G., Eds., Plenum Press, New York, 1986, 191.

190. **Boxer, D. H., Jenkins, R. E., and Tanner, M. J. A.,** The organization of the major protein of the human erythrocyte membrane, *Biochem. J.,* 137, 531, 1974.

191. **Williams, D. G., Jenkins, R. E., and Tanner, M. J. A.,** Structure of the anion-transport protein of the human erythrocyte membrane. Further studies on the fragments produced by proteolytic digestion, *Biochem. J.,* 181, 477, 1979.

192. **Jennings, M. L., Adams-Lackey, M., and Denney, G. H.,** Peptides of human erythrocyte band 3 protein produced by extracellular papain cleavage, *J. Biol. Chem.,* 259, 4652, 1984.

193. **Jennings, M. L. and Adams, M. F.,** Modification by papain of the structure and function of band 3, the erythrocyte anion transport protein, *Biochemistry,* 20, 7118, 1981.

194. **Brock, C. J., Tanner, M. J. A., and Kempf, C.,** The human erythrocyte anion-transport protein, *Biochem. J.,* 213, 577, 1983.

195. **Tanner, M. J. A., Williams, D. G., and Kyle, D.,** The anion-transport protein of the human erythrocyte membrane. Studies on fragments produced by pepsin digestion, *Biochem. J.,* 183, 417, 1979.

196. **Jenkins, R. E. and Tanner, M. J. A.,** The structure of the major protein of the human erythrocyte membrane, *Biochem. J.* 161, 139, 1977.

197. **Markowitz, S. and Marchesi, V. T.,** The carboxyl-terminal domain of human erythrocyte band 3. Description, isolation, and location in the bilayer, *J. Biol. Chem.,* 256, 6463, 1981.

198. **Mueller, T. J. and Morrison, M.,** Detection of a variant of protein 3, the major transmembrane protein of the human erythrocyte, *J. Biol. Chem.,* 252, 6573, 1977.

199. **Ramjeesingh, M., Gaarn, A., and Rothstein, A.,** The amino acid conjugate formed by the interaction of the anion transport inhibitor 4,4′-diisothiocyano-2,2′-stilbenedisulfonic acid (DIDS) with band 3 protein from human red blood cell membranes, *Biochim. Biophys. Acta,* 641, 173, 1981.

200. **Cousin, J.-L. and Motais, R.,** Inhibition of anion transport in the red blood cell by anionic amphiphilic compounds. I. Determination of the flufenamate-binding site by proteolytic dissection of the band 3 protein, *Biochim. Biophys. Acta,* 687, 147, 1982.

201. **Kopito, R. R. and Lodish, H. F.,** Primary structure and transmembrane orientation of the murine anion exchange protein, *Nature (London),* 316, 234, 1985.

202. **Demuth, D. R., Showe, L. C., Ballantine, M., Palumbo, A., Fraser, P. J., Cioe, L., Rovera, G., and Curtis, P. J.,** Cloning and structural characterization of a human nonerythroid band 3-like protein, *EMBO J.,* 5, 1205, 1986.

203. **Brock, C. J. and Tanner, M. J. A.,** The human erythrocyte anion-transport protein. Further amino acid sequence from the integral membrane domain homologous with the murine protein, *Biochem. J.,* 235, 899, 1986.

204. **Kyte, J. and Doolittle, R. F.,** A simple method for displaying the hydropathic character of a protein, *J. Mol. Biol.,* 157, 105, 1982.

205. **Holzwarth, G.,** Ultraviolet spectroscopy of biological membranes, in *Membrane Molecular Biology,* Fox, C. F. and Keith, A. D., Eds., Sinauer Associates, Stamford, CT, 1972, 228.

206. **Greenfield, N. and Fasman, G. D.,** Computed circular dichroism spectra for the evaluation of protein conformation, *Biochemistry,* 8, 4108, 1969.

207. **Oikawa, K., Lieberman, D. M., and Reithmeier, R. A. F.,** Conformation and stability of the anion transport protein of human erythrocyte membranes, *Biochemistry,* 24, 2843, 1985.

208. **Chen, Y.-H., Yang, J. T., and Chau, K. H.,** Determination of the helix and beta form of proteins in aqueous solution by circular dichroism, *Biochemistry,* 13, 3350, 1974.

209. **Kopito, R. R., Andersson, M., and Lodish, H. F.,** Structure and organization of the murine band 3 gene, *J. Biol. Chem.,* 262, 8035, 1987.

210. **Appell, K. C. and Low, P. S.,** Evaluation of structural interdependence of membrane-spanning and cytoplasmic domains of band 3, *Biochemistry,* 21, 2151, 1982.

211. **Bjerrum, O. J., Selmer, J. C., Larsen, F. S., and Naaby-Hansen, S.,** Exploitation of antibodies in the study of cell membranes, in *Investigation and Exploitation of Antibody Combining Sites,* Reid, E., Cook, G. M. W., and Morre', D. J., Eds., Plenum Press, New York, 1985, 231.

212. **Rao, A. and Reithmeier, R. A. F.,** Reactive sulfhydryl groups of the band 3 polypeptide from human erythrocyte membranes. Location in the primary structure, *J. Biol. Chem.,* 254, 6144, 1979.

213. **Salhany, J. M. and Cassoly, R.,** Kinetics of *p*-mercuribenzoate binding to the sulfhydryl groups of the isolated cytoplasmic fragment of band 3 protein. Effect of hemoglobin binding on the conformation, *J. Biol. Chem.,* 264, 1399, 1989.

214. **Bunn, H. F. and Forget, B. G.,** *Hemoglobin: Molecular, Genetic and Clinical Aspects,* W.B. Saunders, Philadelphia, 1986.

215. **Knauf, P. A. and Rothstein, A.,** Chemical modification of membranes. I. Effects of sulfhydryl and amino reactive reagents on anion and cation permeability of the human red blood cell, *J. Gen. Physiol.,* 58, 190, 1971.

216. **Ramjeesingh, M., Gaarn, A., and Rothstein, A.,** The sulfhydryl groups of the 35,000 dalton C-terminal segment of band 3 are located in a 9000-dalton fragment produced by chymotrypsin treatment of red cell ghosts, *J. Bioenerg. Biomembr.,* 13, 411, 1981.

217. **Ramjeesingh, M., Gaarn, A., and Rothstein, A.,** The locations of the three cysteine residues in the primary structure of the intrinsic segments of band 3 protein, and implications concerning the arrangement of band 3 protein in the bilayer, *Biochim. Biophys. Acta,* 729, 150, 1983.

218. **Lukacovic, M. F., Verkman, A. S., Dix, J. A., and Solomon, A. K.,** Specific interaction of the water transport inhibitor, pCMBS, with band 3 in red blood cell membranes, *Biochim. Biophys. Acta,* 778, 253, 1984.

219. **Yoon, S. C., Toon, M. R., and Solomon, A. K.,** Relation between red cell anion exchange and water transport, *Biochim. Biophys. Acta,* 778, 385, 1984.

220. **Toon, M. R., Dorogi, P. L., Lukacovic, M. F., and Solomon, A. K.,** Binding of DTNB to band 3 in the human red cell membrane, *Biochim. Biophys. Acta,* 818, 158, 1985.

221. **Reithmeier, R. A. F.,** Inhibition of anion transport in human red blood cells by 5,5'-dithiobis(2-nitrobenzoic acid), *Biochim. Biophys. Acta,* 732, 122, 1983.

222. **Tanner, M. J. A., Williams, D. G., and Jenkins, R. E.,** Structure of the erythrocyte anion transport protein, *Ann. N.Y. Acad. Sci.,* 341, 455, 1980.

223. **Ramjeesingh, M., Gaarn, A., and Rothstein, A.,** Pepsin cleavage of band 3 produces its membrane-crossing domains, *Biochim. Biophys. Acta,* 769, 381, 1984.

224. **Lieberman, D. M., Nattriss, M., and Reithmeier, R. A. F.,** Carboxypeptidase Y digestion of band 3, the anion transport protein of human erythrocyte membranes, *Biochim. Biophys. Acta,* 903, 37, 1987.

225. **Wieth, J. O., Bjerrum, P. J., Brahm, J., and Andersen, O. S.,** The anion transport protein of the red cell membrane. A zipper mechanism of anion exchange, *Tokai J. Exp. Clin. Med.,* 7, 91, 1982.

226. **Jay, D. and Cantley, L.,** Structural aspects of the red cell anion exchange protein, *Annu. Rev. Biochem.,* 55, 511, 1986.

227. **Kleinfeld, A. M., Lukacovic, M., Matayoshi, E. D., and Holloway, P.,** Conformation of membrane proteins determined from the spatial distribution of tryptophan, *Biophys. J.,* 37, 146a, 1982.

228. **Pradhan, D. and Lala, A. K.,** Photochemical labeling of membrane hydrophobic core of human erythrocytes using a new photoactivable reagent 2-[³H] Diazofluorene, *J. Biol. Chem.,* 262, 8242, 1987.

229. **Kopito, R. R. and Lodish, H. F.,** Structure of murine anion exchange protein, *J. Cell. Biochem.,* 29, 1, 1985.

230. **Lodish, H. F.,** Multi-spanning membrane proteins: how accurate are the models?, *Trends Biochem. Sci.,* 13, 332, 1988.
231. **Anjaneyulu, P. S. R., Beth, A. H., Sweetman, B. J., Faulkner, L. A., and Staros, J. V.,** Bis(sulfo-*N*-succinimidyl) [¹⁵N,²H₁₆]Doxyl-2-spiro-4′-pimelate, a stable isotope-substituted, membrane-impermeant bifunctional spin label for studies of the dynamics of membrane proteins: application to the anion-exchange channel in intact human erythrocytes, *Biochemistry,* 27, 6844, 1988.
232. **Johnson, R. M., McGowan, M. W., Morse, P. D., and Dzandu, J. K.,** Proteolytic analysis of the topological arrangement of red cell phosphoproteins, *Biochemistry,* 21, 3599, 1982.
233. **Conrad, M. J. and Penniston, J. T.,** Resolution of erythrocyte membrane proteins by two-dimensional electrophoresis, *J. Biol. Chem.,* 251, 253, 1976.
234. **Findlay, J. B. C.,** The receptor proteins for concanavalin A and lens culinaris phytohemagglutinin in the membrane of the human erythrocyte, *J. Biol. Chem.,* 249, 4398, 1974.
235. **Golovtchenko-Matsumoto, A. M. and Osawa, T.,** Heterogeneity of band 3, the major intrinsic protein of human erythrocyte membranes, *J. Biochem. (Tokyo),* 87, 847, 1980.
236. **Tsuji, T., Irimura, T., and Osawa, T.,** The carbohydrate moiety of band-3 glycoprotein of human erythrocyte membranes, *Biochem. J.,* 187, 677, 1980.
237. **Tsuji, T., Irimura, T., and Osawa, T.,** The carbohydrate moiety of band 3 glycoprotein of human erythrocyte membranes. Structures of lower molecular weight oligosaccharides, *J. Biol. Chem.,* 256, 10497, 1981.
238. **Steck, T. L. and Dawson, G.,** Topographical distribution of complex carbohydrates in the erythrocyte membrane, *J. Biol. Chem.,* 249, 2135, 1974.
239. **Fukuda, M. N., Fukuda, M., and Hakomori, S.,** Cell surface modification by endo-beta-galactosidase. Change of blood group activities and release of oligosaccharides from glycoproteins and glycosphingolipids of human erythrocytes, *J. Biol. Chem.,* 254, 5458, 1979.
240. **Fukuda, M., Dell, A., and Fukuda, M. N.,** Structure of fetal Lactosaminoglycan. The carbohydrate moiety of band 3 isolated from human umbilical cord erythrocytes, *J. Biol. Chem.,* 259, 4782, 1984.
241. **Fukuda, M., Dell, A., Oates, J. E., and Fukuda, M. N.,** Structure of branched Lactosaminoglycan, the carbohydrate moiety of band 3 isolated from adult human erythrocytes, *J. Biol. Chem.,* 259, 8260, 1984.
242. **Jay, D. G.,** Glycosylation site of band 3, the human erythrocyte anion-exchange protein, *Biochemistry,* 25, 554, 1986.
243. **Ideguchi, H., Matsuyama, H., and Hamasaki, N.,** Heterogeneity of human erythrocyte band 3 analyzed by two-dimensional gel electrophoresis, *Eur. J. Biochem.,* 125, 665, 1982.
244. **Ross, A. H. and McConnell, H. M.,** Reconstitution of the erythrocyte anion channel, *J. Biol. Chem.,* 253, 4777, 1978.
245. **Waxman, L.,** The phosphorylation of the major proteins of the human erythrocyte membrane, *Arch. Biochem. Biophys.,* 195, 300, 1979.
246. **Dekowski, S. A., Rybicki, A., and Drickamer, K.,** A tyrosine kinase associated with the red cell membrane phosphorylates band 3, *J. Biol. Chem.,* 258, 2750, 1983.
247. **Flockhart, D. A. and Corbin, J. D.,** Regulatory mechanisms in the control of protein kinases, *CRC Crit. Rev. Biochem.,* 12, 133, 1982.
248. **Tao, M.,** Mechanism of activation of a rabbit reticulocyte protein kinase by adenosine 3′,5′-cyclic monophosphate, *Ann. N.Y. Acad. Sci.,* 185, 227, 1971.
249. **Tao, M. and Hackett, P.,** Adenosine Cyclic 3′:5′-Monophosphate-dependent protein kinase from rabbit erythrocytes, *J. Biol. Chem.,* 248, 5324, 1973.
250. **Simkowski, K. W. and Tao, M.,** Studies on a soluble human erythrocyte protein kinase, *J. Biol. Chem.,* 255, 6456, 1980.
251. **Tao, M., Conway, R., and Cheta, S.,** Purification and characterization of a membrane-bound protein kinase from human erythrocytes, *J. Biol. Chem.,* 255, 2563, 1980.
252. **Phan Dinh Tuy, F., Henry, J., Rosenfeld, C., and Kahn, A.,** High tyrosine kinase activity in normal nonproliferating cells, *Nature (London),* 305, 435, 1983.
253. **Phan Dinh Tuy, F., Henry, J., and Kahn, A.,** Characterization of human red blood cell tyrosine kinase, *Biochem. Biophys. Res. Commun.,* 126, 304, 1985.
254. **Habib-Mohamed, A. and Steck, T. L.,** Band 3 tyrosine kinase. Association with the human erythrocyte membrane, *J. Biol. Chem.,* 261, 2804, 1986.
255. **Lu, P.-W. and Tao, M.,** Phosphorylation of protein tyrosine by human erythrocyte casein kinase A, *Biochem. Biophys. Res. Commun.,* 139, 855, 1986.
256. **Vasseur, C., Piau, J. P., and Bursaux, E.,** Cation dependence of the phosphorylation of specific residues in red cell membrane protein band 3, *Biochim. Biophys. Acta,* 899, 1, 1987.
257. **Hillsgrove, D., Shores, C. G., Parker, J. C., and Maness, P. F.,** Band 3 tyrosine kinase in avian erythrocyte plasma membrane is immunologically related to pp60(c-src), *Am. J. Physiol.,* 253, C286, 1987.
258. **Low, P. S., Allen, D. P., Zioncheck, T. F., Chari, P., Willardson, B. M., Geahlen, R. L., and Harrison, M. L.,** Tyrosine Phosphorylation of band 3 inhibits peripheral protein binding, *J. Biol. Chem.,* 262, 4592, 1987.

259. **Soong, C.-J., Lu, P.-W., and Tao, M.,** Analysis of band 3 cytoplasmic domain phosphorylation and association with ankyrin, *Arch. Biochem. Biophys.,* 254, 509, 1987.

260. **Bursaux, E., Hilly, M., Bluze, A., and Poyart, C.,** Organic phosphates modulate anion self-exchange across the human erythrocyte membrane, *Biochim. Biophys. Acta,* 777, 253, 1984.

261. **Boivin, P., Galand, C., and Bertrand, O.,** Protein band 3 phosphotyrosyl phosphatase purification and characterization, *Int. J. Biochem.,* 19, 613, 1987.

262. **Pontremoli, S., Sparatore, B., Salamino, F., De Tullio, R., Pontremoli, R., and Melloni, E.,** The role of calpain in the selective increased phosphorylation of the anion-transport protein in red cell of hypertensive subjects, *Biochem. Biophys. Res. Commun.,* 151, 590, 1988.

263. **Springer, M. S., Goy, M. F., and Adler, J.,** Protein methylation in behavioural control mechanisms and in signal transduction, *Nature (London),* 280, 279, 1979.

264. **Koshland, D. E., Jr.,** *Bacterial Chemotaxis as a Model Behavioral System,* Raven Press, New York, 1980.

265. **Paik, W. K. and Kim, S.,** *Protein Methylation,* John Wiley & Sons, New York, 1980, 255.

266. **Kim, S.,** S-adenosylmethionine: protein-carboxyl methyltransferase from erythrocyte, *Arch. Biochem. Biophys.,* 161, 652, 1974.

267. **Galletti, P., Paik, W. K., and Kim, S.,** Methyl acceptors for protein methylase II from human-erythrocyte membrane, *Eur. J. Biochem.,* 97, 221, 1979.

268. **Terwilliger, T. C. and Clarke, S.,** Methylation of membrane proteins in human erythrocytes. Identification and characterization of polypeptides methylated in lysed cells, *J. Biol. Chem.,* 256, 3067, 1981.

269. **Lou, L. L. and Clarke, S.,** Carboxyl methylation of human erythrocyte band 3 in intact cells. Relation to anion transport activity, *Biochem. J.,* 235, 183, 1986.

270. **Hsu, L. and Morrison, M.,** A new variant of the anion transport protein in human erythrocytes, *Biochemistry,* 24, 3086, 1985.

271. **Swanson. M. L., Keast, R. K., Jennings, M. L., and Pessin, J. E.,** Heterogeneity in the human erythrocyte band 3 anion-transporter revealed by Triton X-114 phase partitioning, *Biochem. J.,* 255, 229, 1988.

272. **Anderson, D. R., Davis, J. L., and Carraway, K. L.,** Calcium promoted changes of the human erythrocyte membrane. Involvement of spectrin, transglutaminase, and a membrane-bound protease, *J. Biol. Chem.,* 252, 6617, 1977.

273. **Golovtchenko-Matsumoto, A. M., Matsumoto, I., and Osawa, T.,** Degradation of band 3 glycoprotein in vitro by a protease isolated from human erythrocyte membranes, *Eur. J. Biochem.,* 121, 463, 1982.

274. **King, L. E., Jr. and Morrison, M.,** Calcium effects on human erythrocyte membrane proteins, *Biochim. Biophys. Acta,* 471, 162, 1977.

275. **Murachi, T.,** Calpain and calpastatin, *Trends Biochem. Sci.,* 8, 167, 1983.

276. **Tarone, G., Hamasaki, N., Fukuda, M., and Marchesi, V. T.,** Proteolytic degradation of human erythrocyte band 3 by membrane-associated protease activity, *J. Membr. Biol.,* 48, 1, 1979.

277. **Nickson, J. K. and Jones, M. N.,** The degradation of band 3 protein in Triton X-100 extracts of the human erythrocyte membrane, *Biochem. Soc. Trans.,* 8, 308, 1980.

278. **Morrison, M., Grant, W., Smith, H. T., Mueller, T. J., and Hsu, L.,** Catabolism of the anion transport protein in human erythrocytes, *Biochemistry,* 24, 6311, 1985.

279. **Jardetzky, O.,** Simple allosteric model for membrane pumps, *Nature (London),* 211, 969, 1966.

280. **Singer, S. J.,** Thermodynamics, the structure of integral membrane proteins, and transport, *J. Supramol. Struct.,* 6, 313, 1977.

281. **Salhany, J. M. and Sloan, R. L.,** Direct evidence for modulation of porter quaternary structure by transport site ligands, *Biochem. Biophys. Res. Commun.,* 159, 1337, 1989.

Chapter 3

FUNCTIONAL CHARACTERISTICS AND MECHANISM OF BAND 3 ANION EXCHANGE

I. INTRODUCTION

Jardetzky's[1] idea for oligomeric porter function differs from Singer's[2] more complex models. Jardetzky proposed that an association of monomers forms a multicharged dimeric common channel (Figure 20B of Chapter 2) where intersubunit conformational changes serve as a "lock in overland waterways" to change the potential energy of the transported species. This mechanism should yield hyperbolic transport kinetic plots since the sites are tightly coupled. Singer[2] discussed this type of model, but he also mentioned a homotropic porter dimer where "...2 ligand binding sites would be present related to the twofold rotation axis..." (see Figure 5B of Chapter 1). He stated "...These sites might exhibit cooperativity of either positive or negative type..." Although Singer's model was also a common channel model, separate channels could exist with each having an independent transport activity and with superimposed homotropic allosteric interaction energies. The distinction between various models is subtle but discernible. Since each monomer contributes "half of a site" to the porter function in a Jardetzky-type model, dissociation of the dimer would cause a loss of porter function. Furthermore, selective labeling of the monomeric half-site should completely inhibit transport. There is no other outcome since each half-site must be available for the porter to work. This is not the case for Singer's homotropic porter dimer. In that model, monomers have inherent transport activity. They can either function as a unit or be uncoupled and function independently.

The best characterized anion-exchange porters are oligomers which show complex kinetics (Chapter 1). Band 3 porter shows complex transport kinetics and exists in the membrane as at least a stable dimer (Chapter 2) with one active site or class of active sites per monomer. New cross-linking studies have shown that transport site ligands induce a reversible change in the band 3 quaternary structure between dimer cross-linkable (DC) and tetramer cross-linkable (TC) states (Chapter 2). These functional and structural results seem to favor an allosteric theory. This chapter will offer an allosteric interpretation of band 3 porter transport kinetics. We will study a growing body of complete kinetic patterns to see if they are recognizable as those of a classical allosteric homotropic dimer or tetramer.[3] We will also study the effect of inhibitors on pattern type, both in velocity vs. substrate plots and in activity-labeling correlation plots. New ligand distribution experiments will be presented which identify the allosteric interactions as predominantly intermonomeric. Evidence will be given to explain how intermonomeric allosterism can be consistent with linear inhibition by the stilbene disulfonates by showing that the latter uncouple the intermonomeric allosteric interactions. In addition, we will discuss evidence challenging the idea that stilbene disulfonates are pure competitive inhibitors. The issue of the exact site on band 3 for stilbene disulfonate binding has come into sharper focus with the discovery discussed in Chapter 2, that they modulate an allosteric equilibrium between two band 3 porter quaternary structures. Since many reviews exist which describe the details of the band 3 transport literature,[4-22] this review will be selective in its presentation of the data with the attempt of a new synthesis.

II. EVIDENCE THAT ANION EXCHANGE IS THE PREDOMINANT MODE OF RED CELL ANION TRANSPORT

Anion transport through the proteins of a lipid bilayer could occur by two general pathways. The first would be simple conductance (i.e., diffusion of a charged species) through a membrane protein pore or channel while the second would involve a porter mechanism (Chapter 1).[23] Although band 3 is often called a "chloride channel", the use of the name is probably too loose and certainly misrepresents the main mode of chloride transport.

The distinction between the function of band 3 as an anion-exchange porter and its ability to function as an anion-conducting channel is significant. The first distinction is that net anion flow is very much slower than anion exchange.[19,21] In order to measure net anion flow it is first necessary to somehow "uncouple" the movement of cations from their rate-limiting status. The advent of cation ionophores has allowed such uncoupling by providing a pathway for rapid cation permeability. Chappell and Crofts[24] and Harris and Pressman[25] first used cation ionophores. The latter authors concluded that true chloride permeability must be lower than halide self-exchange. These results were subsequently confirmed and similar conclusions were drawn.[26-28] Hunter[29,30] measured the permeability coefficient for the net movement of chloride and found a number of 2×10^{-8} cm-sec^{-1}. Brahm[31] then made chloride equilibrium exchange measurements at pH 7.4 and 37°C and found a number of 5×10^{-8} mole-cm^{-2}-sec^{-1}. The flux for the equilibrium exchange experiment can be calculated,[19] and it should be 2.2×10^{-12} mole-cm^{-2}-sec^{-1}. However, this is fully four orders of magnitude different from that measured by Brahm.[31] Thus, for every 10,000 chloride ions which cross the membrane through the exchange pathway, only one chloride ion crosses the membrane by a mechanism which carries charge. The predominance of the exchange pathway for the chloride transport mechanism is quite the opposite from what one might expect for a simple channel or channel-like pore such as protein P (Chapter 1).

The related feature which distinguishes porter-mediated transport from channel-mediated transport is the so-called *trans* (opposite side of the membrane) acceleration.[23] *Trans* acceleration is an increase in the influx rate of an external anion consequent to an increase in the concentration of the *trans* coanion. Gunn and Fröhlich,[32] Salhany and Rauenbuehler,[33] and Hautmann and Schnell[34] have all performed the experiment for the red cell band 3 system and have shown that increasing the *trans* anion concentration does indeed increase the velocity of transport. This finding is inconsistent with a simple channel model in which occupancy of *trans* channel sites should inhibit anion influx.

The results just described suggest that the influx of one anion is very tightly coupled to the efflux of the other. Yet, despite its apparent insignificance, the low permeability pathway is a major conductance pathway of the red cell since the flux rate is high with respect to cation flow. Chloride conductance is about two orders of magnitude larger than the conductances of either potassium or sodium. Therefore, membrane potential is essentially determined by the chloride equilibrium potential, and intracellular and extracellular chloride are at electrochemical equilibrium due to the high chloride conductance of the membrane.[35-37]

There are two significant pathways for chloride conductance in the membrane. One is inhibited by the covalent inhibitor of anion exchange known as DIDS (4,4′-diisothiocyano-2,2′-stilbene disulfonate) or the related compound H$_2$DIDS (4,4′-diisothiocyano-1,2-diphenylethane-2,2′-disulfonate), while the other pathway is apparently not.[38-41] It was suggested that the stilbene-sensitive portion of conductive flux involves band 3, while the stilbene-insensitive component is due to simple electrodiffusion. This hypothesis was tested by studying the temperature[40] and pH[41] dependencies of net flux. H$_2$DIDS-sensitive net flux was independent of pH over the same range where equilibrium chloride exchange showed no dependence, while the H$_2$DIDS-insensitive net flux was pH dependent over that range. These differences led to the further support of bipartite diffusion processes, one through band 3 and one elsewhere on the membrane. However, site assignment based on the ability of H$_2$DIDS to inhibit one component of conductive anion flux over the other may have a shortcoming if an anion pathway on band 3 exists which is incompletely or allosterically blocked by H$_2$DIDS. Recent chloride nuclear magnetic resonance (NMR) anion-binding data[42] suggest that DIDS may incompletely block chloride binding to sites on band 3 despite the ability of DIDS to totally inhibit transport (see

Section IV.E.3, below). This point is raised only as a caveat, since it is simpler to assume that one site is on band 3 and the other somewhere else. The interpretation does, nevertheless, depend on how the exact mechanism by which DIDS or H_2DIDS inhibits band 3 anion transport is viewed, a topic for a later discussion.

Aside from site assignment problems, it is clear that at least one component of anion diffusion involves a band 3-mediated pathway. However, the mechanism is very different from the faster anion-exchange pathway.[43] It is relevant to an understanding of the mechanism of anion exchange to briefly consider current views on the mechanism of band 3-mediated anion conductance. In a porter system where solute exchange is much faster than solute net movement (e.g., band 3), the maximum velocity for the zero-*trans* net efflux of an anion (i.e., efflux into a virtually solute-free medium) should be limited by the movement of the unloaded porter. This is called "slippage" to indicate recycling of the empty porter. Slippage, because it does not involve the bound anion, should be independent of the type of transported anion actually used in the experiments.[23] However, Fröhlich[44] found that there can be a considerable difference in the flux depending on anion type. To explain this, he proposed a new mechanism called "tunneling"[45,46] where the anion is transported without a conformational change in the carrier.

Although there is a good deal of circumstantial evidence favoring the tunneling hypothesis,[46] other mechanisms are possible, and some have been discussed recently by Fröhlich.[46] One interesting interpretation of this effect has been given by Stein.[23] He points out that the rates of net transport and of equilibrium exchange are not compatible with the simple carrier model since V_{max}/K_m of the simple model must be the same for the zero-*trans* and the equilibrium exchange experiments, yet they differ by a factor 10^4.[39] An alternative (and he suggests simpler) model is proposed which is the same mechanism proposed by Salhany and Rauenbuehler[33] for band 3 anion exchange and later by Aronson[47] for sodium-proton exchange. In those models (unlike the Ping-Pong model of Chapter 1), the release of one anion occurs only after the binding of a second anion to the exchanger (i.e., in association with formation of a ternary complex). Gottipaty and Fröhlich[48] have recently discovered a second anion binding site which is involved in anion conductance and which is apparently not mutually exclusive with the stilbene disulfonate site.

In summary, it is seen that the role of the *trans* anion is different for the two functional modes of band 3. Increasing the concentration of extracellular chloride hyperbolically reduces the stilbene disulfonate-sensitive net efflux of chloride,[40] while it accelerates exchange flux.[32-34] Thus, net flux through band 3 is affected by *trans* chloride as if band 3 were a channel, while *trans* chloride affects equilibrium exchange flux as if band 3 were a porter. The porter functional mode dominates. For a more comprehensive discussion of band 3 anion conductance, consult References 19 and 46.

III. CHARACTERISTICS OF THE BAND 3 ANION EXCHANGE FUNCTION WHICH ARE INDICATIVE OF MECHANISM

A. KINETIC PATTERNS FOR BAND 3 PORTER

1. Introduction

Certain characteristics of any mediated transport process are expected. Mediation of solute transport should involve a finite number of membrane entities and, consequently, saturation phenomena in plots of transport velocity vs. substrate concentration. This distinguishes mediated transport from general diffusion through the lipid. If there are mediators, there should be agents which will bind to the mediation element and prevent transport. These prerequisites should yield the following characteristic patterns: (1) hyperbolic or Henri-Michaelis-Menten kinetics, (2) pure competitive inhibition for substrates or substrate analogues, and (3) linear 1:1 stoichiometric inhibition for the covalent binding of the inhibitor to the single active site of the mediator. The last could also be observed through the *covalent* 1:1 stoichiometric binding of a noncompetitive inhibitor. If the porter unit is a protein monomer, then one active site inhibitor will bind per monomer. If the porter unit is a dimer with half-site reactivity, then the covalent inhibitor will bind with a 1:2 inhibitor to monomer stoichiometry. Either the inhibitor could cross-link both monomeric half-sites simultaneously or it could bind to one or the other half-site and turn off all of transport. Covalent inhibition studies, although they indicate nothing about the mechanism of inhibition (competitive vs. noncompetitive), can reveal a great deal about the presence or absence of interactions between porter subunits. For example, half-site reactivity associated with hyperbolic transport kinetics implies a Jardetzky-type dimeric porter unit with tight coupling between monomeric sites. Linear (1:1 per monomer) covalent activity-labeling correlation plots associated with hyperbolic substrate kinetics imply a monomeric porter functional unit. However, if substrate kinetics are nonhyperbolic, then at least two sites are present which may interact, assuming that the nonhyperbolic kinetics are not arising for trivial reasons. Such reasons could include the existence of more than one pathway for transport, such as simple diffusion plus mediated transport or two transport mediators, one specific and one nonspecific. If a covalent inhibitor exists and all of transport is turned off by binding to a specific membrane component, complex kinetic patterns may then be assigned to that membrane component.

How should nonhyperbolic transport kinetic patterns be approached when simple diffusion can be neglected and when there is clear evidence for the existence of only one porter entity in the membrane? The most unrestrictive way to proceed is to consider kinetic pattern types and then to ask if these are recognizable. Although such general inspection of kinetic patterns alone cannot unequivocally distinguish the operative mechanism, it has the possible advantage of helping to decide which mechanisms *not* to consider.

Pattern recognition is facilitated by considering the calculus of complex kinetics in terms of empirical rate laws. One can generally describe nonhyperbolic kinetic patterns by the following equation:

$$y = (a_1x + a_2x^2 + ... a_nx^n) / (b_0 + b_1x + b_2x^2 ... b_nx^n) \tag{1}$$

where the a's and b's are positive coefficients, y is the velocity, and x the varied anion concentration. Bardsley and his co-workers[49,50] have presented a detailed analysis of the calculus of polynomials for velocity vs. substrate curves. Their discussion distinguishes between the general equation for a two-site interactive mechanism (the so-called 2:2 function) and the modifier site mechanism (the so-called 1:2 function). Equation 2, can be used to describe a wide variety of two-site mechanisms.

$$y = (a_1x + a_2x^2) / (1 + b_1x + b_2x^2) \tag{2}$$

This function has four possible distinct shapes in the y vs. x plots or y^{-1} vs. x^{-1} plots of Figure 1A. Depending on the relative values of the a/b coefficients of x, observed patterns may include: hyperbolic-partial substrate inhibition, I(ii), sigmoid-partial substrate inhibition, II(ii), negative cooperativity as shown in one of the double reciprocal plots, I(i), and pure sigmoidal II(i).

The behavior of the 1:2 function is that of the classical "modifier site" model involving classic "dead-end" substrate inhibition. Because it can account for substrate inhibition without abandoning the single transport site concept, it has been a popular mechanism to explain the anomaly of substrate inhibition for band 3 anion exchange, as was illustrated in Figure 15 of Chapter 1.[51] The idea is that a noncompetitive inhibitory site (which does not affect the affinity of the transport site) "simply" prevents the "carrier" from "turning" when occupied. Because the basic active site does not involve a second anion binding site, the nonhyperbolic nature of this mechanism arises solely due to a squared term in the denominator and so is called a 1:2 function (Equation 3):

$$y = (a_1x) / (1 + b_1x + b_2x^2) \tag{3}$$

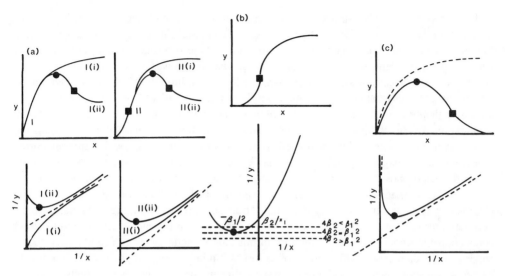

FIGURE 1. Possible shapes for the 2:2 function (Equation 2 of the text). (a) Pattern I, $a_2 < a_1b_1$: I(i), $a_1b_2 < a_2b_1$; I(ii), $a_1b_2 > a_2b_1$. Pattern II, $a_2 > a_1b_1$: II(i) $a_1b_2 < a_2b_1$; II(ii) $a_1b_2 > a_2b_1$. Note that when $a_1b_2 = a_2b_1$, y/x has no maximum and (1/y)/(1/x) has zero gradient at the origin. Also, when $a_2 = a_1b_1$, the y/x behavior is as for case I, but the (1/y)/(1/x) asymptote passes through the origin. (b) $a_2, b_1, b_2 > 0$, but $a_1 = 0$. y/x must be sigmoid (y′ = 0 at the origin) and can have no maximal. (1/y)/(1/x) is a parabola as indicated. (c) $a_1, b_1, b_2 > 0$, but $a_2 = 0$. The dashed line is the same function but also with $b_2 = 0$. This is the equation of dead-end substrate inhibition (1:2 or "modifier site" function), which looks superficially like the 2:2 function with a maximum (partial substrate inhibition, see case I[ii] above). The functions can be distinguished since y/log × is *symmetrical* for the 1:2 case but *asymmetrical* for the 2:2 case. Also, (1/y)/x has no inflection for the 1:2 case but can have one inflection for the 2:2 case. (From Bardsley, W. G. and Childs, R. E., *Biochem. J.*, 149, 313, 1975. With permission.)

Although both 2:2 and 1:2 functions can yield substrate inhibition-type plots, the discriminating feature worth noting is that the 1:2 function will always yield symmetrical y vs. log x plots.[49] Deviation from symmetrical behavior implies a higher-degree rate law. This is a consequence of the fact that raising the concentration to high levels in pure dead-end modifier mechanisms (1:2 functions) must drive the velocity to zero (Figure 1C), while 2:2 functions will approach some constant nonzero value lying below the maximum (Figure 1A). In addition to this distinction, 2:2 functions can account for many more complexities of a system that cannot be explained by the 1:2 function (Figure 1). In other words, if one observes patterns like those in Figure 1A for a system, even if the exact mechanism is not known, the final form of the equation will look like the 2:2 function with concentration-squared terms in both the numerator and the denominator. The recognition of such patterns requires that data be collected over the broadest ranges possible, for restricting data collection to a narrow (even physiological) range would make even the most complex pattern look simple.

2. What Type of Kinetic Patterns Are Observed for Band 3 Porter?

When the red cell chloride exchange was initially characterized, the kinetic patterns suggested the presence of a saturation phenomenon.[52] Then Cass and Dalmark[53] showed that the chloride exchange is not hyperbolic, but shows partial substrate inhibition when data are collected at higher anion concentration (see Figure 15 of Chapter 1). One of the first questions to ask about the partial substrate inhibition is if it is an artifact of high ionic strength. If the transport curve is arbitrarily divided into two parts (which, of course, may have no mechanistic significance), then one could at least experimentally ask if the "transport" function and the "substrate inhibition" function both show competitive-like behavior when other anions are added. This question presumes that specific anion-binding sites are involved for each function. Dalmark[51] showed that both chloride transport and substrate inhibition functions are competitive with bicarbonate. He also showed that the concentration dependence of these effects was different for the various halides, further suggesting that partial substrate inhibition was not due to ionic strength. Schnell and co-workers[54] showed that the substrate inhibition phenomenon was also pH dependent, as if some specific group on a protein was being titrated.

Can any single site model explain partial substrate inhibition? The answer would be affirmative in the case where the so-called "ion-hopping" rates of a Läuger-type kinetic model are faster than the conformational fluctuations of the protein (Chapter 1). This could be an explanation for the behavior of chloride self-exchange, but it seems to fail to explain the observation of substrate inhibition with anions such as sulfate and iodide, which are transported several orders of magnitude more slowly than either chloride or bicarbonate.[19] Nevertheless, Tanford[55] has proposed an approach site concept which is an expansion of Läuger's kinetic model but with the addition of the specific assignment of a function to the additional sites. The model once again preserves the idea of a single "transport site" by assuming that kinetic effects between approach sites and the transport site are responsible for substrate inhibition at high anion concentration. Experimental support for this kinetic model of the self-inhibition effect is lacking. Indeed, recent NMR studies of chloride binding[56] suggest that anion binding to exofacial transport sites on band 3 is at rapid equilibrium precluding kinetic effects.

If kinetic effects can be ruled-out as an explanation for substrate inhibition, then there may be a physically distinct "second site" involved. It has been proposed that partial substrate inhibition arises from the existence of a so-called modifier site.[51] Although this may be a possible explanation, it is not supported by the observed partial inhibitory character of the pattern in Figure 15 of Chapter 1. Partial substrate inhibition contradicts expectations from a modifier site model and favors an allosteric interpretation. When first considered, the modifier site was believed to be an exofacial site.[19,21] However, recent studies by Knauf and Mann[57] clearly show that raising internal but not external chloride leads to the same type of substrate inhibition pattern seen in the usual experiment in which anion concentrations are raised on both sides of the membrane simultaneously. If there is an external substrate inhibition function, its affinity would have to be even lower than the site(s) which are responsive at the inner surface.

Because the anion-exchange system depends on both external and internal anion concentration, it is necessary to systematically study the curves as a function of one anion at various constant *trans* anion concentrations. Salhany and Swanson[58] performed such an experiment using a dithionite-sulfate exchange system. The experimental principle is shown in Figure 2. Intact red cells or resealed ghosts are treated so that the internal hemoglobin is converted to the methemoglobin (metHb) form. This form of hemoglobin directly and stoichiometrically reacts with internal dithionite to yield deoxyhemoglobin and SO_2 gas. The reaction is associated with a major change in color which is followed in the dual wavelength stopped-flow apparatus, on-line to a computer. The theory of ion trapping in this "zero-*trans*" heteroexchange experiment has been extensively discussed.[58] The advantage of the method over the use of radio-labeled tracers is its extreme accuracy and the ability to easily vary *trans* anion concentration independent of the outside anion concentration. Since the internal consumption reaction is several orders of magnitude faster than membrane transport, one observes the internal reaction, but the rate is limited either by diffusion or by a mediated process.

Dithionite-sulfate heteroexchange shows saturation-like behavior (Figure 3). However, when the data are plotted in Lineweaver-Burk form, a distinct negative cooperative pattern is evident (Figure 3C).[58] The negative cooperativity in dithionite-sulfate exchange could arise from three sources. One possible source of negative cooperative-appearing patterns would be the presence of a combination of band 3-mediated anion exchange and diffusion. The second source would be the presence of band 3 exchange plus dithionite transport via some other mediated pathway. Finally, the complexity could be an inherent property of band 3 porter itself. Both negative cooperativity and substrate inhibition imply the existence of a low affinity, alternate pathway for anion transport, and they can be related to each other in certain complex allosteric kinetic models.[3]

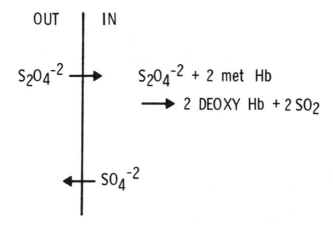

1) COLOR CHANGE $\equiv$ met Hb $\rightarrow$ Hb
2) RATE DETERMINED BY
$S_2O_4^{-2}$ - SO_4^{-2} EXCHANGE
ACROSS THE MEMBRANE

FIGURE 2. Principle of the dithionite-sulfate exchange experiment. Intra-cellular dithionite stoichiometrically reduces metHb to yield deoxy Hb which causes a color change. However, the rate-limiting step is dithionite-sulfate exchange across the red cell membrane because the internal dithionite consumption rate is many orders of magnitude faster than divalent anion exchange across the membrane.

In order to rule out the first two possibilities, Salhany and co-workers titrated band 3 in intact red cells with covalent DIDS.[59] If there is a significant second pathway for dithionite influx, it would be impossible to inhibit transport fully. Figure 4 shows the graph of DIDS titration of intact red cells and of resealed ghosts derived from the same intact cells.[60] It is clear that in both cases transport is totally inhibited. This indicates that there are no significant alternate pathways for dithionite transport. Salhany took the test a step further. He fully labeled intact red cells with DIDS and then added dithionite to levels in excess of 1 M. In unlabeled metHb cells there was an immediate color conversion from the characteristic brown to the deep purple color of deoxy-hemoglobin. Yet even at such abnormally high dithionite concentrations, the DIDS-treated cells did not turn color until more than 36 h later at room temperature. This very slow change must represent the diffusion component for dithionite. Such slow diffusion requiring extremely high dithionite concentration for intact red cells cannot contribute to any of the transport kinetics which have been published. From these studies it seems clear that the negative cooperativity in dithionite transport is a real feature of band 3.

It is worth noting that Shoemaker and co-workers[61] have found a phosphate/sodium co-transport pathway which is apparently insensitive to addition of the reversible stilbene disulfonate DNDS (4,4'-dinitrostilbene-2,2'-disulfonate) added at 37°C. This pathway accounts for 20% of phosphate transport, while the DNDS-sensitive pathway accounts for 70%. The DNDS-insensitive pathway is apparently not used at 20°C since under those conditions the authors see virtually complete inhibition of anion transport by DNDS.[61] Although there is no evidence as to whether or not sulfate or dithionite could use this pathway, because of its temperature dependence it would not be operative in the dithionite-sulfate exchange experiments which were performed at 25°C or less. In addition, it is important to realize that the DNDS-

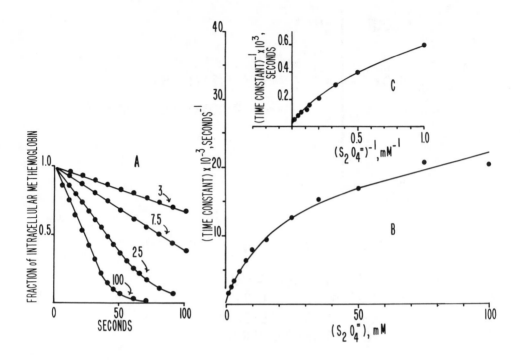

FIGURE 3. Intracellular methemoglobin reduction as a function of extracellular dithionite concentration. (A) Computer corrected, normalized time courses at 3, 7.5, 25, and 100 mM extracellular dithionite after the mix. (B) Plot of the time constant (equivalent to velocity) from the linear portion of curves in (A) vs. extracellular dithionite concentration. (C) Double-reciprocal or Lineweaver-Burk plot of the data in B. Note the negative cooperative appearance of the Lineweaver-Burk plot. (From Salhany, J. M. and Swanson, J. C., *Biochemistry,* 17, 3354, 1978. With permission.)

insensitive pathway is functionally defined using a reversible inhibitor. It is not known if a covalent inhibitor such as DIDS would also inhibit only 70% of total phosphate transport or if it would inhibit all of phosphate transport even at 37°C.

The observation of negative cooperativity with an unconventional method like the dithionite-sulfate assay requires confirmation by a more conventional technique. Schnell and co-workers[34,62] performed an extensive series of studies on the complete concentration dependence of sulfate, phosphate, and chloride anion exchange. We consider these to be among the most extensive kinetic results available on the band 3 transport system in terms of the completeness of data collection. The findings shed considerable light on the mechanism. First, the authors found that both phosphate and sulfate equilibrium self-exchange show positive cooperativity at the low end of the curve (Figure 5). (Note that positive cooperativity cannot be explained by the existence of a second, high affinity transport pathway.) Since partial substrate inhibition is a well-established feature at the top of the curve, divalent anion equilibrium exchange may be characterized as following sigmoidal-partial-substrate inhibition kinetics. This result is totally inconsistent with a 1:2 modifier site formalism and strongly supports a 2:2 kinetic rate law for the band 3 system.[49,50]

The complexity of the kinetics was further revealed by the efflux and influx exchange experiments,[62] which were performed under analogous conditions to the Salhany-Swanson[58] experiment. Schnell and Besl[62] found that when internal anion concentration is held constant and external anion concentration varied, the kinetics present a negative cooperative pattern (Figure 6) in full agreement with the results of Salhany and co-workers.[58,63,64] Interestingly, when the same experiment is performed in the opposite direction (in to out) using sulfate or phosphate, hyperbolic patterns are seen (Figure 7).[62] It would appear that the shape of the kinetic pattern is

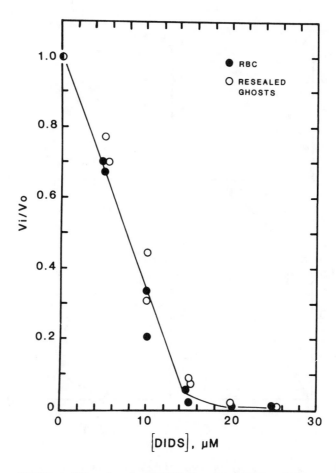

FIGURE 4. Effect of covalent DIDS binding on the inhibition of dithionite transport in intact red cells and resealed ghosts derived from the same red cells. (From Salhany, J. M., Rauenbuehler, P. B., and Sloan, R. L., *J. Biol. Chem.*, 262, 15974, 1987. With permission.)

a manifestation of some type of membrane mechanistic asymmetry in the transport of divalent anions.

Monovalent anion exchange has been extensively characterized by Hautmann and Schnell[34] in a manner similar to that used for divalent exchange. Their equilibrium exchange results are shown in Figure 8. The data in this study were not extended to ranges where substrate inhibition is seen. The Lineweaver-Burk plot shows that the lower portion of the curve does follow an initially hyperbolic function. Thus, monovalent anion exchange can be characterized in equilibrium self-exchange as hyperbolic-partial substrate inhibition which, because of the partial character of substrate inhibition, is inconsistent with a 1:2 modifier site function but would rather be consistent with a general 2:2 function.

Hautmann and Schnell[34] also investigated the kinetic patterns by varying the concentration of chloride on each side of the membrane independently. There are two potentially significant findings shown in Figure 9. First, when velocity vs. *cis* chloride curves are constructed and plotted vs. various constant *trans* chloride concentrations, these Lineweaver-Burk plots are not parallel. We will discuss the significance of this finding in Section VII.D.2. Second, when internal chloride is lowered, a negative cooperative curve seems to develop. The authors discussed this deviation but elected to draw a straight line through some of the data points. Although it may appear that there is only one point off the line, quantitative analysis (given the

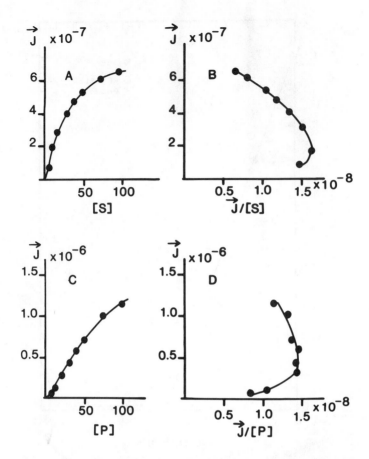

FIGURE 5. Concentration dependence of the sulfate and the phosphate *equilibrium* self-exchange flux. J (mol × min⁻¹) is unidirectional self-exchange flux; [S], 2 to 100 m*M,* is the sulfate; and [P], 5 to 100 m*M,* is the phosphate concentration. Figures A and C are flux/concentration curves of sulfate and phosphate, respectively. Figures B and D are corresponding Woolf-Augustinsson-Hofstee plots. This pattern is characteristic of positive cooperativity. Conditions were 10% suspension of resealed erythrocyte ghosts, 30 m*M* K-citrate, sorbitol substitution, pH 7.3, and 25°C. (From Schnell, K. F. and Besl, E., *Pfluegers Arch., 402,* 197, 1984. With permission.)

small error bars shown) would suggest that a negative cooperative curve should give a better fit. The reality of the effect is evident in that negative cooperativity occurs only at the extracellular surface for all anions and is not observed at the inner surface over the same range of concentrations. More work of this type needs to be performed with monovalents, preferably by using a *trans* kinetic trapping method for chloride like that used for dithionite.

The answer to the question raised in this section is that the transport kinetic patterns look very much like those seen for homotropic, allosteric proteins (Figure 1). This behavior would fit with the fact that the protein exists as an oligomer and that transport site ligands modulate the porter quaternary structure between two states (Chapter 2). If each monomer has the inherent capacity to exchange anions, then the ingredients for homotropic allosterism are in place.

3. Influence of Pattern Shape on the Interpretation of Transport Kinetic Parameters (An Important Aside)

Regardless of the insight which may be gained about mechanism, there are, nevertheless, some important and practical implications of the kinetic results just discussed. These implications should significantly impact on future kinetic studies with band 3 protein.

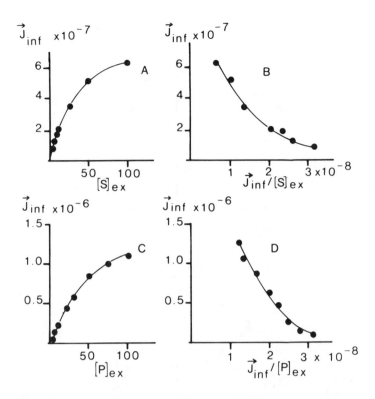

FIGURE 6. Concentration dependence of the *inward* homoexchange-fluxes of sulfate and phosphate. J_{inf}(mol × min^{-1} × g cells^{-1}) is the inward, unidirectional homoexchange flux; $[S]_{ex}$, 2 to 100 mM, is the extracellular sulfate; and $[P]_{ex}$, 2 to 100 mM, the extracellular phosphate concentration. The intracellular concentrations of sulfate or phosphate were 100 or 110 mM, respectively. Figures A and C are flux/concentration curves for sulfate and phosphate respectively. Figures B and D are corresponding Hofstee plots. The shapes of the Hofstee plots are characteristic of negative cooperativity. There was a 2% suspension of red cell ghosts. The conditions in A and B were K-citrate substitution, while those in C and D were sorbitol substitution, pH 7.3, and 25°C. (From Schnell, K. F., and Besl, E., *Pfluegers Arch.*, 402, 197, 1984. With permission.)

Most approaches to quantitative analysis of band 3 anion transport assume hyperbolic kinetics as a "first approximation" and proceed to extract and compare V_{max} and K_m by standard methods.[3] The justification for this approach in the case of chloride or bicarbonate transport data is that at the low end of the curve the data appear hyperbolic, while the substrate inhibition effect seems to be half saturated at 330 mM. However, quantitative analysis of a 1:2 function indicates that K_m and V_{max} cannot be determined accurately unless data are collected over a very broad concentration range. Then it is necessary to actually fit the data to a 1:2 function. This is because the data at the low end of the curve only approach the "true" hyperbolic function asymptotically (see Figure 1C, dashed line).

If quantitative analysis of monovalent anion exchange is complex, simple analyses of transport parameters for divalent anions is fraught with major pitfalls. If the equilibrium self-exchange experiment is used, the unfortunate fact must be noted (on the basis of the extensive work of Schnell and Besl[62]) that measurements of V_{max} and K_m for the transporter are meaningless. The reason is very clear. There is a sigmoidal dependence at the bottom of the curve and substrate inhibition at the top. That means that most data in the literature collected over a narrow concentration range and fit to a hyperbolic function actually represent a tangent to a curving Lineweaver-Burk plot. These considerations raise questions about the interpretation of

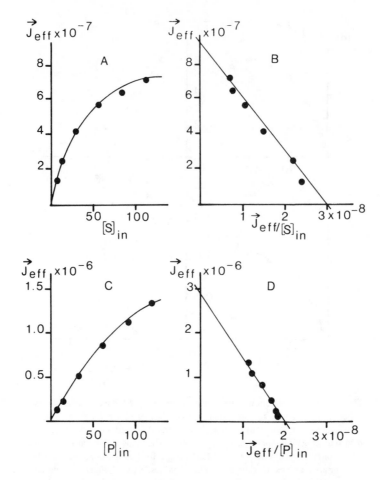

FIGURE 7. Concentration dependence of the *outward* homoexchange flux of sulfate and phosphate. J_{eff} (mol × min^{-1} × g cells^{-1}) is the outward unidirectional homoexchange flux; $[S]_{in}$, 5 to 100 mM, and $[P]_{in}$, 5 to 120 mM, are the intracellular concentrations of sulfate and phosphate. The extracellular sulfate and phosphate concentrations were 100 mM. Figures A and C are flux/concentration curves and Figures B and D are the corresponding Hofstee plots which are hyperbolic. There was a 2% suspension of resealed ghosts in K-citrate substitution, pH 7.3, and 25°C. (From Schnell, K. F. and Besl, E., *Pfluegers Arch.*, 402, 197, 1984. With permission.)

reversible inhibition studies in which site assignments are made based on such kinetic measurements.

B. THE EFFECT OF STILBENE DISULFONATES AND BIS(SULFOSUCCINIMIDYL)SUBERATE ON THE SHAPE OF THE TRANSPORT KINETIC PATTERN

1. Introduction

The impression of red cell anion-exchange kinetics obtained from a survey of the transport kinetic patterns would favor a homotropic allosteric porter dimer or tetramer model. The observed pattern complexities cannot be understood in terms of a single site transport function for either divalent or monovalent anions (which both use the same porter).[65]

In addition to showing characteristic kinetic patterns, a homotropic allosteric dimer or tetramer may be affected by inhibitors in several ways which can also serve to identify the

SELF-EXCHANGE

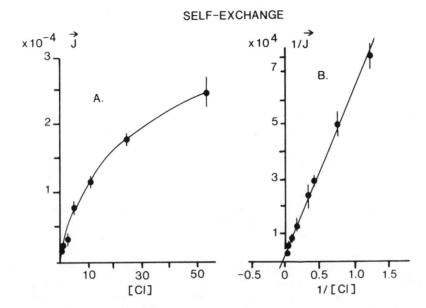

FIGURE 8. Concentration dependence of the chloride *equilibrium* self-exchange flux. (A) Flux/concentration curve. (B) Plot of 1/J versus 1/[Cl]. J, mol/(min × g cells) is the unidirectional chloride flux with [Cl] in millimoles. The incubation solution was 330 mos$M$: 0.25 to 100 mM KCl, 40 mM K-citrate, 0 to 220 mM sorbitol for isoosmotic substitution. There was a 1% suspension of red cell ghosts, pH 7.3, and 0°C. Chloride concentrations on both membrane sides are equal. (From Hautmann, E. K. and Schnell, K. F., *Pfluegers Arch.*, 405, 193, 1985. With permission.)

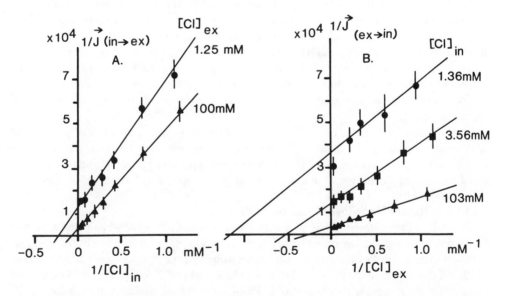

FIGURE 9. Concentration dependence of the chloride homoexchange fluxes in two directions (A and B). (A) Plots of 1/J$_{(in \to ex)}$[mol/(min × g cells)]$^{-1}$ vs. 1/[Cl]$_{in}$, mM^{-1}. (B) Plots of 1/J$_{(ex \to in)}$ vs. 1/[Cl]$_{ex}$, mM^{-1}. [Cl]$_{ex}$ and [Cl]$_{in}$ as indicated in the figures. J$_{(in \to ex)}$ is the outward unidirectional flux, J$_{(ex \to in)}$ the inward unidirectional flux, [Cl]$_{in}$ and [Cl]$_{ex}$ are the intracellular and the extracellular concentrations of chloride. Incubation solution (330 mos$M$): 1 to 100 mM KCl, 40 mM K-citrate, 0 to 220 mM sorbitol for isoosmotic substitution. Either [Cl]$_{in}$ or [Cl]$_{ex}$ was varied, while chloride concentrations at the opposite membrane side were kept constant. The experiments shown in B were performed in bicarbonate-free solutions under N$_2$-atmosphere. There was a 1% suspension of red cell ghosts, 0°C, pH 7.3. Note that the lines are not parallel. (From Hautmann, E. K. and Schnell, K. F., *Pfluegers Arch.*, 405, 193, 1985. With permission.)

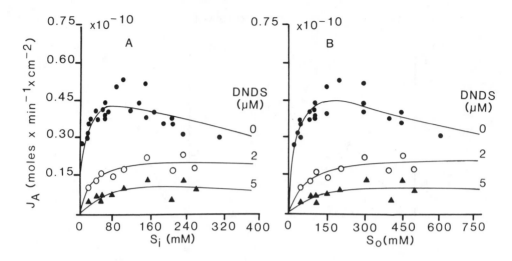

FIGURE 10.   Sulfate self-exchange flux in amphotericin B-treated red blood cells (pH 7.4, 25°C). Ordinate: sulfate self-exchange flux per unit area, J_A (moles $\times$ min^{-1} $\times$ cm^{-2}). Abscissa: (A) internal sulfate concentration, S_i; (B) external sulfate concentration, S_o. The fluxes were performed with 2% cell suspension and the specified concentrations of DNDS. (From Barzilay, M. and Cabantchik, Z. I., *Membr. Biochem.*, 2, 255, 1979. With permission.)

allosteric interactions as homotropic in nature. One effect concerns the influence which inhibitors may have on interactions between porter subunits. Within a homotropic allosteric theory we may expect that certain inhibitors will preserve interactions, while others could destroy or uncouple them. For example, if a covalent inhibitor is bound to one monomer of a homotropic unit and "breaks" the functional connection between monomers of the unit, it would inhibit the function of the newly independent monomer to which it is bound, while the other monomer is now able to function independently. In other words, the mechanism would change by uncoupling the original allosteric interactions. This is only possible for a homotropic allosteric model where each subunit has the inherent potential to function independently even though the native state has concerted subunit functionality. A second effect with which to be concerned is the actual mechanism of inhibition for a given inhibitor for each monomeric anion transport site once the allosteric interactions have been uncoupled (if the inhibitor is an uncoupling agent).

In this section evidence is presented which suggests that stilbene disulfonate binding and other modifications at the stilbene site convert the allosteric kinetic pattern to a simple hyperbolic form, both in reversible binding studies and in partial covalent labeling studies. We also discuss the apparent type of inhibiton seen after uncoupling with surprising results.

2. Effect of Reversible Stilbene Disulfonate Binding

The study of reversible inhibition of anion transport can be useful when entire transport kinetic patterns are studied as a function of inhibitor concentration. Unfortunately, there are few examples available in the literature of such studies using stilbene disulfonates. The only studies which use this approach are those by Barzilay and co-workers[66,67] for DNDS and Salhany and Gaines[63] for the reversible component of SITS (4-acetamido-4'-isothiocyanate-stilbene,2,2'-disulfonate) binding. The Barzilay and Cabantchik[67] results are shown in Figure 10. At zero DNDS the characteristic self-inhibition effect is observed. However, when 2 and 5 μM DNDS are added, two things happen. First, DNDS appears to change the shape of the transport kinetic pattern from complex to hyperbolic. Then higher levels of DNDS seem to lower V_{max}.

How are we to understand these changes in shape? There are two possible explanations. One assumes that DNDS only interacts with the transport site on each monomer and has no allosteric effect on the porter at all. In this view, the substrate inhibition arises from the classic modifier site. Under these circumstances, DNDS would only lower the affinity of the transport site for sulfate and thereby obscure the modifier site function which by definition cannot change its affinity when a ligand binds to the transport site. The second possibility suggests that the original complex transport curve is due to homotropic allosteric interactions and that DNDS eliminates or uncouples those interactions leading to the resulting hyperbolic plots. As seen in Chapter 2, there is now clear evidence that "transport site ligands", including DNDS, change the quaternary structure of band 3 from a form cross-linkable by bis(sulfosuccinimidyl)suberate (BS^3) to dimers (the DC-state) to a form cross-linkable to tetramers (the TC-state). Thus, the assumption that DNDS would only block the transport site with no allosteric effects on other band 3 sites is clearly not supportable. Furthermore, the pure noncompetitive inhibitory modifier site concept cannot explain the partial nature of the substrate inhibition in the first place.

If the conversion from complex to hyperbolic patterns seen in Figure 10 involves allosteric uncoupling, then within the frame work of hyperbolic kinetics, the decrease in velocities near saturation with increasing DNDS suggests that DNDS lowers V_{max}. This is characteristic of a noncompetitive inhibitor, not a competitive inhibitor. It may be concluded that the dual effect of DNDS (uncoupling of allosteric effects and noncompetitive inhibition of the transport activity of the uncoupled monomer) has been mistaken for competitive inhibiton in other analyses where less sensitive kinetic analyses are employed (e.g., Dixon plots). We will discuss in greater detail below more data on the ability of stilbene disulfonates to uncouple intersubunit interactions and on whether or not the stilbene disulfonate site on a monomer is in fact the transport site. The fact that DNDS changes the quaternary structure of band 3 (Chapter 2) reopens this important issue.

Salhany and Gaines[63] made a quantitative stopped-flow analysis of the effect of reversible SITS binding on initial velocities of dithionite-sulfate exchange. They found that the degree of negative cooperativity was dependent on the concentration of stilbene disulfonate present. This finding is analogous to the results in Figure 10 where DNDS appears to change the shape of the transport curve with increasing concentration. Based on these data Salhany and co-workers[63,64] suggested that the most likely interactions responsible for the change in the shape of the transport kinetic curve were intersubunit interactions within the band 3 dimer. Salhany and Gaines[63] specifically state in that 1981 paper: "...the relevant kinetic question is whether half-saturation of band 3 protein dimer by covalently binding stilbene disulfonates eliminates the substrate inhibition pattern always seen in the equilibrium isotope exchange studies. Our results suggest that substrate inhibition should be eliminated or severely attenuated under these conditions since stilbene disulfonate binding affects the shape of the kinetic curves..."

3. Does Partial Covalent Labeling of Band 3 with Stilbene Disulfonate Change the Shape of the Transport Kinetic Pattern?

The effect of reversible inhibitors on curve shape can be revealing, but effects of partial covalent modification on curve shape are easier to understand. In principle, loss of complex kinetic behavior is expected if an inhibitor covalently labels one monomer and eliminates intermonomeric interactions. Salhany and Swanson[58] showed that partial covalent labeling with SITS converted the inhibitory pattern from negative cooperative to hyperbolic. Since full labeling with DIDS completely inhibits dithionite transport, the residual flux cannot be due to the existence of an alternate transport mediator.

Others have tried the same type of experiment and have arrived at conclusions which support the view that even though the monomers are tightly associated and use conformational changes to exchange anions, one monomer functions independently of the other. For example, one widely cited paper is the report of Macara and Cantley[68] on the effect of partial covalent BIDS (4-benzamido-4'-isothiocyanostilbene-2,2'-disulfonate) on divalent anion exchange. The authors attempted to test the dimer hypothesis as an explanation for substrate inhibition. They correctly reasoned that if there are intersubunit interactions, then covalently labeling 50% or

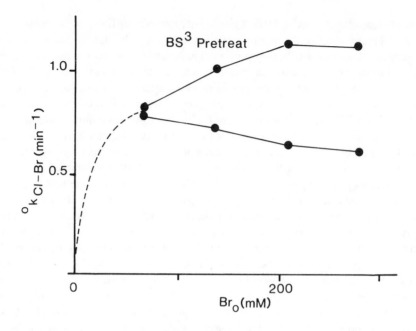

FIGURE 11.   Effect of BS[3] on self-inhibition of Cl-Br exchange vs. extracellular Br concentration. Cells were pretreated and loaded with tracer, and the tracer flux was measured in a hypertonic medium containing 70 to 280 mM KBr, varied at the expense of gluconate. All media were buffered at pH 6 with 10 mM phosphate. The shrinkage of the cells in the hypertonic medium has no effect on monovalent anion exchange. Each data point represents the mean of three to six measurements. The dashed line was inserted into the original figure to note the point of origin only. (From Jennings, M. L., Monaghan, R., Douglas, S. M., and Nicknish, J. S., *J. Gen. Physiol.*, 86, 653, 1985. With permission.)

more of the band 3 monomers with a stilbene disulfonate should change K_m. V_{max} is expected to decrease with irreversible inhibition due to the reduction in the total number of working transporters. Macara and Cantley[68] fitted a straight line through control sulfate-transport data and one through the BIDS-reacted data. However, based on the results of Schnell and Besl[62] the straight line drawn through the control data in the Macara and Cantley[68] paper has no quantitative significance. In fact, it seems that the BIDS-reacted curve in their paper is indeed hyperbolic and that partial covalent labeling of band 3 changes the shape of the curve.

4. Effect of Covalent Modification of Band 3 with BS[3]

BS[3] forms both intra- and intermonomeric covalent cross-links between lysine residues of the band 3 dimer.[69,70] The final covalent product is not charged. BS[3] is a very large and impermeant molecule and so it should not reach internal sites.[69] BS[3] is thought to form its intramonomeric cross-links at the DNDS site.[70] Its effect on the shape of the monovalent transport curve is shown in Figure 11 from a paper by Jennings and co-workers.[71] Not only does this modification cause the curve to become hyperbolic, but this is accomplished through an activation of the velocities in the substrate inhibition region of the curve. If the substrate inhibition effect like all of the complex band 3 kinetic patterns comes from allosteric interactions between subunits of band 3 dimer, then BS[3] modification has uncoupled those interactions based on the change in curve shape. However, unlike DNDS, BS[3] does not inhibit transport of the uncoupled monomers (Figure 11). A pure uncoupling agent should relieve the conformational constraints between monomers but not actually inhibit transport at the active site, according to the homotropic dimer allosteric theory. This would be consistent with the effects of BS[3] chemical modification.

C. CONCLUSIONS

When band 3 porter kinetics are viewed from the most unrestrictive perspective possible, the observed kinetic patterns are recognizable as those of a classic homotropic allosteric dimer or tetramer. The idea that deviations from simple expectations of hyperbolic behavior are due to modifier sites is at least not consistent with generally accepted mathematical requirements for the behavior of such sites. The substrate inhibition effect is incomplete for band 3 porter and sigmoidal behavior is usually considered the hallmark of allosterism. All of the band 3 transport kinetic data can be explained using a general 2:2 kinetic rate law. A 1:2 rate law is inadequate to represent the data. More telling than this is the fact that reversible DNDS binding (Figure 10), BS^3 covalent modification of sites mutually exclusive with the DNDS (Figure 11), partial covalent SITS binding,[58] and reversible SITS binding[63,64] all change the shape of the transport kinetic patterns from complex to hyperbolic. As also seen in Chapter 2, DNDS changes the quaternary structure of band 3 and BS^3 forms intermonomeric cross-links which could serve to "freeze" all allosteric transitions while allowing the monomeric active site to function independently in the unnatural, uncoupled state. DNDS does lower transport velocities further by apparently lowering V_{max}. These findings indicate that the BS^3 reaction uncouples allosteric interactions, while the stilbene disulfonates are both uncouplers and noncompetitive on allosteric inhibitors (see addenda to this chapter and to the book).

IV. IS THE STILBENE DISULFONATE BINDING SITE ON BAND 3 THE TRANSPORT SITE?

A. INTRODUCTION

The ability of DNDS to change the shape of the transport curve in Figure 10 suggests a change in mechanism. This functional change can be generally correlated with the ability of DNDS to change the quaternary structure of the porter from the DC-state to the TC-state (Chapter 2). Thus, allosteric effects of DNDS must be separated from any direct inhibitory effects since it is possible for DNDS to bind to a site and inhibit transport through the allosteric transition which has been identified. If the transition from complex to hyperbolic patterns in Figure 10 indicates a change in state, then the further apparent effect of DNDS on V_{max} may be considered a direct effect of the inhibitor within the TC-state. Under conditions where hyperbolic kinetics obtain, increasing DNDS concentration decreases V_{max}. This effect raises the question: do stilbene disulfonates bind to a monomeric transport site?

In this section, the evidence will be reviewed to see if stilbene disulfonates bind to the transport site. First, the effects of proteolysis will be studied. If the stilbene site is the transport site, then destroying that site through the action of proteases should also diminish substrate binding and inhibit transport. Since DIDS covalent binding involves lysines, evidence concerning small chemical modifications of the lysines will be discussed to see if they are directly involved in substrate binding, and evidence that arginine residues are directly involved at the transport site will be discussed. After this, the only evidence in the literature on the kinetics of direct reversible stilbene binding to band 3 to see if it follows a simple rate law as a function of chloride concentration will be discussed. Finally, to be discussed are the assumptions of the chloride NMR line-broadening experiment which has been used to measure substrate binding. Ultimately, direct inhibitor and substrate binding to the isolated porter should provide answers about substrate stoichiometry and interactions between multiple sites if they exist. In all studies, means to clearly define the quaternary state or transitions in state must also be considered in order to properly interpret the data.

B. EFFECT OF PROTEOLYSIS

Passow[72] first used pronase to see if membrane proteins were involved in anion transport. He observed that proteolysis affected the rate of anion exchange. His paper opened the field for much of the structure-function work which followed. Several papers have addressed the question of the effect of different proteolytic enzymes on the structure and reactivity of band 3 protein.[73-79] Neither external nor internal chymotrypsin or trypsin seem to alter anion transport.[73,74,76,80] However, full transport curves are usually not analyzed to see if the mechanism has changed. Despite this shortcoming, the evidence has been used to rule out a role for the cytoplasmic domain in transport. Yet, experiments with a genetically engineered version of band 3, of which the cytoplasmic domain has been removed, show altered transport.[81]

Unlike trypsin and chymotrypsin, papain when added to intact cells leads to substantial (but never complete) inhibition of anion transport.[74,75,82,83] Jennings and Adams[75] studied the effect of exofacial papain digestion on anion transport and on reversible stilbene-disulfonate binding. They found that under equilibrium exchange conditions transport was inhibited, but the unidirectional influx of sulfate, phosphate, or chloride was unaffected. To explain the reduction in the equilibrium exchange velocity in the absence of a change in unidirectional influx. velocities, the authors suggested that the outward translocation step had been altered. If this interpretation is correct, it might be further concluded that the exofacial part of the protein being cut by papain is intimately involved in the protein conformational changes and that the anion transport site should not be altered. Indeed, Jennings and Adams[75] found that the apparent K_m for sulfate transport was unaffected by proteolysis, while that for chloride was increased. However, the complexity of the sulfate curve makes interpretations based on K_m comparisons quantitatively suspect, but perhaps qualitatively passable in the present situation. Nevertheless, what was clear was that mild exofacial papain proteolysis reduced reversible DNDS binding by one order of magnitude. The authors suggested that the DNDS site may involve parts of the protein not intimately involved in substrate binding. Perhaps the substrate site is more integral and cannot be reached by the large DNDS molecule after exofacial papain digestion. Perhaps the stilbene disulfonate site is not the transport site.

Consider further the results of Matsuyama and co-workers[83] and of Jennings and co-workers[82] who found that it was the action of papain on CH35 yielding P7 and the 28-kDa subfragment (Chapter 2) which seemed to account for the partial inhibition of anion transport and the large reduction in the binding of DNDS. Does CH35 contain a high affinity allosteric site? There is some evidence favoring this interpretation. Cousin and Motais[77,78] studied flufenamate, which is one of the most potent reversible binding, but apparently noncompetitive inhibitors of anion transport known. They found that degradation of the outer surface of CH35 with papain inhibited the binding.[77] Significantly, flufenamate binding to ghosts was blocked by prelabeling with SITS.[77] In other words, the stilbene disulfonate binding site overlaps or interacts with a site on CH35 which binds a potent, apparently noncompetitive inhibitor.

In summary, papain digestion of CH35 has a very large effect on stilbene binding without significantly affecting function at the transport site. Surely, if the stilbene site were exactly coincident with the transport site, then papain should have lowered sulfate affinity 12-fold as it does DNDS binding, at least according to a simple model. The stilbene site could be on or near CH35 which binds several diverse chemicals.

C. EFFECT OF METHYLATION OF LYSINE AMINO GROUPS ON STILBENE DISULFONATE BINDING

Methylation, like the BS^3 treatment, blocks lysine residues at or near the stilbene disulfonate site among other sites. However, methylation introduces sterically small groups into the protein while BS^3 is a large molecule. Jennings[84] found that reductive methylation blocks the covalent reaction of H_2DIDS with CH17 and CH35 lysines, while not affecting reversible stilbene disulfonate binding. Methylation only partially inhibits transport without affecting substrate (bromide) binding, at least based on kinetic measurements.[84] The partial inhibitory effect seems to correlate with methylation of CH35.[84] Partial inhibition is not consistent with formation of the substrate binding site by lysine residues. Based on the methylation and the BS^3 data, it would appear that the exofacial lysines are very important in modulation of porter conformation, but that they do not seem to be intimately involved in substrate binding.

D. EFFECT OF ARGININE-SPECIFIC REAGENTS ON ANION TRANSPORT AND STILBENE-DISULFONATE BINDING

The stilbene site can be digested by proteases or chemically modified without greatly altering transport. Certain characteristics of the transport curves may change as seen in the BS^3 study, but the basic transport function seems intact. If lysines are not involved in direct substrate binding, another likely candidate is the guanidino group of arginine. Bjerrum and co-workers[85-87] and Zaki and co-workers[88-94] carried out extensive studies with arginine specific reagents in order to establish whether or not arginine residues form the substrate binding site. If arginines are located at the transport site, then expected as a minimum would be that covalent modification of arginines should totally inhibit transport.

Phenylglyoxal (PG) reacts with the guanidino group with a 2:1 PG stoichiometry and is very specific for arginine residues.[95] There are two components to the reaction of PG with band 3. One is reversible. This is followed by an irreversible step.[86] PG is not charged, and so it cannot be considered an affinity probe. Therefore, it may react with any accessible arginine residue at any membrane location. Arginines at the active site should be chloride competitive, while other arginines may not be directly so. Wieth and co-workers[85] demonstrated the chloride and pH dependence of the rate of irreversible PG inactivation of anion transport. As the chloride concentration increases, so too does the pK of the single titration.

The increase in pK of PG inhibition with increasing chloride seems consistent with a competitive mechanism at a single arginine. However, there are several complicating factors which detract from such an interpretation. At physiological pH, the reversible component of the PG reaction inhibits exactly 50% of anion exchange.[85] When the pH is raised to 10, the reversible component of PG binding causes nearly complete inhibition. This is an unusual pH dependence, since the incomplete reactivity at physiological pH is not expected if we have reacted the single transport site. To complicate matters further, Zaki[90] found that the irreversible component of the PG reaction inhibits transport about 50% in chloride below pH 10; however, when the same reaction conditions are used, this time in sulfate medium, nearly total inhibition ensues. Despite these uncertainties, Zaki and Julien[92] tried to establish whether or not arginine residues could be chloride binding sites in a series of well-executed studies where time and PG concentration were used to establish kinetic rate laws. Although competitive-like behavior was observed, it was impossible to exclude allosteric effects because a transport assay was used.

If there are uncertainties as to whether arginines are direct substrate-binding sites, there seems to be little doubt that stilbene disulfonates and the arginine-specific reagents are not mutually exclusive. The rate of transport inactivation by PG in physiological chloride is totally unaffected by the presence of up to 1 mM DNDS (a concentration far above its apparent micromolar transport inhibitory constant).[85] When the same reactions were studied at pH 10, this time in sucrose-citrate, Wieth and co-workers[85] did observe some competitive effect of DNDS. Julien and Zaki[93] also found that the stilbene-disulfonate binding was not mutually exclusive with arginine-specific reagents, but that there is some type of interaction of an unknown nature.[94]

In summary, attempts to identify either the stilbene-disulfonate site or arginine sites as being directly involved in transport are inclusive at best. The use of a transport assay to judge simple competitive inhibition in a conformationally active protein is a fundamentally flawed method. This is clear in the case of DNDS where inhibition could be due to the change in quaternary structure, to binding to a specific monomeric site, or to both. Still, it does appear that the stilbene disulfonates are not mutually exclusive with band 3 arginine-reactive reagents. These may be the direct substrate-binding residues, but it is not known for certain.

E. REVERSIBLE STILBENE-DISULFONATE AND CHLORIDE BINDING TO BAND 3

1. Introduction

If transport kinetic interpretations on the location of a given site are ambiguous, then direct measurements of inhibitor and chloride competitive binding to band 3 might be less so. However, here too, control of quaternary structure is needed. In this section the direct binding of stilbene disulfonate and chloride to band 3 in unsealed ghosts is studied. The fundamental question is whether stilbene disulfonate and chloride compete by a simple mechanism or whether multiple interacting chloride-binding sites exist which interact allosterically with the stilbene disulfonate site.

2. Reversible Stilbene-Disulfonate Binding

Several studies have been published on reversible stilbene-disulfonate binding to band 3.[68,96-103] However, the only kinetic studies have come from Solomon's laboratory with Dix and Verkman principally.[100,102,103] The equilibrium binding studies have variably shown apparent negative cooperativity. Fröhlich[96] studied DNDS binding to cell suspensions using a centrifugation method and found apparent hyperbolic binding. Schnell and co-workers[97,101] synthesized a stilbene-disulfonate spin label and found that its reversible binding could be directly measured. Binding followed a hyperbolic function, in agreement with Fröhlich's findings with DNDS. Yet, both Lieberman and Reithmeier[104] and Macara and Cantley[98] found evidence for negative cooperativity with BADS (4-benzamido-4′-aminostilbene-2,2′-disulfonate) binding. Furthermore, labeling 80% of the band 3 monomers with BIDS, reduced the apparent affinity of the remain stilbene sites for $H_2(NBD)_2DS$ (4,4′-*bis*-[4-nitro-2,1,3-benzoxadiaoly]dihydrostilbene-2,2′-disulfonate),[98] consistent with a cooperative binding hypothesis.

All of the reversible stilbene-disulfonate binding data just described come from static binding studies. Kinetic information is needed in order to confirm the mechanism. Fortunately, Dix and co-workers[103] have provided a detailed kinetic analysis of DBDS (4,4′-dibenzamidostilbene-2,2′-disulfonate) binding to band 3. They also presented static binding measurements as a function of chloride, which offer a unifying view of the mechanism. The details of the fluorescence temperature-jump method are given in the paper by Verkman and co-workers.[102] When Dix and co-workers[100] first reported the appearance of negative cooperativity in DBDS binding, it was suggested by some that steric hindrance was responsible. Two facts speak against that interpretation. First, a very significant new result by Anjaneyulu and co-workers[105] suggests that the distance between monomeric stilbene disulfonate sites is >16 Å. This is too great to support steric hindrance arguments. Second, the results of Dix and co-workers[103] shown in Figure 12 indicate that the absence or presence of negative cooperativity depends on the concentration of chloride at otherwise constant ionic strength. These facts do not fit a simple steric hindrance argument. Apparently, ligation of chloride sites influences the degree to which the stilbene sites interact or to which that interaction is detectable. Dix and co-workers[103] proposed that there must be two interconvertible states of the band 3 dimer. The chloride-free state would demonstrate site-site interactions in DBDS binding, while the chloride-bound state would not. This is an interesting suggestion since these functionally defined states might be assignable to the two quaternary states discovered recently by Salhany and Sloan (the DC-state and the TC-state, Chapter 2).

Dix and co-workers[103] then presented a revealing study of the dependence of static K^{app} for DBDS binding on chloride concentration. They took data over a very wide concentration range, which is necessary to reveal the mechanism. It is clear from the findings in Figure 13 that K^{app} is a nonlinear function of chloride concentration. The data fit a simple rectangular hyperbola. The nonlinear dependence of K^{app} on chloride is inconsistent with the simple competition hypothesis expected for the single-site "Ping-Pong" mechanism. The hyperbolic function comes from a saturable model where DBDS and chloride each possess separate but interacting

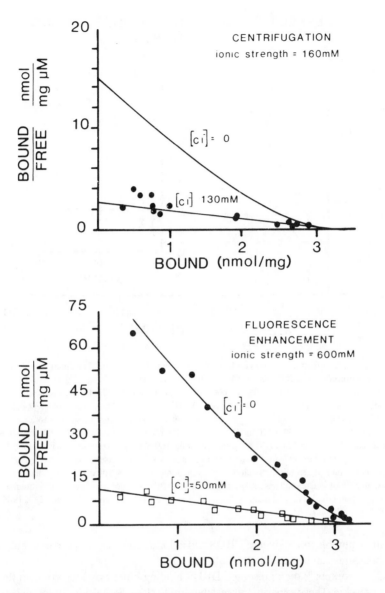

FIGURE 12. Effect of chloride on DBDS binding to red cell ghost membranes. (Top) Binding data using the centrifugation method. Known concentrations of ghosts and DBDS were incubated for 30 min at 25°C, pH 7.4, in buffer consisting of 0 or 130 mM NaCl and Na citrate at 160 mM constant ionic strength. The quantity of bound DBDS was determined from the difference between total DBDS and unbound supernatant DBDS measured by absorbance or by fluorescence upon addition of ghosts (excitation = 350 nm; emission = 420 nm) after centrifugation. Results are shown in the form of a Scatchard plot. The curve for [Cl] = 0 is that given previously by Verkman and co-workers[102] for a two-site sequential binding mechanism which characterizes DBDS binding in the absence of chloride (stoichiometry 3.2 ± 0.3 nmol/mg ghost protein). The [Cl] = 130 mM curve is a least-squares fit to a single-site model with K_{eq} = 1.2 ± 0.2 μM, and stoichiometry = 3.3 ± 0.3 nmol/mg ghost protein (r = 0.97). (Bottom) Binding data obtained using the fluorescence enhancement technique for 0 and 50 mM chloride at a constant 600 mM ionic strength are displayed in the form of a Scatchard plot. The fitted curve for [Cl] = 0 is a fit to the two-site sequential binding mechanism, and the curve for [Cl] = 50 mM is a single site fit. (From Dix, J. A., Verkman, A. S., and Solomon, A. K., *J. Membr. Biol.*, 89, 211, 1986. With permission.)

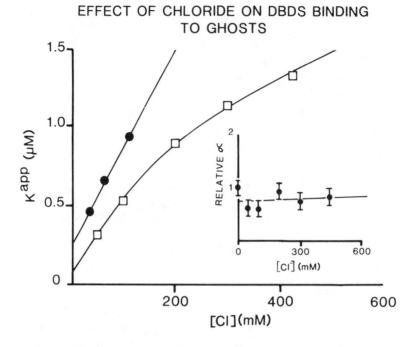

FIGURE 13.   Effect of [Cl] on equilibrium DBDS binding to ghosts. The fitted equilibrium dissociation constants, K^{app}, obtained by the fluorescence enhancement technique are plotted as a function of [Cl] for 160 mM (●) and 600 (❑) mM ionic strength. The 160 mM ionic strength data were fitted to a straight line with slope = 0.0062 ± 0.0002 μM/mM and y-intercept 0.25 ± 0.02 μM. The 600 mM ionic strength data were fitted by nonlinear least squares to a single, saturable site model. $K^{app} = A[Cl]/(K^*_{Cl} + [Cl]) + B$, with A = 2.7 ± 0.7 μ$M$, B = 0.067 ± 0.008 μ$M$, and K^*_{Cl} = 450 ± 50 mM. The x-intercept for the 160-mM ionic strength data is 40 ± 4 mM; the x-intercept for the 600-mM ionic strength data is 11 + 3 mM. (Insert) The relative quantum yield of bound DBDS (alpha) is plotted as a function of [Cl]. The fitted line was obtained by weighted least squares and has a slope of $(1.4 ± 4.7) × 10^{-4}$ mM^{-1}, not significantly different from zero. (From Dix, J. A., Verkman, A. S., and Solomon, A. K., *J. Membr. Biol.*, 89, 211, 1986. With permission.)

comes from a saturable model where DBDS and chloride each possess separate but interacting sites, and both sites can be occupied simultaneously.[103]

Dix and co-workers[103] then presented DBDS binding kinetics which confirm this site-site interaction proposal. These experiments test the simple "Ping-Pong" idea of mutual competition between a single chloride ion and a single stilbene disulfonate.[22,96] Figure 14 shows relaxation "tau" values for DBDS binding to band 3 at different chloride concentrations. The authors infer that if chloride and DBDS were to simply compete for a single binding site, each line in Figure 14 should have the same intercept on the y axis. This was not the case.[103] Furthermore, at any DBDS concentration "tau" values should increase with increasing chloride rather than decrease as they clearly do in Figure 14.

In summary, the results of Dix and co-workers[103] seem to show unequivocally that the mechanism of chloride and reversible stilbene disulfonate binding to band 3 involves separate but interacting sites. This is not consistent with simple competitive kinetics expected for the single site "Ping-Pong" model where either one chloride or one stilbene occupies the single band 3 site. The conclusion from these findings is that the simple model is not supported. There is clear evidence for the formation of a ternary complex between band 3, DBDS, and chloride. Although the stoichiometry of chloride binding is not known, multiple, interacting sites are required to explain the data. This would be consistent with the observation of complex kinetics and with the

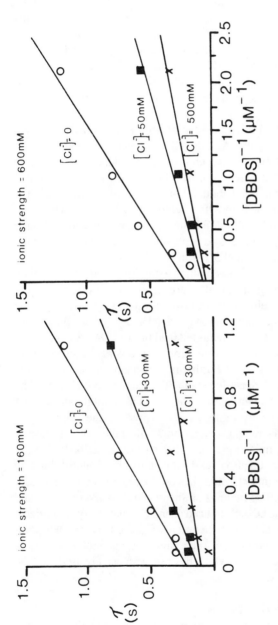

FIGURE 14.   Effect of Cl on band 3/DBDS binding kinetics. Plots are of concentration dependence of stopped-flow time constants for DBDS binding to ghost membranes vs. inverse DBDS concentration. The ordinate is the fitted single exponential time constant obtained from the measured time course of DBDS binding to ghosts. Each point is an average of experiments performed in quadruplicate; errors (not shown) were in the range of 10 to 20%. (Left) Data are shown for 0, 30, and 130 mM [Cl] at 160 mM ionic strength. (Right) Data are shown for 0, 50, and 500 mM [Cl] at 600 mM ionic strength. (From Dix, J. A., Verkman, A. S., and Solomon, A. K., $J.$ $Membr.$ $Biol.$, 89, 211, 1986. With permission.)

complex way in which reversible stilbene disulfonates seem to inhibit anion exchange (e.g., Figure 10).

3. Chloride-Binding Measurements by the NMR Line-Broadening Method
a. Introduction

Until recently, one of the major drawbacks in band 3 research was the lack of data on the binding and/or stoichiometry of chloride or bicarbonate to isolated band 3. One approach to this problem has been the application of chloride NMR to the study of chloride binding to band 3.[42,56,79,106-110] Chloride NMR line broadening was first applied to the band 3 problem in 1977 by Shami and co-workers.[109] They showed that Triton X-100 extracted band 3 and unsealed ghosts were able to broaden the chloride NMR line width, an effect indicative of binding (see the paper by Falke and co-workers[56] for a detailed discussion of the theory and some assumptions of this experiment).

The main purpose for using the chloride NMR line-broadening approach is to provide a probe of the transport site using the physiological ligand. Although this seems like a good approach in principle, there is one very fundamental problem which needs to be addressed. If multiple chloride-binding sites exist, how are we to tell which chloride-binding site is the transport site? This question is raised to make a very simple point about all of the chloride NMR data in the literature. In that body of work, authors were dealing with a heterogeneous system in the form of unsealed ghost preparations. Many possible chloride-binding sites may exist, both on band 3 and perhaps elsewhere on the membrane. Yet there is no work with isolated band 3, except the paper by Shami and co-workers[109] with a crude band 3 Triton X-100 extract.

Falke and co-workers[42,56,79,106-108,110] accept DNDS as binding to the "transport site", and then further assume implicitly that DNDS binding has no allosteric effect on the other chloride-binding sites which probably exist on the protein. In other words, they use DNDS to identify the transport site. However, in light of the clear demonstration that DNDS changes the quaternary structure of band 3 (Chapter 2), how can NMR experiments tell if addition of DNDS has directly or allosterically lowered chloride affinity? It cannot. Site assignment problems are suggested in the kinetic experiments of Dix and co-workers.[103] Furthermore, Shami and co-workers[109] showed that although Triton X-100 extracts (containing about 80% band 3) could broaden the chloride line, covalent DIDS pretreatment of intact cells (enough to totally inhibit transport and therefore cover all of the transport sites) only inhibited about 50% of the original line broadening. Where does the residual chloride binding come from? Is the other 50% of chloride binding due to interactions with the diluted lipid or glycophorin? This seems unlikely. In light of the Dix paper[103] it seems likely that stilbene disulfonates do not totally block chloride binding to isolated band 3 because all of the interacting chloride sites on the protein are not mutually exclusive with the stilbene-disulfonate site. The findings of Shami and co-workers,[109] Dix and co-workers,[103] and the recent evidence on the DNDS-induced change in quaternary structure all challenge the very nature of the fundamental interpretation of the chloride NMR line-broadening experiments with respect to the problem of site assignment and multisite interactions. Still, this is a potentially important technique which has been extensively used, and the experimental results are worth careful study.

b. Inhibitors Which Lower Chloride Affinity to Ghosts

Figure 15 shows experiments where the observed chloride NMR line broadening is plotted vs. the total ghost protein present and the effect of DNDS is tested.[56] As ghost protein increases, the number of binding sites increases and line broadening increases linearly, in accordance with theory.[56] However, when saturating concentrations of DNDS (1 mM) are added under the conditions used, the authors observe that no more than 50% of the line broadening is prevented. On the basis of DNDS and chloride concentration dependent studies, the authors proposed that the DNDS-sensitive sites were the hypothetical competitive transport site on band 3 and that the

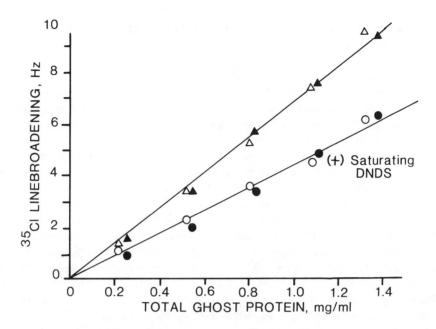

FIGURE 15. The relationship between the $^{35}Cl^-$ NMR line broadening and the ghost membrane concentration. The $^{35}Cl^-$ line broadening of samples containing leaky ghost membranes with ($\bigcirc$, $\bullet$) or without ($\triangle$, $\blacktriangle$) DNDS, 1 mM total concentration. The solid lines are least squares best fit straight lines (y = Mx) that have slopes of 6.87 ± 0.04 Hz/mg/ml of total ghost protein. The buffers used were 250 mM NH$_4$Cl, 5 mM NaH$_2$PO$_4$, 20% D$_2$O, pH to 8.0 with NH$_4$OH ($\blacktriangle$, $\bullet$); or 220 mM NaCl, 30 mM glycylglycine HCl, 2.5 mM NaH$_2$PO$_4$, 20% D$_2$O, pH to 8.0 with NaOH ($\triangle$, $\bigcirc$). Spectral parameters: 8.8 MHz, 3°C, and standard assay parameters. (From Falke, J. J., Pace, R. J., and Chan, S. I., *J. Biol. Chem.*, 259, 6472, 1984. With permission.)

low affinity sites were located somewhere else on the membrane. There may be enough positively charged phospholipid to bind chloride, but this hypothesis has not been directly tested. Rather, the results of Dix and co-workers[103] and Shami and co-workers[109] suggest that the low affinity chloride sites may be located on band 3 and that their low affinity could very well be a result of stilbene disulfonate binding.[103] In neither case does fully covering all of the "transport sites" on band 3 with stilbene disulfonates totally block chloride binding. Although there seems to be little question that chloride binding to ghosts followed apparently competitive patterns with DNDS, iodide, bicarbonate, and fluoride,[42,56] the results do not rule out allosteric "competition" or a combination steric-allosteric competition between two sites, which was one of the models proposed Dix and co-workers.[103] Since DNDS changes band 3 quaternary structure (Chapter 2) allosteric effects must be controlled before data can be interpreted.

One of the most unusual aspects of the interpretation of the chloride NMR data which seems to fit a multisite allosteric theory is the problem of the difference between the ability of DNDS and DIDS to inhibit chloride binding to ghosts. Falke and Chan[42] found that DNDS was a more complete inhibitor than covalent DIDS binding (keep in mind that it does not inhibit all of the sites on ghosts [Figure 15]). This is a very remarkable result. How can this be explained? The basic principle upon which these inhibitors are used is the principle of the affinity probe. The affinity groups on these molecules come from the two sulfonic acid groups. There is no difference between DIDS and DNDS in this respect. Yet, considerable differences are observed. DIDS not only blocks fewer sites than DNDS in the chloride NMR studies, but also the remaining sites have a lower affinity. That means that sites which had an originally high affinity in the absence of DIDS or DNDS are now not actually blocked by DIDS, yet they have their chloride affinity lowered by DIDS. Falke and Chan[42] suggested partial blockade by DIDS, but allosteric effects seem at least equally plausible, if not likely, in light of the detailed kinetic work of Dix and co-workers.[103]

F. CONCLUSION

The fact that covalent DIDS binding to band 3 totally inhibits anion transport is irrelevant to its mechanism of inhibition under reversible binding conditions. When full transport curves are analyzed as a function of reversible stilbene disulfonate concentration, the originally complex transport kinetic patterns become hyperbolic and V_{max} seems to be lowered. This implies that stilbene disulfonates have a bipartite mechanism of inhibition. In the first part, the interactions between sites responsible for the complex curves are uncoupled. BS^3, the final covalent product of which is uncharged but which covers the stilbene lysines, seems to purely uncouple interactions leading to hyperbolic curves. However, when we look at stilbene reversible binding with direct kinetic methods, simple competitive kinetic laws totally fail to be observed. This failure would be expected if the stilbene site is not coincident with the chloride-binding transport site(s) as suggested by the reversible inhibiton studies with stilbene disulfonates. The results of Barzilay and Cabantchik[67] (Figure 10), those of Dix and co-workers[103] (Figures 12 to 14), and the other evidence presented above together all suggest that DNDS and probably all reversible stilbene disulfonates are noncompetitive uncoupling agents. Their initial binding stops the allosteric interactions between sites, while they inhibit noncompetitively by binding to a nonmutually exclusive site on each uncoupled monomer. The stilbene site may be exofacial to a more deeply placed transport site. Stilbenes may block monomeric conformational changes at that transport site in addition to stopping allosteric interactions between monomers, all without actually directly binding to the amino acids of the transport site within each channel. The transport site(s) within each channel may be composed of arginine residues, but this has to be absolutely proven, and until allosteric effects are controlled it cannot be proven. The question remaining is if uncoupling of interactions is such a dominant part of the stilbene inhibitory effect, are those interactions intermonomeric in nature between monomers of a band 3 dimer or tetramer? In the next section, direct evidence to support an intermonomeric interaction hypothesis will be presented.

V. EVIDENCE FOR SUBUNIT INTERACTIONS OR OTHER ALLOSTERIC EFFECTS WITHIN A BAND 3 DIMER OR TETRAMER

A. INTRODUCTION

Band 3 certainly is at least a stable dimer within the intact membrane and probably further associates to tetramers due to interactions with the cytoskeleton (Chapter 2). The folded structure of the monomer seems to depend on the dimeric state of association, as does stilbene disulfonate binding (Chapter 2). The structural inference is that there are strong energies of interactions between monomers. Inspection of the transport kinetic patterns favors homotropic allosterism, since they are recognizable as those of a dimer or tetramer with multiple active sites under homotropic allosteric control (by analogy with well-established enzyme kinetic patterns).[3] This view was strengthened through demonstration that partial covalent stilbene-disulfonate binding or even reversible inhibitor binding or chemical modification of the stilbene site by BS^3, all caused the transport kinetic patterns to change from complex to hyperbolic, as if homotropic allosteric interactions had been uncoupled. Furthermore, direct stilbene-disulfonate binding data suggest separate but interacting chloride and stilbene binding sites. Finally, there is now direct evidence that ligands can modulate porter quaternary structure. Taken together, the results could be explained if the two monomers of a band 3 dimer interact within a tetrameric porter according to Singer's homotropic allosteric porter model.[2]

If allosteric interactions exist, it is essential to show that the interacting sites (be they competitive or noncompetitive) are separated in space and that the activity and/or affinity of one depends on the ligation of the other site. Spatial separation of monomeric sites is strengthened by the finding that the distance between the stilbene-disulfonate binding site on each monomer is greater than 16 Å.[105] Although it is impossible to make site assignments based on covalent inhibition data alone, covalent inhibition studies can be used to identify the presence or absence of subunit interactions through the study of activity-labeling correlation plots. In this case, the actual mechanism of inhibition is unimportant as long as it involves total inhibition.

DIDS covalent activity-labeling correlation plots are the most well known, and until recently, almost the only such data available in this field. DIDS binds with a 1:1 stoichiometry and inhibits transport linearly. Yet, the linear inhibition seems puzzling in light of the complex kinetic curves, but, then, stilbenes seem to change the transport kinetic pattern. If stilbene disulfonates are uncoupling agents, perhaps linear inhibition is a manifestation of such uncoupling of interactions. Support for the uncoupling hypothesis would require that an inhibitor be found for comparison where the conformational coupling was preserved. The inhibitor to be studied is pyridoxal 5′-phosphate (PLP), which shows allosteric interactions in covalent activity-labeling correlation plots. It will be demonstrated that addition of DNDS uncouples those interactions, just as DNDS and partial covalent labeling at the stilbene site convert complex transport kinetic plots to a hyperbolic form.

B. DISTINCTION BETWEEN STILBENE DISULFONATE TRANSPORT INHIBITION AND INHIBITION BY THE TRANSPORTABLE ANION AND AFFINITY PROBE PYRIDOXAL 5′-PHOSPHATE (PLP)

1. Stilbene-Disulfonate Inhibition of Anion Exchange: A Nontransportable, Linear Inhibitor

a. Establishing the Stoichiometry with Activity Labeling Correlation Plots

The earliest attempt to correlate anion transport inhibition with modification of membrane proteins was made in 1943, using tannic acid.[111] The work with amino reactive reagents and with proteolytic enzymes began in earnest in the late 1960s and early 1970s.[72,112-115] The stilbene disulfonates were first synthesized by Maddy[116] in the form of SITS, mainly to obtain a fluorescent, nonpenetrating label for the outer cell surface. They are now the most widely used and, some may argue, the most important probes of the so-called "transport site" on band 3. SITS was initially used by Knauf and Rothstein[114] because of its ability to react covalently with amino groups on the red cell membrane, but they found that it was a potent inhibitor of anion exchange. This discovery opened the field of inhibition kinetics to quantitative analysis. The usefulness of this inhibitor to red cell physiology increased greatly in 1974, when Cabantchik and Rothstein[73,117] showed that the predominant stilbene-disulfonate binding site is located on the band 3 protein of the red blood cell membrane.

Having identified band 3 as the predominant location for DIDS, the next step was to correlate transport inhibition with the number of covalent DIDS molecules bound per copy of band 3. It should be kept in mind that at the time this research was being carried out, Steck[118] had already shown that band 3 may exist in the membrane as a noncovalently associated dimer. Some of the kinetic complexities of the system were also known, but there was no published suggestion that the complex curves could be related to the existence of the dimer or higher oligomers of band 3 in the membrane.

It was important to learn the exact stoichiometry of DIDS binding to band 3. Cabantchik and Rothstein[117] showed that there was a linear relationship between loss of activity and covalent DIDS binding to band 3. Although there was some technical problem in the determination of the exact stoichiometry, this was corrected in a later paper[119] and in a paper by Lepke and co-workers.[120] The results of Lepke and co-workers[120] is shown in Figure 16. They confirm the linearity of the activity-labeling correlation plots and show a 1:1 stoichiometry with band 3 polypeptide (Figure 16B). The difference between Figures 16A and B is thought to be due to

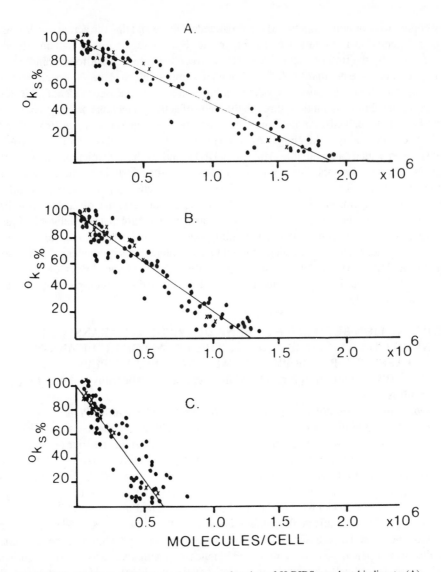

FIGURE 16. Sulfate equilibrium exchange as a function of H$_2$DIDS covalent binding to (A) whole cells, (B) the protein in band 3, (C) binding sites other than those in band 3 (difference between [a] and [b]). The data points have been obtained in 15 different experiments. *Ordinate:* rate constant for sulfate equilibrium exchange in percent of control value measured in the absence of H$_2$DIDS. *Abcissa:* H$_2$DIDS binding in molecules per cell. The straight lines in (A) and (B) represent maximum-likelihood estimates as calculated on the assumption that both variables contain error. The result of the calculations was affected to within less than 1% when the correlation between the errors of measured rates of sulfate movement (ordinate) and binding (abcissa) was varied between −1 and +1 and when the rate of the variances of ordinate and abcissa was varied between 0.8 and 1.25. The abscissas of this figure were modified by the authors to account for improved determinations of the number of band 3 protein present. (From Lepke, S., Fasold, H., Pring, M., and Passow, H., *J. Membr. Biol.*, 29, 147, 1976. With permission.) I thank Professor Herman Passow for providing this new figure.

those DIDS molecules which bind to glycophorin, since they may be removed by extracellular proteolysis with trypsin.[19]

b. Confirmation of the 1:1 Stoichiometry of DIDS Binding to the Band 3 Monomer
Since DIDS is a bifunctional affinity probe containing two *trans* sulfonates and two

isothiocyanate groups, it can react with more than one protein amino group. Band 3 can be cleaved into two integral subdomains (CH35 and CH17) through preparation of unsealed ghosts followed by bilateral digestion with chymotrypsin (Chapter 2). The two subdomains are integral to the membrane and are candidates for housing the transport function of the protein. If certain proteolytic enzymes are added to the outside of intact cells, two products are formed, CH35 and CH65, with the latter containing the CH17 subdomain. Cabantchik and Rothstein[73] digested DIDS-labeled band 3 protein into its integral parts to see which subdomain contained the DIDS molecule. They found DIDS on CH65. From the proteolytic studies discussed in Chapter 2, it is now seen that CH65 must traverse the membrane, since it can be cleaved into an integral CH17 subdomain and an N-terminal, water-soluble, 42-kDa cytoplasmic fragment.

Although the results strongly suggest that there is a 1:1 stoichiometry between DIDS and the band 3 monomer, the conclusive evidence was published in a paper in 1979 by Jennings and Passow.[74] They showed that under conditions of mild proteolysis of intact red cells, chymotrypsin cleaves the two integral subdomains of band 3 without affecting transport. When Jennings and Passow[74] added DIDS at neutral pH (the usual conditions), they saw predominant labeling at CH65. However, raising the pH to 9.5 led to the formation of DIDS cross-links between CH35 and CH65. The authors ran several controls to establish that the cross-links were not arising from any intermonomeric interactions between neighboring subdomains. They drew the important conclusion that one DIDS molecule is in contact with both integral chymotryptic subdomains of one band 3 monomer.

Later, Kampmann and co-workers[121] reported that the Jennings-Passow effect could also be observed at more acidic pH values, but at a much slower rate. They used this fact to perform a series of very interesting kinetic studies on the rate of intramolecular cross-linking of band 3 monomers. At pH 8, there was a slow but progressive increase in CH65 labeling with time, followed by the appearance of label on the intact 95-kDa monomer. The eventual decrease in the CH65 band was then observed as it was cross-linked to CH35 to form the 95-kDa band. The authors studied the reaction at several pH values and found that regardless of pH, the CH65 fragment always formed the uncross-linked covalent product faster than any covalent reaction of DIDS with CH35. The kinetic data mandated a model with two different states for the H_2DIDS binding site. Furthermore, the transition from one state to the other was related to changes in the CH65 subdomain or to both subdomains simultaneously. An analysis of the pH dependence of the thiocyanylation of the CH35 lysine residue(s) gave an apparent pK value of about 10, close to the value for an epsilon-amino group of lysine in an aqueous environment.

In summary, the linear inhibition of anion transport by DIDS and the 1:1 stoichiometry demonstrated directly and through intramonomeric cross-linking suggest that when DIDS is bound to one monomer, the other monomer can transport anions. There seems to be little doubt that each monomer can function independently within the band 3 dimer or tetramer when DIDS is bound to its neighbor. The fact that DIDS only binds to monomers when they are associated to dimers (Chapter 2) does not contradict this conclusion. It only means that either the DIDS site requires a dimeric niche or the folded structure of the active site changes significantly upon monomerization (Chapter 2). Still, partial covalent labeling with stilbene disulfonates changes the shape of the transport kinetic curve. If monomers of a band 3 dimer are functionally uncoupled by DIDS, could they be conformationally coupled in the absence of DIDS when a transportable anion is covalently bound?

2. PLP: A Biphasic Inhibitor Which Is Also a Transported Anion
a. Establishment of the Biphasic Activity-Labeling Correlation Plot
i. Stoichiometry

Although stilbene disulfonates bind to band 3 with a 1:1 stoichiometry, there is every reason to believe that because of their size and impermeability, they either directly or indirectly affect several subsites or subdomains of the protein. Salhany and co-workers[122] investigated the labeling of the two well-defined chymotryptic subdomains of the integral 52-kDa domain using the transportable affinity probe PLP.[60,122-129] Both reversibly bound and covalently fixed (with borohydride) PLP totally inhibit anion exchange,[124] and they inhibit to the same degree at concentrations below saturation.[122,124] This is an important point to keep in mind because it suggests that the fraction of ligand bound to the transport site after borohydride fixation is the same as the amount reversibly bound prior to the addition of the reducing agent. Furthermore, if a PLP molecule could bind to an inhibitory site but not be fixed to an adjacent lysine, it would be impossible to totally inhibit transport by covalent fixation alone. Therefore, one may use the fraction of PLP covalently fixed to band 3 to determine binding isotherms.

As might be expected for a transportable probe, PLP binding appears competitive with chloride, and its binding can be totally blocked by DIDS covalent binding.[122,124,130,131] Since there are several lysine residues on band 3 which could be directly or indirectly involved, it was first necessary to establish the correlation between transport activity and the amount or fraction of PLP bound to band 3. This approach required that PLP be covalently fixed to band 3 in red cells at various concentrations (using constant borohydride, since it is a competing anion). After fixation some of the cells from each condition were used to measure dithionite-sulfate exchange. The remainder of the cells were used to extract and isolate purified band 3.

PLP has a very strong fluorescence, and when enough labeled band 3 is present, the optical absorbance of the PLP-bound protein can be measured. The extinction coefficient for the PLP-bound protein is well established,[122] and this, in combination with the fluorescence, was used to measure the amount of PLP bound to the isolated porter.[122] These measurements are shown in Figure 17 since they are so important to the establishment of the stoichiometry. First, it will be noted that the relationship between fluorescence and PLP-bound porter is linear at each PLP. As the concentration of PLP increases at the cellular reaction step, the slope of the line increases, due to the increase in the amount of bound probe. Slope replots show saturation behavior. Extrapolation of the top of the curve gives the maximal slope value in terms of PLP fluorescence units per milligram per milliliter of band 3 protein. From the absorbencies of several samples it was possible to calculate the number of moles of PLP bound per mole of band 3 monomer at saturation;[122] this is about 4 mol. Reaction of purified band 3 in Triton X-100 with PLP showed about 16 mol of PLP bound per mole of band 3 monomer.[122]

A stoichiometry of 4:1 for reaction at exofacial sites seems large for a single transport site. However, it is likely that these sites line a single, funnel-shaped monomeric channel (Chapter 2). We might then expect these sites to behave as a canonical set. When the channel is open, all sites can bind PLP. When the channel is closed or partially occluded, very high PLP concentrations would be required to achieve ligation. All sites could be blocked from exofacial reaction with PLP by one inhibitor if that inhibitor is large enough (e.g., DIDS) to occlude the entrance to the channel. Any one or all of these channel sites could contribute to the inhibitory potency. The problem is then to map protein subdomains to determine the distribution of PLP. After mapping studies are complete, one can then attempt to establish the relationship between PLP subdomains and the binding sites for other inhibitors, especially the stilbene disulfonates. Finally, the labeling of the whole of the exofacial PLP sites and the sites on each subdomain can be correlated with transport activity of the same cells. This can be performed for cells labeled in the absence and presence of other inhibitors which may protect certain subdomains from being labeled, thereby suggesting the possible location of inhibitory sites.

The subdomain distribution of PLP was determined by isolating the membranes of labeled red cells and performing bilateral chymotrypsin digestion plus alkali stripping followed by SDS gel electrophoresis. Slicing slab gels and extracting proteins allowed measurement of the corresponding fluorescence characteristic of the PLP label. Figure 18 shows the gel pattern for uncut band 3. These were 10% acrylamide gels, and band 3 migrates nearer the top in the uncut

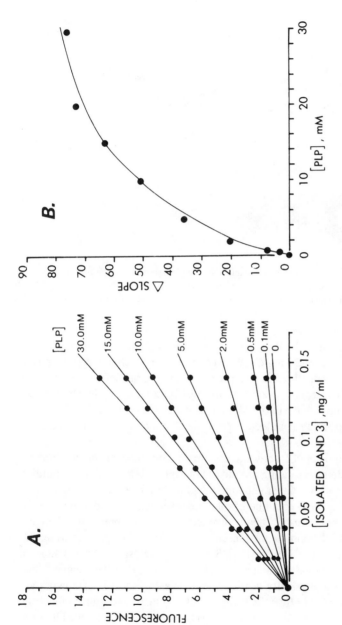

FIGURE 17. PLP band 3 fluorescence for isolated band 3 derived from red cells labeled at different PLP concentrations. Intact red cells were labeled and fixed with sodium borohydride under controlled conditions at various PLP concentrations. (A) Plot of measured fluorescence (exitation wavelength = 394 nm; emission wavelength = 323 nm) vs. measured protein concentration for isolated band 3 derived from cells which were labeled and fixed at various PLP concentrations. (B) Plot of delta slope values from A vs. the concentration of PLP present in the extracellular medium at the time of fixation with borohydride. The stoichiometry for PLP labeling of the exofacial sites was calculated and found to be 4.2 mol of PLP per mole of band 3 monomer. This is about 25% of the total observed labeling sites when the "naked" protein was reacted with PLP in Triton-X-100. (From Salhany, J. M., Rauenbuehler, P. B., and Sloan, R. L., *J. Biol. Chem.*, 262, 15965, 1987. With permission.)

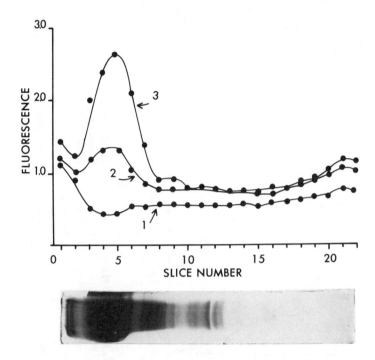

FIGURE 18.   Fluorescence gel slicing experiment for alkali-stripped membranes derived from PLP-labeled intact red cells. Band 3 is the predominant protein and increasing the concentration of PLP present at the time of labeling and fixation increases the amount of fluorescence present at the band 3 region. These are 10% acrylamide gels.

form. Increasing the concentration of PLP present at the time of cellular fixation leads to increased probe fluorescence in the band 3 region. When band 3 is cut by chymotrypsin and the same amount of total protein applied, all of the fluorescence moves to the defined positions of CH35 and CH17, showing that the label is associated with these porter subdomains (Figure 19). The label is evenly distributed between the two subdomains of the transport site. Since the total stoichiometry was determined to be 4 PLP molecules per mole of monomer, there must be 2 mol of PLP per mole of subdomain.

The apparently equal distribution of PLP between subdomains could result from PLP binding to a singular site on a lone subdomain rotating around the phosphate bond within the binding pocket so as to be linked to a lysine on either subdomain. Although the transport site may be located on one of the subdomains, both could be labeled nearly equally. In order to see if the labeling of the two subdomains represents physically distinct sites or overlapping sites, Salhany and co-workers[122] performed PLP labeling in the presence of DNDS, DIDS, NAP-taurine, and chloride. Figure 20 shows the effect of DNDS. DNDS seems to exclusively protect sites on CH35 (in agreement with other findings[125]), but it increases labeling to CH17. This suggests that each PLP labeling subdomain is a physically distinct site. If DNDS and PLP CH35 sites are mutually exclusive and CH35 and CH17 PLP sites are mutually exclusive, no simple model can explain how addition of DNDS can lead to an increase in CH17 labeling through steric blockade of a singular site. Thus, PLP does not bind to a single site and simply covalently attaches to either CH17 or CH35.

Since DNDS is a reversibly binding inhibitor, each subdomain can actually be titrated with PLP in the absence and presence of DNDS as in Figure 21. The closed circles confirm that PLP labeling of each subdomain is virtually identical. Clearly, DNDS is only apparently competitive with CH35 sites, but it consistently causes the exposure of additional sites on CH17. In fact, the saturation point for CH35 with DNDS present is also greater to about the same degree as CH17.

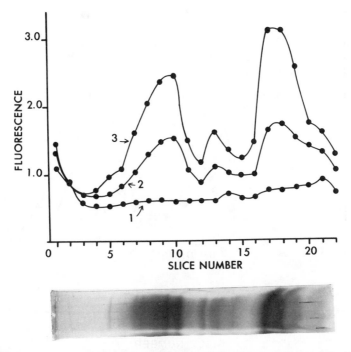

FIGURE 19. Fluorescence gel-slicing experiment for alkali-stripped membranes derived from the same group of cells as in Figure 18 after bilateral chymotrypsin digestion. The total fluorescence is two times greater because the same amount of total protein is on the gel. Since the cytoplasmic domain (accounting for about one half of the mass of band 3) is cleaved here, there are twice the number of band 3 integral domains added to this gel as compared to Figure 18.

We can conclude that the addition of DNDS either exposes new CH17 and CH35 labeling sites or it increases the affinity of otherwise low affinity sites on each subdomain.

The relationship of the PLP labeling sites to the DIDS binding site was investigated next. DIDS binding is more complex than DNDS, since it initially binds in a reversible fashion and then reacts covalently with a CH17 lysine under the conditions of the experiment. Because alkali stripping is used in the analysis of the labeled membranes, we could not quantitatively analyze results where DIDS pretreatment of red cells was used because of the tendency of DIDS to cross-link the two subdomains at alkaline pH. Instead DIDS was added with PLP and the PLP reaction stopped at different times by addition of borohydride (Figure 22). PLP binds similarly to both subdomains with time in the absence of DIDS (Figure 22B), but with DIDS present, the amount of PLP bound to each subdomain decreased with time (Figure 22A). Thus, covalent reaction of DIDS with a CH17 lysine leads to diminution in PLP labeling to both subdomains through either direct or allosteric effects in agreement with two other such findings.[124,130]

Why does DNDS only block PLP labeling of CH35, while DIDS blocks labeling to both subdomains? The ultimate answer to this question requires a more detailed knowledge of the three-dimensional structure of the band 3 monomer than is currently available. If both subdomains form a single monomeric channel, the CH35 PLP sites could be somewhat more exofacial, while the CH17 sites could be deeper, or there could be adjacent and deeper sites on a funnel-shaped channel. DIDS, because it is known to react covalently with a CH17 lysine, may have a more drastic effect on channel structure then does DNDS binding. The isothiocyanate group may also reach a spot which is inaccessible by DNDS.

Salhany and co-workers[122] also looked at the effects of NAP-taurine and chloride on PLP labeling patterns, and they found that NAP-taurine had no effect under the conditions used, despite the fact that it is thought to be mutually exclusive with the stilbene-disulfonate site.

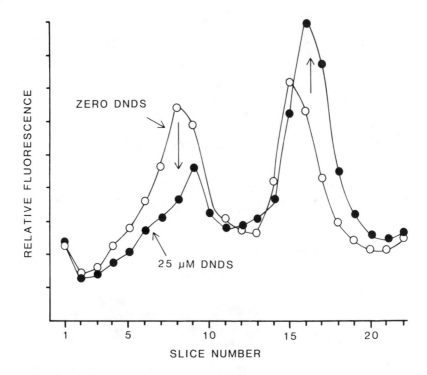

FIGURE 20. Fluorescence measurements from gel-slicing experiments for chymotrypsin-digested membranes from cells labeled with constant PLP in the presence and absence of DNDS. Cells were labeled with 10 mM PLP in the presence and absence of 25 μM DNDS. After electrophoresis, the gels were sliced, the protein extracted, and fluorescence was measured. There is a diminution in PLP labeling at CH35, but an increase in PLP labeling at CH17. The Coomassie-Blue staining patterns for both gels were identical, based on measurement of integrated peak areas of gel scans. (From Salhany, J. M., Rauenbuehler, P. B., and Sloan, R. L., *J. Biol. Chem.*, 262, 15965, 1987. With permission.)

Increasing chloride at constant ionic strength led to a decrease in PLP labeling to both subdomains.[122] The subdomain labeling map of Figure 23 shows a summary of their findings. Each subdomain of the transport site is believed to bind the transported anions PLP and chloride. DNDS reversible binding occurs at CH35, but it allosterically exposes new sites on CH17. DIDS can reach lysine sites on CH17 due to its ability to react covalently with that subdomain, and perhaps for other chemical reasons that are related to the presence of the isothiocyano groups. NAP-taurine does not protect either site at the concentration used, but has been shown in other studies to overlap both DNDS and DIDS sites.[19,21]

ii. Correlation of Transport Activity with Labeling

The mapping experiments just described raise several issues which need careful study and consideration. Which subdomain contains the transport site, or are both transport inhibitory? What is the significance of the apparent increase in PLP labeling to both subdomains with reversible DNDS addition? To investigate some of these and other questions, Salhany and co-workers[122] correlated the transport activity of PLP-labeled cells with the fraction of PLP bound to the whole of the exofacial sites on the integral domain (Figure 17) and to the fraction of label bound to each subdomain (Figure 21), with cellular labeling and fixation step performed in the absence and presence of DNDS.

To interpret the results, expectations for activity-labeling correlation plots need to be reviewed first. Consider that two classes of equivalent PLP labeling sites exist. Suppose one

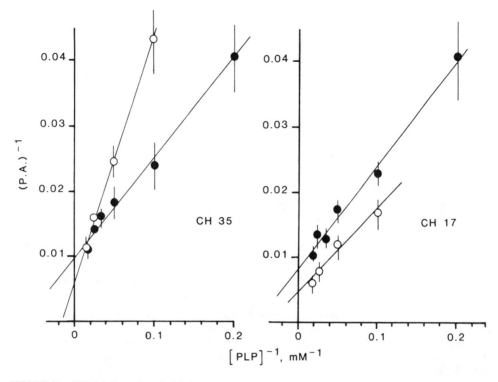

FIGURE 21. PLP labeling of exofacial sites on CH17 and CH35 of band 3 as a function of extracellular PLP concentration present at the time of fixation with sodium borohydride. The binding data are presented in double reciprocal form as integrated peak area of fluorescence (P.A.) vs. PLP concentration present at the time of cellular fixation. The integrated peak area is proportional to the amount of PLP bound to each domain and shows apparent hyperbolic binding over the concentration ranges accessible in gel-slicing studies. The saturable nature of these plots is reflected by the linearity of the double reciprocal plots over the range studied. The solid circles are for control and show that PLP labels both integral subdomains equivalently. The open circles are for labeling experiments in the presence of the reversible inhibitor DNDS. DNDS apparently competitively protects CH35, but uniformly allosterically increases CH17 labeling. However, since DNDS is a reversible inhibitor, it is displaced from CH35 and the extrapolated saturation value is similarly higher for this subdomain as well. Thus, addition of DNDS actually exposes additional labeling sites on both subdomains of the monomer. See the original paper for quantitative analysis (From Salhany, J. M., Rauenbuehler, P. B., and Sloan, R. L., *J. Biol. Chem.*, 262, 15965, 1987. With permission.)

class of sites is a high affinity transport inhibitory site (T) and that the other is a noninhibitory site (N) with low PLP affinity. For whole porter exofacial labeling studies we expect to see a 50:50 biphasic plot like curve B of Figure 24. PLP would label the high affinity transport site first and completely inhibit transport activity, following which the lower affinity N sites would become labeled to yield the biphasic curve. If labeling is performed in the presence of a selective protecting molecule (D) several possible outcomes could be observed. If D binds to an N site, the curve B plot would not change much. It would just require higher PLP concentrations to saturate the N site to the same degree. However, this would not influence correlation plots which are concentration independent. On the other hand, if D binds to the T site of a T-N pair with higher affinity than PLP, then the N site will be preferentially labeled initially, and there should be a transition in the plot from curve B to curve A. The lag in curve A occurs because filling the N sites first has no effect on transport by definition. The curve eventually turns down as higher PLP concentration begins to displace D from the T site.

Now suppose the two classes of sites are interacting T sites (T_1 and T_2). Binding to one lowers the affinity and diminishes the activity of the other. Two sites interacting with such negative cooperativity would give a B pattern in the absence of DNDS. However, unlike the T-N model, addition of D to protect a T site will yield a linear correlation plot (curve C) no matter how high

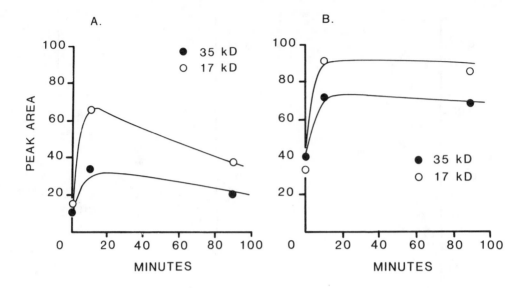

FIGURE 22.   Plots of peak area of fluorescence from gel electrophoretic slicing experiments vs. time for control cells and cells simultaneously mixed with DIDS and PLP. (A) 50 μM DIDS and 20 mM PLP were mixed simultaneously with washed red cells at a 5% hematocrit as described; (B) control cells were mixed with 20 mM PLP in the absence of DIDS. (From Salhany, J. M., Rauenbuehler, P. B., and Sloan, R. L., *J. Biol. Chem.*, 262, 15965, 1987. With permission.)

the DNDS concentration is raised. Thus, pattern conversions in activity correlation plots can discriminate between a T-N two-site model and a two-interacting transport-inhibitory site model. Keep in mind that although it is possible to tell if a site is inhibitory, one cannot tell what type of inhibitory site it is from covalent labeling studies alone.

With this background consider now the results of Figure 25. Here transport activity of red cells is plotted vs. the fraction of PLP bound to band 3 isolated from the same cells. Figure 25A shows clear evidence for the biphasic nature of this correlation. However, increasing the concentration of DNDS present at the cellular PLP labeling and fixation step causes the conversion of the plot to linear (Figure 25C). Since DNDS reversibly protects CH35 sites, the findings suggest the both subdomains contain PLP transport inhibitor sites and that the original biphasicity results from interactions between sites. That DNDS leads to linear correlation plots offers direct evidence that it uncouples the interactions between sites which were responsible for the original biphasic correlation plot (Figure 25A). It is important to realize that this conversion of the pattern from biphasic to linear is associated with the exposure of new labeling sites on both subdomains (Figure 21). These effects taken together seem to support an uncoupling hypothesis where the initial constraints which lower the affinity of coupled sites are broken, thus raising the affinity of the low affinity sites.

Salhany and co-workers[122] carried the study further by adding excess DNDS and selectively titrating CH17. Since the correlation plot for the whole molecule is linear (Figure 25C), interactions are absent and sites can be assigned as transport inhibitory. Figure 26 shows the titration of CH17. It is clear that they were able to titrate CH17 to the 80% level while suppressing CH35 titration to <5%. The CH17 data exactly follow the 1:2 correlation line showing that full coverage of CH17 leads to 50% inhibition of transport with interactions absent. Coverage of CH35 inhibits the other 50%.

The correlation plots of Figures 25 and 26 have some deeper meanings which need to be explored. First, the linearity of Figure 25C and the 1:2 correlation of Figure 26 for CH17 suggest that with interactions absent all PLP sites are transport inhibitory. The simplest way to understand this lack of stoichiometry in inhibition is to suppose that filling the PLP sites blocks anion flow through a channel to deeper sites.

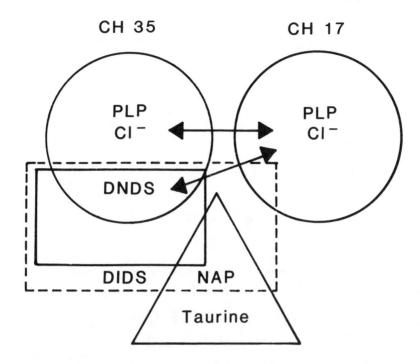

FIGURE 23. Schematic diagram showing the relationship of the various substrate and inhibitor binding domains on band 3. The circles represent the PLP labeling domains on CH17 and CH35. The apparent competitive effect of chloride on PLP labeling of both domains suggests that both domains contain chloride binding sites. The arrow drawn between the two chloride domains indicates possible allosteric interactions between domains (either intramonomeric, intermonomeric, or both). The solid box indicates that DNDS is apparently mutually exclusive with CH35 PLP sites. The arrow indicates that DNDS binding to its site allosterically affects the labeling pattern at nonoverlapping sites on CH17. The dashed box indicates that DIDS is able to block labeling to PLP sites at both chymotryptic domains. Finally, the triangle represents the NAP-taurine binding site which is known to overlap the stilbene-disulfonate binding site, but it does not block substrate binding to sites within the transport domain. It is suggested that the band 3 transport domain contains multiple, interacting PLP labeling subdomains composed of CH17 and CH35. Both of these subdomains are transport inhibitory and interact with chloride and the stilbene-disulfonate binding site, but are not part of the high affinity NAP-taurine modifier site. (From Salhany, J. M., Rauenbuehler, P. B., and Sloan, R. L., *J. Biol. Chem.*, 262, 15965, 1987. With permission.)

Another point to discuss is how each subdomain can have virtually identical labeling patterns in the absence of DNDS, while the correlation plot for the whole molecule is biphasic. This situation would imply that the interactions between sites must be intermonomeric in nature. That is, at 50% saturation, two subdomains on one monomer must be preferentially labeled due to the lowered affinity of the subdomains on the adjacent monomer. The demonstration that half saturation of band 3 with PLP changes the quaternary structure (Figures 3 and 4 of Chapter 2) is direct evidence to support an allosteric interpretation of the biphasic plots in Figure 25A. With DNDS bound, those interactions would be functionally uncoupled, thus raising the affinity of both subdomains on the adjacent monomer. This would explain the increased labeling of both subdomains seen in Figure 21 at saturation with DNDS present. Because it also selectively protects CH35 at low PLP, labeling CH17 "locks" the protein in the uncoupled state, and neither monomer can return to the low affinity (i.e., empty) coupled state.

To demonstrate conformational coupling in the form of negative intermonomeric cooperativity as suggested by the biphasic activity-labeling correlation plot in Figure 25A, Salhany and co-workers[128] have recently studied the distribution of the PLP label between band 3 monomers

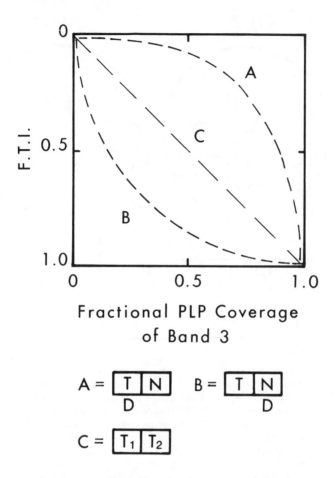

$$A = \boxed{T \mid N} \quad B = \boxed{T \mid N}$$
$$D \qquad\qquad D$$

$$C = \boxed{T_1 \mid T_2}$$

FIGURE 24. Hypothetical activity-labeling correlation plots. Fractional transport inhibition (F.T.I.) is plotted vs. fractional covalent PLP coverage of isolated band 3 derived from labeled red cells. Three models are shown. For two of the models, two populations of sites are considered. Half of the sites are transport inhibitory (T) sites, while the other half are nontransport inhibitory (N). The third model considers the presence of two interacting transport inhibitory sites (T_1 and T_2). D is DNDS, a reversible binding inhibitor.

as a function of fractional PLP covalent coverage. They also analyzed Hill plots of the affinity binding isotherm from data like that in Figure 17. The label distribution studies can be understood by considering the models shown in Figure 27. Key species are shown for a two-site (CH35 and CH17 are considered as canonical binding sites in this study) random, monomeric model (Figure 27A) and a nonrandom, cooperative, dimeric model (Figure 27B). There are four kinds of species present in the random monomer labeling model. They are the unloaded monomer, the two kinds of half-labeled "hybrid" species shown in Figure 27A, and the fully labeled monomer. The fraction of unlabeled monomer for the two-site random model can be calculated using the following equation:

$$\left[\frac{B_0}{B_{tot}}\right] = \left\{\frac{1}{[1 + 2(P/k) + (P/k)^2]}\right\}$$

where B_0 is the unlabeled monomer and B_{tot} is the total of band 3 species present. The constant k is the overall dissociation constant. Fractional PLP saturation of sites (Y) is

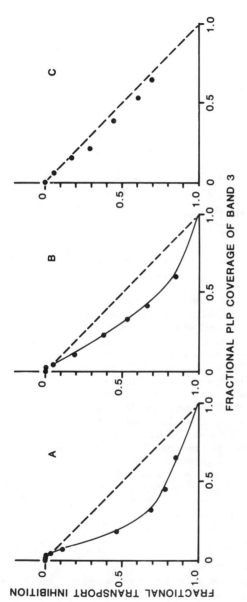

FRACTIONAL PLP COVERAGE OF BAND 3

FIGURE 25. Correlation of fractional transport inhibition due to covalently bound PLP with fractional covalent PLP coverage of isolated band 3 derived from labeled red blood cells. Panel A shows results from control red cells where labeling was performed as described in the text. Panels B and C show correlation plots for 10 and 25 μM DNDS, respectively. The labeling conditions were 150 mM chloride, 50 mM bisTris, pH 6.6. In the absence of DNDS the correlation plot was nonlinear. The full saturation value corresponds to 4.2 mol of PLP per mole of band 3 (see Figure 17). Addition of saturating DNDS during PLP labeling caused the plots to become linear. DNDS also increased the number of exofacial sites available for labeling. The value in C for saturating DNDS at full coverage with PLP is about 7.4 mol of PLP per mole of band 3. (From Salhany, J. M., Rauenbuehler, P. B., and Sloan, R. L., *J. Biol. Chem.*, 262, 15965, 1987. With permission.)

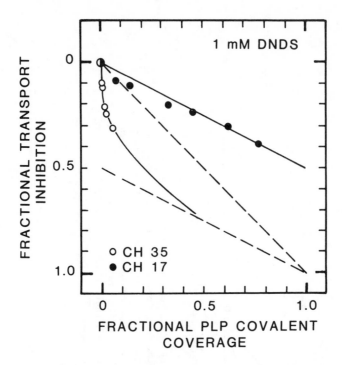

FIGURE 26. Correlation of fractional transport inhibition vs. fractional PLP covalent coverage of CH17 and CH35 with PLP labeling performed in the presence of 1 m*M* DNDS. The conditions were chosen so as to favor DNDS displacement of PLP from CH35 sites. Labeling was performed at 20 m*M* chloride (balance 153 m*M* citrate with 50 m*M* bisTris, pH 6.6) where the DNDS binding constant is reported to be near 100 n*M*. Fractional PLP coverage of each domain was determined as described previously, using quantitative fluorescence gel electrophoretic and slicing methods. As can be seen, CH35 labeling only reaches about 6% saturation while CH17 reaches near 80% saturation at the highest PLP. Furthermore, the CH17 data follows the 1:2 correlation line showing that all of the CH17 sites account for exactly one half of PLP transport inhibition. The curve drawn for the CH35 data points intersects the other hypothetical 1:2 correlation line at about 75% inhibition, as expected if CH17 and CH35 each contained independent inhibitory sites under labeling conditions where interactions between domains were absent. It is estimated that full coverage of each domain is equivalent to the binding of 3.7 mol of PLP per mole of domain at the DNDS concentration used in the labeling studies. (From Salhany, J. M., Rauenbuehler, P. B., and Sloan, R. L., *J. Biol. Chem.*, 262, 15965, 1987. With permission.)

$$(P/k) = \frac{Y}{1 - Y}$$

Figure 27B shows one species of a nonrandom cooperative labeling model where a second class of canonical PLP labeling sites on a given monomer are labeled before the adjacent conformationally coupled monomer becomes liganded. Preferential labeling could arise from intermonomeric negative cooperativity, intramonomeric positive cooperativity, or both.

The disappearance of the unlabeled monomer with increasing fractional PLP ligation can be directly measured using the Jennings-Passow effect: the ability of DIDS to cross-link CH35 to CH17 after chymotrypsin digestion. DIDS and PLP are mutually exclusive with each other at both chymotryptic subdomains. Thus, prelabeling with PLP and reaction with DIDS at alkaline pH in the absence of free PLP will lead to exclusive cross-linking of the unlabeled subdomains.

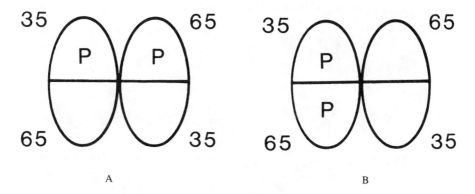

FIGURE 27.   Distribution of PLP (P) between subdomains of a band 3 monomer for intermediate species of a random labeling model (A) vs. a nonrandom labeling model (B). One canonical PLP site is shown per chymotryptic subdomain. There are four molecular species for a two-site random-labeling monomer model: the unlabeled and fully labeled monomeric species (not shown) and two half-labeled intermediate "hybrid" monomers. The two "hybrid" species are shown as a noninteracting dimer in A. One hybrid has PLP on the CH35 subdomain, while the other has PLP on the CH65 subdomain. This model is contrasted with one intermediate species from a model proposing the preferential, nonrandom labeling of one mono-mer. This could arise from intramonomeric positive cooperativity, intermonomeric negative cooperativity (or steric hindrance), or mixed cooperativities. The basic experiment to be performed in Figures 28 to 31 uses the fact that covalent DIDS and PLP labeling are mutually exclusive at both subdomains. Intramon-omeric DIDS cross-linking of the two subdomains can then be used as a direct measure of the fraction of PLP-free monomers along the ligation manifold. Random labeling and steric hindrance models predict a rapid loss of DIDS cross-linkability along the ligation manifold, while cooperative labeling models predict linear correlation plots.

If hybrid species form, they will not be cross-linked by DIDS. Fractional DIDS cross-linking is then a direct measure of the fraction of unlabeled monomer present along the PLP ligation manifold. Fractional DIDS cross-linking can be plotted vs. the fraction of PLP labeling to each subdomain measured in the same experiment using the fluorescence gel-slicing methodology discussed earlier. Cross-correlation of these two measurements will be linear if cooperativity is present.

Random labeling and steric hindrance models can be distinguished from cooperative labeling models in these experiments. In the random model, there is an early increase in "hybrid" labeled species. Since they are not DIDS cross-linkable, the fraction of cross-linkable, unlabeled monomer would decrease. Similarly, if PLP labeling of the first monomer sterically blocks PLP labeling of the second, it will also block DIDS cross-linking of the second because they are mutually exclusive sites. There will be less DIDS cross-linking, and the plot will look like a random labeling model. Recent electron spin resonance (ESR) evidence[105] suggests that the DIDS (and therefore the PLP) sites on each monomer are too far apart for intermonomeric steric hindrance arguments to be entertained. Cooperative models lead to preferential labeling of one monomer without blocking the DIDS cross-linking of the second monomer. Therefore, there will be relatively more DIDS-cross-linkable material present at a given fractional PLP in cooperative labeling models and the correlation plot will be a straight line.

Figure 28 shows the change in the DIDS cross-linking of band 3 on alkali-stripped membranes as a function of increasing PLP present at the time of the cellular fixation step. DIDS cross-linking was performed on PLP-modified cells as described by Jennings and Passow[74] in the absence of free PLP. Increasing fractional PLP covalent coverage decreases the fraction of DIDS cross-linkable material present near the top of the gel. Lanes E show unlabeled, chymotrypsin-treated band 3 without addition of DIDS. Lanes A show the extent of DIDS cross-linking on PLP-free band 3. The quantitative analysis of the loss of DIDS cross-linkable material

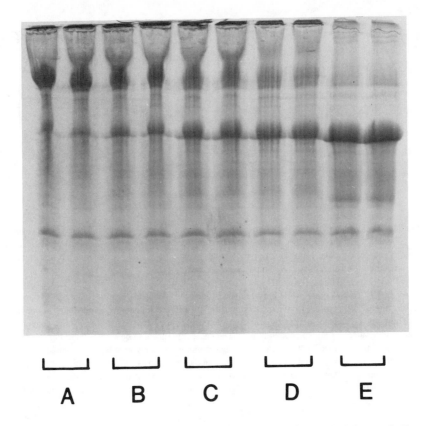

FIGURE 28.   DIDS cross-linking of chymotrypsin-digested band 3 labeled within intact red cell membranes at various PLP concentrations. Ten percent polyacrylamide gels were run for NaOH-stripped membranes derived from cells reacted with the various PLP concentrations and fixed with borohydride, then treated with chymotrypsin and DIDS as described in the text. The gel shown here demonstrates the disappearance of the 100-kDa cross-linked band 3 fragments (top major band) with the appearance of the uncross-linked fragments represented by the second major visible band. Each sample was run on duplicate lanes. The following PLP and DIDS concentrations were present: A, 0 mM PLP, 100 μM DIDS; B, 2 mM PLP, 100 μM DIDS; C, 10 mM PLP, 100 μM DIDS; D, 30 mM PLP, 100 μM DIDS; and E, 0 mM PLP and 0 μM DIDS.

is shown in Figure 29 as a single reciprocal plot. The linearity of this plot indicates that the fraction of unlabeled species decreases hyperbolically with increasing PLP concentration. The relationship of this decrease to increasing fractional PLP coverage of each subdomain required measurement of that quantity independently in fluorescence gel-slicing experiments (Figure 30). The fraction of DIDS cross-linkable material is then cross-correlated with the fraction of PLP coverage of each subdomain in Figure 31. The correlation is linear, indicating that at 50% coverage of each subdomain of the band 3 monomer, half of the monomers are empty, while half are fully labeled with PLP. Expected correlations for a two- and four-site random labeling model is shown in Figure 31. It should also be noted that there is no disproportion in the appearance of each subdomain in Figure 30, and no PLP fluorescence was seen in the DIDS cross-linked region of the gel, despite the fact that at 30 mM PLP there is a substantial amount of cross-linkable material present (Figure 28).

   In order to see what type of cooperativity accounts for the preferential labeling of one monomer, Hill plots were quantitatively analyzed according to the methods of Cornish-Bowden and Koshland,[132] treating each subdomain of a cooperative dimer as a single *canonical* class of sites. The data come from results like those in Figure 17B and in Figure 32. The solid line in Figure 32 comes from a fit to the fourth-power Hill equation given in the paper by Cornish-

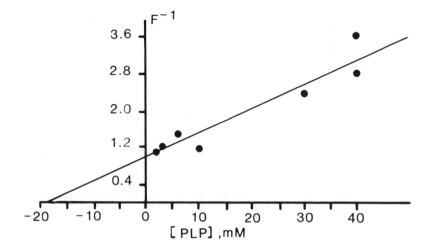

FIGURE 29.   Single reciprocal plot of the fractional integrated peak area for the 100-kDa cross-linked fragment from gels like those shown in Figure 28. The peak area was determined as described in the text and the data shown come from a total of four independent gels. The line is the best fitting linear least-squares fit of the data. The value of the half-inhibition association constant was $5.0 \pm 0.004 \times 10^{-2} \, M^{-1}$. The correlation coefficient was 0.9497.

Bowden and Koshland,[132] with the constants listed in the figure legend. In combination with the distribution results of Figure 31, we can assign K_1' and K_2' to labeling of the subdomains on the first monomer, with K_3' and K_4' being assigned to labeling of the subdomains on the second monomer. This analysis shows that preferential labeling arises from a 20-fold lower PLP affinity of the second monomer ($K_3' \ll K_1'$, association constants). There is some indication for the existence of positive intramonomeric cooperativity in the analysis.

b. Ligation Manifolds for PLP and Stilbene-Disulfonate Binding

The results with PLP show that this transported ligand of band 3 binds to the dimer with strong intermonomeric negative cooperativity and inhibits the anion exchange activity biphasically. However, these interactions can be uncoupled by performing the labeling experiments in the presence of DNDS. Since both of these ligands convert the porter to the TC-state, the differences in functionality must be a consequence of substates within a *liganded* quaternary structure of the porter. These substates and various mechanisms are illustrated by the ligation manifolds in Figure 33. The square substates are considered to be active substates in transport and they have a high ligand affinity, while the triangular substates have a low ligand affinity and are inactive in transport. Another possible way to consider these substates is to assign the square state as an open channel and the triangular state to a partially occluded channel. When the channel is open, all four PLP sites (two per subdomain) can bind. When the channel is partially occluded, none of the PLP sites on that monomer bind PLP at low concentration. The biphasic activity-labeling correlation plot of Figure 25A arises from preferential PLP labeling of the active monomer of the conformationally coupled dimer. Coverage of that monomer inhibits its transport, but preserves the coupling of the second inactive, low-affinity monomer. This accounts for the greater than expected fractional inhibition of transport. At high enough PLP concentration, the low affinity (partially occluded) monomer becomes labeled, but transport is already inhibited, and this additional labeling accounts for the biphasic appearance of the curve (Figure 25A).

The effect of addition of DNDS during PLP labeling is shown in Figure 33 as the D' ligation manifold. Since DNDS is added under affinity conditions ([ligand] >> [sites]) and since it has a high affinity for band 3, it will bind to both monomers and offer protection to CH35 sites.

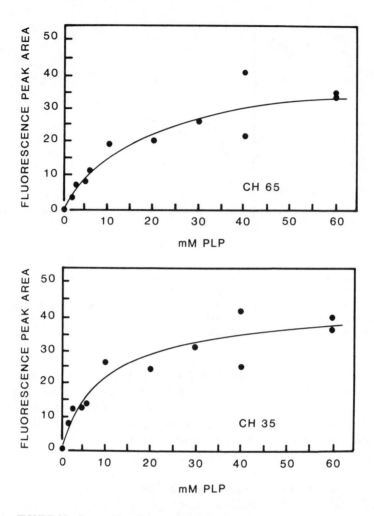

FIGURE 30. Integrated peak area of PLP fluorescence as a function of PLP concentration present during labeling and fixation for the CH65 and CH35 peaks. The peak area of PLP fluorescence was determined as described in the text. The data are from four independent experiments and the line drawn through the data is a weighted, robust fit to a hyperbolic function. The apparent half-labeling constant for CH65 was 16.7 ± 5.3 mM, while the maximum fluorescence peak area was 49.4 ± 5.7. The apparent half-labeling constant for CH35 was 10.3 ± 3.3 mM with a maximum fluorescence peak area of 43.7 ± 4.2.

However, it is important to realize that if it did not also uncouple the interactions and raise the affinity of the nonmutually exclusive CH17 sites on the low affinity monomer, those subdomains would not be labeled at lower PLP. Yet, we saw that addition of DNDS increased CH17 labeling (Figures 20 and 21). Since the second monomer has an originally lower affinity, this change must be due to the rise in the affinity of the sites on that monomer associated with the conformational uncoupling event. Increased labeling of CH17 is clearly an allosteric effect and it correlates with the resulting conversion of the PLP activity-labeling correlation plot from biphasic to linear (Figure 25 C). Once CH17 is labeled in the uncoupled state, it is apparent from the ligand distribution shown in the DNDS-PLP ligation manifold of Figure 33 that it is impossible for either monomer to relax to the conformationally coupled state. This explains why the PLP activity-labeling correlation plots are linear, even though DNDS was not present during the transport measurements.

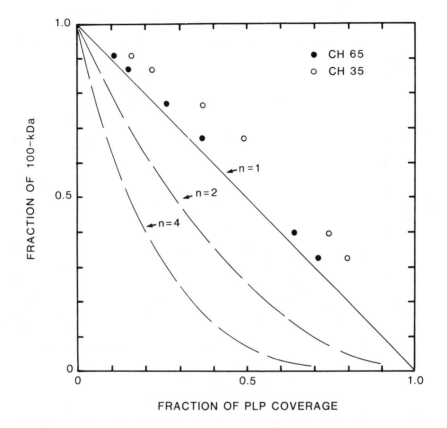

FIGURE 31. Correlation of the calculated fraction of 100-kDa DIDS cross-linked material vs. the fraction of PLP coverage of CH65 and CH35 subdomains. The calculated values for both axes came from the best fits of the primary data in Figures 29 and 30. The two curves shown were calculated based on a two-site (n = 2) and four-site (n = 4) random-labeling monomer model. Contrary to expectations of a random-labeling model, the data follow the 1:1 correlation line (n = 1) for both subdomains. The results suggest that PLP labels one band 3 monomer preferentially due to some type of cooperativity.

What is the significance of this functional difference between the PLP-bound vs. the DNDS-bound (or the CH17-PLP-labeled) quaternary substates? Both are in the same quaternary structure based on the BS³ cross-linking results of Chapter 2, yet they are functionally quite different. The functional difference may reflect certain of the liganded species expected to exist along a complete transport cycle. The stilbene-bound substate could be an "outward-facing", liganded quaternary substate, while the PLP-bound substate (because PLP is transportable) could be a true intermediate, perhaps an "inward-facing", liganded quaternary structure. The possible role of various substates will be discussed later as a possible mechanism for the complete transport cycle is considered.

C. SIGNIFICANCE OF THE ALLOSTERIC UNCOUPLING HYPOTHESIS TO THE INTERPRETATION OF OTHER DATA
1. The Linear DIDS Activity-Labeling Correlation Plot Revisited
We saw in the beginning of this section that DIDS binds 1:1 with a band 3 monomer and linearly inhibits transport. This suggests monomeric functional independence. On the other hand, PLP, which binds to apparently mutually exclusive sites on the channel, inhibits transport biphasically. The biphasic inhibition was shown to arise from intersubunit allosteric (or intermonomeric, "channel-channel") interactions such that when one channel is labeled at both

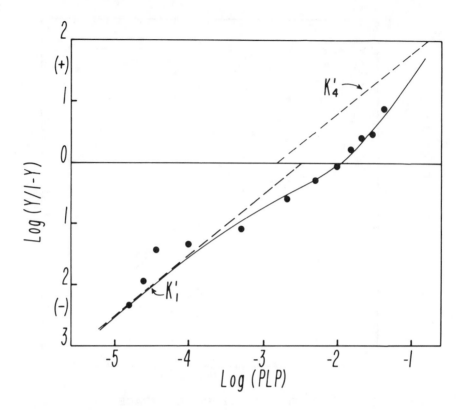

FIGURE 32. Hill plot of fractional PLP bound to isolated band 3 derived from labeled red blood cells. Band 3 was labeled in intact red cells at various PLP concentrations over a broad range. The protein was then isolated in pure form and the amount of PLP bound was determined. This data was then used to calculate fractional saturation which, in turn, was used to construct the plot. The number of moles of PLP bound per mole of band 3 monomer was determined to be 4.2, at saturation. The solid line is a computer fit to a fourth-power Hill equation[132] where each site is a canonical site within a four-site dimer model. The four association constants are fit: $K_1' = 300\ M^{-1}$; $K_2' = 100\ M^{-1}$; $K_3' = 15\ M^{-1}$; and $K_4' = 700\ M^{-1}$.

subdomains with PLP, the other allosterically coupled monomeric channel of the dimer is partially occluded and does not bind PLP at low concentration. The allosterically coupled channel is also inactive in transport. Thus, PLP may preserve a native intersubunit allosteric coupling, while DIDS binding to one monomer shows no evidence for conformational coupling. That DIDS as a stilbene disulfonate actually uncouples interactions between monomers is strongly suggested in experiments showing that addition of DNDS during PLP labeling both linearizes the activity-labeling correlation plot and exposes new labeling sites on both subdomains. The ligand distribution studies showed an original preferential monomeric labeling, suggesting that the newly exposed sites labeled with DNDS-induced uncoupling are on the adjacent low-affinity or partially occluded monomer. Thus, stilbene disulfonates can uncouple intersubunit allosteric interactions on band 3, and this may explain why DIDS inhibits anion transport linearly when all of the functional evidence for the native state (i.e., no inhibitor bound) suggests that there are interactions between sites. Furthermore, PLP is a transported anion and it shows interactions which can be uncoupled.

2. Target Molecular Weight Measurements

The ultimate question in our comparison of the mechanism of PLP vs. DIDS covalent inhibition of anion transport is, which inhibitor do we believe is faithfully indicating the state of coupling between band 3 monomers in the native state with physiological anions bound. Our

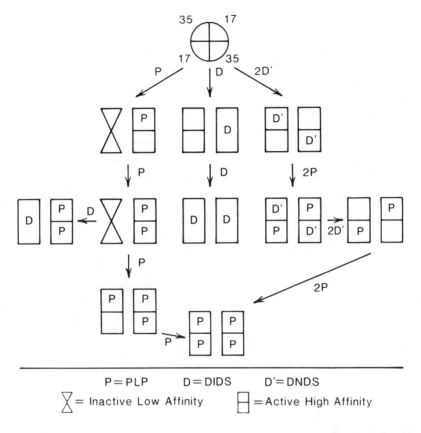

FIGURE 33. Ligation manifolds for covalent PLP labeling of band 3. The ligation manifolds for PLP (P) and DIDS (D) covalent binding are shown. The change in the PLP ligation manifold when the reversible inhibitor DNDS (D′) is present is also shown. The meanings of the different states of the monomer are shown in the figure and discussed in the text.

argument is that the allosteric-like kinetics of the system suggest that conformational coupling is the natural state and that DIDS is an uncoupling agent which also inhibits. The fact that DNDS uncouples the intersubunit interactions of PLP strongly supports the hypothesis. Still, results with all inhibitors are, in the last analysis, an extrapolation. A direct measure of the molecular weight of the active unit of band 3 is needed. Jung and co-workers[133,134] have used the interesting technique of radiation inactivation to assess the molecular weight of the basic functional unit. In this method, high-intensity radiation is used to eliminate the given activity which is correlated with the molecular weight associated with that activity. If the entire band 3 monomer contributes to target size and if the dimer is the natural functional unit, we should see a 200-kDa molecular weight. If only the integral domain contributes, the dimer target size would be 100 kDa, while a tetrameric functional unit would yield a target size of 200 kDa (i.e., four integral domains). In their first paper, Cuppoletti and co-workers[133] found a target molecular weight based on an anion transport assay of 200 kDa. Either a band 3 dimer or a tetramer is the basic native functional unit. In a later paper Verkman and co-workers[134] showed that the target molecular weight determined by a stilbene disulfonate binding assay was lower giving a target size to 59 kDa (one monomeric integral domain). The suggested native functional unit is the band 3 tetramer or a tetramer of two dimers. In the coupled form, a single band 3 monomer does not transport anions alone. This is the state sensed by the transport assay without inhibitors present. If stilbenes can bind to a good monomer of a "crippled" pair, the target molecular weight would be lower. What is needed, are experiments where target molecular weight measurements are made using a transport assay for control cells, DIDS half-labeled band 3 cells and PLP half-labeled band 3 cells. The prediction is that the DIDS half-labeled band 3 will give a target molecular weight which is reduced compared to control based on the anion transport assay, while PLP half-labeled band 3 will have either the same target molecular weight as control or possibly a higher value.

D. SUMMARY

We have seen that there is a clear distinction between DIDS activity-labeling correlation plots and PLP plots. DIDS shows linearity, and one molecule covers or affects several sites on one monomer. But the activity of the neighboring monomer seems unaffected. This either means it was originally uncoupled or DIDS binding uncouples interactions originally present. By contrast, covalent PLP binds to several sites which either overlap the DIDS site or are allosterically affected by DIDS covalent binding on one monomer. PLP activity-labeling plots indicate the presence of conformational coupling between band 3 monomers. The adjacent monomer has a 20-fold lower PLP affinity and is inactive in transport. Stilbene disulfonates uncouple subunit interactions within the native porter oligomer. The ability of DNDS to convert the PLP activity-labeling correlation plot from biphasic to linear while exposing new sites on CH17 and CH35 (or by raising the affinity of those sites) supports this contention. The fact that transport curves for physiological anions show complex patterns which can be converted to hyperbolic by partial covalent labeling with stilbene disulfonate binding supports this contention. The conversion of the PLP activity-labeling correlation plot from biphasic to linear is then equivalent to the conversion of the transport curves from complex to hyperbolic and both indicate that interactions on band 3 have been uncoupled. The target molecular weight based on an anion transport assay may also support an oligomeric functional unit.

VI. EXAMPLES OF OTHER ALLOSTERIC EFFECTS ON BAND 3

A. INTRODUCTION

If molecules like PLP preserve an original conformational coupling, surely other molecules exist which also preserve coupling. They should show evidence for biphasic activity-labeling correlation plots or other evidence for interactions between CH17 and CH35. Also, homotropic allosterism should be reflected in pH-dependent studies. Under conditions of varying pH, the observed pKs for an activity may not intimately involve the titrating amino acid, but rather a distant allosterically linked group which influences conformation and thereby the activity at the active site. In what follows some notable examples of biphasic inhibitors are given, and the factors influencing the pH titration curve for the anion exchange activity are discussed.

B. PH DEPENDENCE OF ANION TRANSPORT

In a simple diffusional fixed-charge model for anion transport, protonation of an amino acid at a barrier might be expected to facilitate anion transport, while deprotonation would stop or severely attenuate the process. Simple facilitation should yield a single pK; if this is not observed, other possibilities need to be considered. For example, a pH maximum could indicate the involvement of more than one kind of titratable group. As indicated in Chapter 1, there is a glutamate residue at the bicarbonate binding site on crocodilian hemoglobin, so even protein negative charges can participate in anion binding. However, what if the groups at the transport site have pKs which are conformationally dependent? Conversely, what if the groups which titrate are not at the transport site but at distant sites and modulate the activity at the transport site allosterically? One needs to distinguish allosteric pH modulation from a direct pH effect at the transport site, considering the mounting evidence that allosteric interactions may be involved in anion transport.

The pH dependence of red cell anion transport is one of the oldest topics in the study of red cell physiology. Mond[135] was the first to examine the pH dependence of net anion exchange

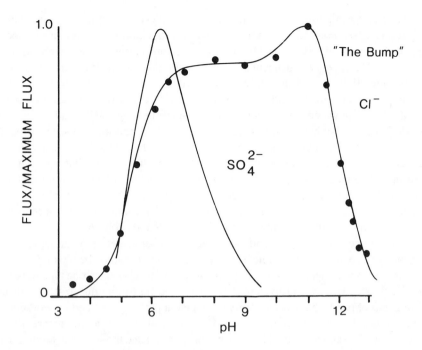

FIGURE 34. The pH dependence of the red cell anion-exchange system. This is a composite normalized to the maximum velocities for chloride and sulfate, respectively. The apparent activation of velocities for chloride prior to the onset of the alkaline branch is called "The Bump" and is discussed in the text.

across the red cell membrane and to relate that response to the dissociation of fixed charges on the membrane. Modern studies of the pH dependence of transport[28,52,54,136-155] focus on a functional interpretation, using expected properties of carriers to explain pH titration curves. Yet, these studies often take the view that the observed titrations involve specific fixed sites on an otherwise rigid protein, despite the fact that the protein is conformationaly active.

Consider the different pH dependencies of sulfate exchange (a divalent anion) vs. chloride exchange (a monovalent anion) (Figure 34). Figure 34 is a composite figure representing studies where pH was varied on both sides of the membrane below pH 8, while above that value only the pH of the extracellular medium was changed. One significant characteristic is that both chloride and sulfate titration curves show pH maxima.[52,54,138,143] That observation seems inconsistent with a simple fixed-charge hypothesis,[156] since one would have expected to observe a single pK with a descending alkaline branch.

Although both sulfate and chloride show pH maxima, there are obvious differences in the titration curves which need to be explained, since both anions exclusively use band 3 porter.[65] Wieth and co-workers[157] interpreted the titration in terms of three apparent pKs. The titration at the acid branch was assigned a pK value of 5.2 to 5.4, at an extracellular chloride of 165 mM. The next major titration of the system occurred with a pK of 12. The pK is chloride dependent and decreases linearly with $\log_{chloride}$ between 150 and 15 mM chloride.[143] The sulfate curve has a similar acid branch but a considerably lower alkaline pK than chloride.

The pH dependence of chloride self-exchange is complicated by a "bump" at around pH 11, which also must have a molecular explanation. The origin of the "bump" in the chloride titration curve was originally assigned to the extracellular modifier site. At the time it seemed reasonable to dissect this portion of the titration curve empirically. Wieth and co-workers[157] found a pK for the activation part of the "bump" to be about 11. Since raising the pH activates the system, it was assumed that protonating this extracellular site inhibited the system, and so the pK was assigned to an extracellular modifier site.[157] Deprotonation of the site with pK 11 caused inhibition by NAP-taurine to be eliminated.[157] Yet the modifier site for chloride self-inhibition depends most strongly on internal chloride.[57] The "bump" in the titration curve, on the other hand, was shown by Knauf and Mann[57] to be dependent on external chloride between 150 and 600 mM at 600 mM *trans* chloride. High external chloride exaggerates the "bump", while lower chloride eliminates the "bump". This contrasts with the apparent chloride competitive-binding constant at the external DNDS site which is less than 50 mM as determined by NMR[56] and is probably closer to 6 mM.[96] Yet, the stilbene disulfonate site and the NAP-taurine site seem to be mutually exclusive.[19,21] Could the extracellular pK 11 titration be related to stilbene-disulfonate binding either through a direct effect or through an allosteric linkage mechanism? The evidence supporting the connection between the pK 11 "bump" and the stilbene-disulfonate binding site is suggested by the Falke and Chan[108] study showing that DNDS-sensitive chloride NMR line broadening has an apparent pK of 11, the same as the extracellular titration for the "bump".[157] The mechanism or whether this may simply be coincidental is obscure.

If the difference in the pH dependence of anion exchange between sulfate and chloride is under allosteric control and is not related to any specifics of the anion being used, then chemical modification of the protein should change the pH titration curve from one type of pattern (e.g., monovalent state) to the other (divalent state). Such state transitions due to seemingly unrelated modifications of band 3 have been observed. For example, Jennings and co-workers[71] showed that intramolecular cross-linking of band 3 lysines with BS[3] at a site apparently mutually exclusive with the extracellular DNDS site not only eliminated the substrate inhibition function (Figure 11), but also changed the pH dependence of monovalent anion exchange to a pH dependence resembling that of divalent anion exchange (Figure 35). Since the apparent pKs are changed between two characteristic titration patterns by chemical modification of the protein, the titration curve may be more dependent on protein conformational state than on any specific difference between the type of anion used. The available evidence would seem to favor allosteric linkage as an explanation of apparent transitions in state.

There are several other examples in the literature which show that chemical modification at diverse protein groups leads to similar characteristic changes in the pH titration pattern which cannot simply be explained by a change at the group being titrated. For example, Legrum and co-workers[144] reported that dansylation of band 3 greatly enhanced the exchange rate for sulfate with little effect on chloride and also converted the pH dependence of sulfate transport from the divalent state pattern to the monovalent state pattern. At pH 8.5, where divalent anion transport is minimal, dansylation increased the exchange rate by about two orders of magnitude. Lepke and Passow[139] reported a similar effect, but reported as well that addition of the transport inhibitor APMB (2-(4-amino-3-sulfophenyl)-6-methyl-7-benzothiazolsulfonate) during dansylation potentiated the effect by at least another order of magnitude (Figure 36). Sulfate anion-exchange velocities were now approaching those of chloride. Yet another difference between the kinetic properties of these two anions seems to be eliminated through protein modification. Berghout and co-workers[145] observed a similar effect for phosphate transport, while Raida and Passow[158] found the same effect with a highly band 3-specific reagent known as PENS-Cl (2-(*N*-piperidine)ethylamine-1-naphthyl-5-sulfonylchloride). Finally, Romano and Passow[153] showed that the pH dependence for sulfate transport in trout red cells was like that of monovalent anions in human red cells with respect to the DIDS-sensitive component of transport.

The evidence presented thus far suggests that the pH dependence of anion exchange could reflect allosteric transitions in which other regulatory groups besides the substrate binding site are pH dependent. Kaufmann and co-workers[97] have presented ESR binding data using a stilbene-disulfonate spin label showing that its binding was virtually independent of pH. Kaufmann and co-workers[97] concluded that the strong pH dependence of chloride and sulfate transport cannot result from a titration at the "substrate site" but rather suggest participation of ionizable regulatory sites for the transport process, in keeping with an allosteric interpretation.

One revealing study recently published by Jennings and Al-Rhaiyel[159] seems to us a classic

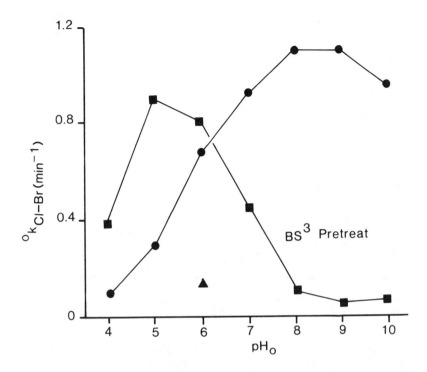

FIGURE 35. Effect of extracellular pH on the rate constant ($^\circ k_{Cl\text{-}Br}$) for ^{36}Cl efflux into 140 mM KBr, buffered with 10 mM gluconate, phosphate, and borate at pH 4 to 10. Control cells (solid circles) were equilibrated with 150 mM KCl (extracellular pH 7) and loaded with tracer immediately before the efflux measurement. BS^3 pretreated cells (squares) were incubated 1 h, 37°C, pH 7.4 in 150 mM KCl medium containing 5 mM BS^3, and then washed and equilibrated with pH 7 medium and loaded with tracer. The triangle refers to cells treated with 10 mM phenlyglyoxal, pH 10, after the BS^3, with the flux subsequently measured at extracellular pH 6 as for the other cells. Each data point represents the mean of two efflux measurements (four time points each) performed on each of at least two preparations of cells. For each data point, the standard error of the mean is not more than 16%. (From Jennings, M. L., Monaghan, R., Douglas, S. M., and Nicknish, J. S., *J. Gen. Physiol.*, 86, 653, 1985. With permission.)

example of the allosteric nature of the pH dependence of anion exchange. They showed that Woodward's K reagent modification changed *both* the external and internal pH dependence of anion transport under conditions where the reagents could not possibly penetrate the membrane. The authors suggested that the same carboxyl group is responsible for both titrations and that it can cross the membrane. Although they mention the possibility of a transmembrane allosteric effect, they favor a so-called "thin-barrier" model. They take the view that the protein is so strongly fixed in the membrane that any external modification which causes a transmembrane effect has, of necessity, to occur through a "thin barrier". Yet, in Chapter 2, we showed that the addition of transport site ligands changes the quaternary structure of band 3. Clearly, band 3 porter molecular biology is at a crossroads. We have "thin barriers" on one hand and allosterism on the other, both seeking to explain the same data. Additional and more conventional points of view concerning the pH dependence of anion transport may be found in some of the original papers and in several reviews.[19-21,141]

C. INHIBITORS WHICH SHOW 50:50 BIPHASIC REACTIONS OR OTHER ALLOSTERIC EFFECTS
1. Effects of 1-Isothiocyanate-4-Benzenesulfonate and Related Compounds
Phenylmonosulfonates and arylisothiocyanates were extensively studied in the earlier phase

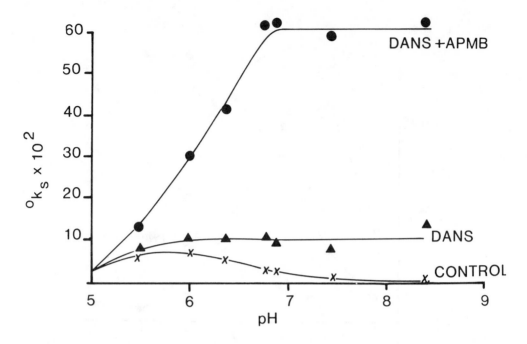

FIGURE 36.   pH dependence of SO_4^{2-} equilibrium exchange in dansylated ghosts. Dansylation in the absence (▲) or presence (●) of 5 mM APMB, compared to control (X). (From Legrum, B., Fasold, H., and Passow, H., *Hoppe Seyler's Z. Physiol. Chem.,* 361, 1573, 1980. With permission.)

of band 3 research.[66,67,160-165] That work showed that CH17 contains a subdomain which when labeled can apparently fully inhibit transport. Zaki and co-workers[160] showed that para-IBS could fully inhibit anion transport. The half-inhibition constant was lower than that of the stilbene disulfonates, but, it can be argued, it is more nearly physiological. Barzilay and co-workers[66] confirmed this effect and separated the reversible from the irreversible components. They showed that para-IBS is a much more potent total inhibitor than meta-IBS.

Ho and Guidotti[161] studied inhibition by total and by covalently bound para-IBS. They were first able to identify the label as being present almost exclusively in the band 3 region of the gel. Interestingly, their plot of percent inhibition of phosphate transport vs. the number of moles of para-IBS bound per mole of band 3 showed virtually complete inhibition at 0.5 mol of reagent per mole of band 3. This represents apparent "half-of-the-sites" reactivity. That is, if the authors had carried their labeling concentrations to higher levels, they may have seen still more labeling of band 3 until saturation was reached, despite the fact that transport was almost completely turned off. From the present perspective, the Ho and Guidotti[161] result is an important finding since it generally supports the biphasic inhibitory plot seen for PLP. However, instead of both subdomains showing equivalent labeling, Drickamer[162] found the label exclusively bound to a 7000-Da hydroxylamine cleavage fragment lying N terminal to the exofacial chymotrypsin cleavage site (i.e., on CH17). That is, the "half-DIDS" molecule para-IBS seems to inhibit completely anion transport with apparent half-of-the-sites reactivity by apparently binding exclusively to CH17. Ho and Guidotti[161] suggested that the 1:2 correlation line was possibly the result of a second protein in the band 3 region. But today we know that there is no other protein present in that region in sufficient number to account for the observed stoichiometry. Indeed, we would suggest that the other "protein" in that region of the gel is the CH35 subdomain of an intact band 3 molecule.

Another example of biphasic inhibition comes from the papers of Sigrist and co-workers.[164-167] In their first paper, the authors reported measurement of the correlation of covalent phenylisothiocyanate binding to band 3 with the percent inhibition of transport. The probe completely inhibited anion transport. However, it was also very clear that the correlation of percent inhibition vs. the coverage of band 3 was biphasic.

In a second important paper, Kempf and co-workers[165] reported that the hydrophobic compound phenylisothiocyanate almost exclusively located in a 10-kDa thermolysin fragment of CH35, with a molar ratio of about 3:1. There was virtually no label in the CH17 subdomain. When these authors prelabeled CH17 with para-IBS and then treated with the hydrophobic probe, they found that the amount of CH35 labeling had decreased by 1 mol/mol of fragment. This is the first indication of an apparent allosteric interaction between CH17 and CH35. Thus, para-IBS binding to CH17 can fully inhibit transport, while phenylisothiocyanate binding to CH35 can also completely inhibit transport; and the subdomains interact with each other.

If allosteric interactions are present on band 3, then how can we assign functions to sites? It seems that CH17 can be fully occupied and turn off transport with a half-site stoichiometry, while CH35, occupied by a similar, but nonionic probe, can completely inhibit transport and also show biphasic activity-labeling correlation plots. Whether these are intermonomeric or intra-monomeric interactions is unclear. In a later paper, the Swiss group, in collaboration with Cacciola and co-workers,[166] investigated the ability of DNDS to protect against the inhibition of anion transport caused by arylisothiocyanate binding to CH35. They found that DNDS could almost completely protect the system from this hydrophobic probe. This result is consistent with DNDS coverage of CH35, in agreement with the PLP studies discussed above.

2. Dinitrophenylation

We have just seen that selective modification of either subdomain by "half-DIDS" molecules can rather completely turn off transport and that there are very probably allosteric interactions between the subdomains. Another chemical modification of band 3 which has been investigated to the same extent is the dinitrophenylation reaction.[19,114,160,168,169] Rudloff and co-workers[169] studied the effect of dinitrophenylation and looked for the distribution of the label between the two chymotryptic subdomains of band 3. Although 1-fluor-2,4-dinitrobenzene can react with several amino acids, Rudloff finds that when transport is inhibited by 80%, two dinitrophenyl groups have been incorporated. One is at CH17 and the other is at CH35, but the correlation plot is biphasic with 95% inhibition obtained with a stoichiometric ratio of 6:1. The subdomain distribution was not reported under those conditions. When DIDS is simultaneously mixed with the reagent, only dinitrophenylation of CH17 is blocked, while, according to the authors, dinitrophenylation of CH35 remains unaffected. Thus, DIDS seems to preferentially block one lysine residue on CH17 from dinitrophenylation.

In order to correlate labeling with function, the authors[169] first studied the effect of DNDS protection of band 3 dinitrophenylation on anion transport. The assumption was that DIDS and DNDS were blocking the same site on CH17. Addition of DNDS was sufficient to completely prevent the inhibition of anion transport by dinitrophenylation of CH17. The authors[169] showed that DNDS reduces the rate of dinitrophenylation of CH17 without affecting the rate of reaction at CH35.[19,169] However, they also showed that dinitrophenylation of CH35 can cause a reduction in the rate of dinitrophenylation of the CH17 lysine. The protective effect of DNDS on the CH17 lysine may be due to its exclusive binding to CH35, just as was seen for PLP. These allosteric effects could be related to uncoupling of intermonomeric interactions.

Passow[19] has discussed the dinitrophenylation reaction as well as some unpublished results in his review. He points out that both lysines are "involved" in transport but in different ways. Dinitrophenylation of CH17 leads to inhibition. However, it is interesting that the rate of reaction depends on whether chloride or sulfate is present under otherwise comparable conditions. Thi is not a direct effect on the CH17 lysine but rather some linked effect.[19] It is worth noting that Passow's results[19] show that dinitrophenylation of CH35 actually leads to a slightly enhanced rate of anion transport.

3. Arginine-Specific Reagents

Since the extent of inhibition by arginine-specific reagents depends on conditions of pH and the type of substrate (chloride vs. sulfate) present in the medium, one might expect the location of the reagent in the protein also to be dependent on those conditions. This is the case.[86,90] When the reaction is carried out at pH 10, there are about 4 million PG molecules bound per red cell, and with a stoichiometry of two PGs per arginine, this gives a value of one reactive arginine per band 3 monomer responsible for maximum inhibition.[86] When PG-treated band 3 is then reacted with chymotrypsin, all of the label is found on CH35. It should be pointed out that transport is not completely inhibited with ligation of this CH35 arginine. At pH 10 there is still some residual flux which is inhibitable by DIDS.[85,86] At physiological pH there is quite a considerable fraction of transport which is not inhibitable by PG in the presence of chloride.[88] When the distribution is investigated at physiological pH in the absence of chloride, Zaki[90] sees near total inhibition of anion transport; however, now the label is found almost exclusively on CH17, with some residual binding to CH35.[91] Furthermore, the total number of PG sites per band 3 is increased by about two arginines (total = 3).

There is another aspect of the PG reaction which needs to be very strongly emphasized. Bjerrum and co-workers[86] showed that cells which had been nearly completely inhibited by PG demonstrated apparent "half-of-the-sites" reactivity toward DIDS; that is, half of the monomers reacted with covalent DIDS while half did not, despite the fact that PG was exclusively bound to all copies of CH35 subdomains (the covalent DIDS site is on CH17). Once again, as we saw with the interactions present for para-IBS and phenylisothiocyanate, we get the distinct impression here that intramonomeric interactions are present (if steric effects can be ruled out).[105] At the same time there must also be some type of intermonomeric interactions, since only half of the copies of the CH17 subdomains are reactive.

In summary, we see that at low chloride and pH 10, where transport is almost totally, but not entirely inhibited, PG is found almost exclusively on CH35 and that there is one arginine involved. At pH 7.4, also at low chloride, there is by contrast, almost three times more labeling of CH17 than CH35 and transport is also nearly totally inhibited. At low chloride and pH 10, where CH35 is labeled, DNDS is protective, while at physiological chloride and at either pH 10 or 7.4, it has absolutely no protective effect towards the PG reaction. What we do not know is what happens to CH17 labeling at physiological pH and increasing chloride. Increasing chloride at physiological pH partially protects the system from PG binding. This may be occurring exclusively at CH17. It is important to find this out because Wieth and co-workers[85] report that establishing a transmembrane chloride gradient, which should recruit a classic Ping-Pong site (see below), had absolutely no effect on the rate of PG binding to the CH35 arginine. Finally, PG shows another clear example of a nonstatistical distribution of label between monomers, since at the point where transport is nearly completely inhibited and PG sits exclusively on CH35, half of the monomers do not react covalently with DIDS at CH17, while the other half of the monomers react covalently.

4. Carboxyl Reactive Reagents

The pK of the acid branch of the titration curve suggests the involvement of an acidic group in the anion transport process. It may be worth recalling the discussion in Chapter 1, on the change in the DPG binding site in crocodile hemoglobin. Crocodile hemoglobin does not bind DPG, but rather has a high affinity for bicarbonate in the deoxy quaternary structure. The X-ray crystallographic work showed that the bicarbonate binds to a lysine residue and to a glutamic acid of one beta-chain. Thus, the involvement of glutamate at a bicarbonate site is expected. Indeed, the same genetic exonic material may code for the bicarbonate binding site on band 3. In any event, it is not surprising to see that reagents directed to carboxyl groups affect anion transport.[87,157,159,170-173]

EAC (1-ethyl-3-(4-azonia-4,4-dimethylpentyl)-carbodiimide) is a carbodiimide compound which inhibits anion transport. It is known to react with carboxyl groups of aspartic and glutamic residues. EAC is not permeant to the erythrocyte membrane. Interestingly, the irreversible inhibition of anion transport is 50:50 biphasic.[87,171] Even more interesting is the fact that at 50% EAC inhibition of transport (the first phase) DIDS is only able to bind to half of the monomers present in the system. Since DIDS inhibits the remainder of transport, those monomers must not have reacted with EAC. Keep in mind that there is no evidence suggesting 50:50 structural heterogeneity in the band 3 population. The biphasic response with EAC seems to offer classic evidence suggesting that band 3 can function as a "half-of-the-sites" reactive, allosteric, dimeric unit in agreement with the findings for PLP. It is interesting to note that Bjerrum[87] was able to show that CH35 was the reacted subdomain under his conditions. The significance of these results has not been strongly emphasized in the literature. They directly suggest that there is extreme negative cooperativity between band 3 monomers with respect to the EAC reaction. This is exactly what was seen in the reaction with PLP. In a recent study, Werner and Reithmeier[173] studied inhibition of a carbodiimide in the presence of citrate. The irreversible inhibition of phosphate transport involved citrate incorporation into CH17. DIDS and DNDS prevented citrate incorporation. Covalent and reversible stilbene binding was reduced.

Jennings and Anderson[172] have recently introduced the use of Woodward's reagent K in the study of band 3 structure and function. This reagent reacts with carboxyl groups. It inhibits anion transport on band 3 by reacting with carboxyl groups on both CH17 and CH35. Labeling of both fragments was found to be sensitive to DIDS covalent binding and DNDS reversible binding.[172] The kinetics of inhibition were not studied. Analysis of an acid hydrolysate of labeled, affinity-purified band 3 revealed that glutamate but not aspartate residues were reacted. This is a potentially important result in light of the participation of a glutamate in the binding of bicarbonate to the anion binding site of deoxy crocodile hemoglobin. Finally, we have already mentioned that this modification of glutamate residues at the exofacial surface changes both the pK at that surface and the internal pK on band 3. These effects were explained by a "thin barrier" model, but allosteric interpretations cannot be ruled out, and both interpretations may be valid.

5. Dipyridamole

Dipyridamole is a very large molecule which inhibits anion transport noncompetitively.[21] Recently, Renner and co-workers[174] presented an interesting series of experiments which strongly suggest that dipyridamole is an allosteric affector of band 3, apparently apart from any effect it may have on the lipid domain. The interesting finding is that dipyridamole is totally ineffective as an inhibitor in the absence of chloride, while with chloride (10 mM) present, this compound inhibits up to 95% of phosphate and sulfate transport. These effects could be related to similar effects of chloride on the observation of negative cooperativity in DBDS binding.[103] If dipyridamole cannot bind to the chloride-free conformation of band 3 but can bind to the chloride-bound form, we expect to see such reciprocal allosteric linkage effects. Dipyridamole changes the chloride inhibition constant from 40 mM in its absence to 0.5 mM, while the dipyridamole inhibition constant decreases from 100 μM with chloride absent to 3 μM at 10 mM chloride. The increasing chloride affinity for band 3 in the presence of a molecule like dipyridamole must reflect some major change in protein conformation. It will be interesting to try to identify such protein conformational changes to see if they extend to several distant locations on the porter.

VII. KINETIC EXPERIMENTS WHICH MAY BE MECHANISTICALLY DISCRIMINATING

A. INTRODUCTION

The demonstration of a possible linkage between the two porter subunits does not in itself suggest how such interactions may be used in a transport cycle. In Chapter 1 some overall transport cycles with emphasis on the classic single-site Ping-Pong model were discussed. There are several features of that model which can be tested because it is so simple. First, pure saturation kinetics are expected. If true saturation kinetics are not observed, the single transport site model does not have to be abandoned, but evidence which will discriminate between a simple and a more complex two-site molecular model must be presented. Second, while kinetic symmetry may or may not be observed in the system, mechanistic symmetry is expected with respect to each side of the membrane. By mechanistic symmetry we mean that the mechanism of anion transport must be exactly the same with respect to variation in anion concentration at each side of the membrane. All Ping-Pong models require this. The essence of the Ping-Pong mechanism is the release of substrate at one side of the membrane before the second substrate can bind. The same mechanism is proposed to occur at each membrane surface.

Kinetic symmetry or asymmetry are terms used to describe the actual values of the constants within the cycle as they influence kinetic measurements with respect to one or the other membrane surface. For example, K_m on the inside may be lower than K_m on the outside of the membrane. This difference is an example of kinetic asymmetry, since it can be explained simply by assigning different values to certain steps in the cycle. The basic mechanism of transport with respect to each membrane surface remains unchanged.

Another discriminating feature of transport systems is the idea that a site has (or sites have) alternating exclusive access to either bathing medium (in or out) as opposed to the other fundamental model where two sites face opposite directions and "move" simultaneously when both are loaded. Alternating access models include both the single-site Ping-Pong model and a class of models where two or more interacting sites "move" back and forth together across the membrane. It should be noted that there is a tendency in the band 3 literature to call any model which "moves back and forth" a Ping-Pong model. However, this is too loose a definition. The essence of a Ping-Pong model is not simply alternating access of sites, but rather the actual release of a substrate from a single site before the addition of a second substrate. This must occur at both membrane surfaces. Of course, the site at either membrane surface need not be the same physical site. There may be two sites, one on either side of the membrane, but they must be allosterically coupled such that when an ion is bound to one, the other is "turned off" (or has a ligand affinity out of the physiological range).

The idea of alternating conformations of the porter implies that sites should be recruitable either by the imposition of transmembrane substrate gradients or by the addition of impermeant inhibitors which act at the transport site. Addition of noncompetitive inhibitors would not be expected to initiate the recruitment event. Otherwise we end up with an "alternating modifier site" model, which is at least a contradiction in terms. Although such an effect can be rationalized by proposing global transport-related conformational changes in the protein, how do we distinguish between transport sites and sites which must be called allosterically linked sites, if ion binding to either affects the "orientation" and affinity of all sites?

Finally, by way of introduction to this section, attention is called to the discussion of kinetic tests of the Ping-Pong model which were mentioned in Chapter 1. The most important of these is the experiment in which anion-exchange velocity is measured with respect to variation in the anion concentration on one side of the membrane (usually the outer surface) at various constant *trans* anion concentrations. The Ping-Pong model predicts that the ratio of "V_{max}" to "K_m" should be constant at all *trans* substrate concentrations (see Chapter 1). That is, lines should be parallel in Lineweaver-Burk plots. A second, but less discriminating experiment is done to learn whether the transmembrane movement of one anion in half of a transport cycle is coupled to or uncoupled from the movement of a *trans* anion. Half-cycle experiments can only rule out one very special class of two-site model, one in which the sites face opposite sides of the membrane and both "turn" when they both become simultaneously loaded.

B. RECRUITMENT EXPERIMENTS

There are basically two kinds of recruitment studies which can be performed. An impermeant probe can be added to one side of the membrane, and its effects on the binding of substrate or of other probes to the other side of the membrane can be monitored. According to the Ping-Pong model, probes which bind to the transport site on one side of the membrane should prevent probes and substrate from binding to the porter on the other side. Alternatively, one can impose a transmembrane anion gradient and either look at the kinetic properties of substrate binding at the opposite side or study the ability of a probe to inhibit transport as compared to the condition where no gradient is imposed. Kinetic constants and probe-binding constants should be altered with the imposition of such gradients.

1. The Effect of Chemical Probes on *Trans* Substrate Binding

There are several examples of addition of chemical probes to the outside of the red cell having an effect on the interaction of substrate or other molecules with the cytoplasmic surface of the membrane.[59,110,175-178] Loading the inside of red cells with PLP reduces external H_2DIDS binding to band 3.[176] Internal APMB (which inhibits anion transport from the inside by some mechanism)[19] reduces the rate of dinitrophenylation of lysine "a" on CH17.[177] Grinstein and co-workers[178] used the fact that NAP-taurine seems to be a competitive inhibitor from the inside of the cell to see how external DIDS affects covalent binding of NAP-taurine at the inner surface. External DIDS reduced the binding of NAP-taurine to band 3, but it also reduced the binding of NAP-taurine to spectrin and other sites. This result raises an essential point that cannot be ignored in the interpretation of any of the data with chemical probes, especially covalent DIDS binding. Covalent reaction of DIDS produces major conformational changes in band 3 which definitely affect the way the protein interacts with hemoglobin[59] and cytoskeletal proteins.[179] The susceptibility to fluorescence quenching of certain cytoplasmic tryptophan residues on the cytoplasmic domain of band 3 is also altered.[175] This is the domain which binds cytosolic proteins and ankyrin (Chapter 4). As we saw above, transmembrane changes in pK occur with external modification of an exofacial carboxyl group.[159] Indeed, there is ample and compelling evidence for the occurrence of major structural changes of the porter upon addition of chemical probes.[180,181] It is interesting that Cacciola and co-workers[166] found that the morphology of red cells was significantly changed with para-IBS which reacts exclusively with CH17, while the noncharged arylisothiocyanates, which react with CH35, do not produce gross changes in erythrocyte shape. CH17 makes the connection to the water-soluble domain which provides one cytoskeletal anchorage site. The new results in Chapter 2 showing that transport site ligands change porter cross-linking patterns may imply that major conformational changes occur with ligand binding.

Since stilbene disulfonates interact directly or allosterically with both integral chymotryptic subdomains of band 3, how can specific recruitment events be separated from global conformational changes? To date none of the chemical recruitment studies that we have read address this important issue. This is especially true of the chloride NMR studies which purport to have actually demonstrated "transport site" recruitment.[110] Falke and co-workers[110] were able to distinguish between internal and external chloride binding sites on the membrane. The authors' assertion that there are fewer transport sites facing out in sealed ghosts, vesicles, or intact cells is based on the fact that there are fewer DNDS-sensitive chloride binding sites in sealed vs. unsealed preparations. Internal chloride binding sites are thought to contribute to the NMR line broadening in the latter but not in the former preparation. This view would seem reasonable and consistent with current views about site "movement" if it were not for the fact that the total number of DNDS-insensitive sites also increases to about the same degree in unsealed vs. sealed preparations. The observation of fewer sites in sealed preparations does not mean they are facing in; it may simply mean that the DNDS-sensitive sites, like the so-called DNDS-insensitive sites, are more buried and inaccessible to chloride. Moreover, these results continue to force us to ask about the validity of site assignment in the chloride-NMR studies.

Addition of DNDS or para-NBS (*p*-nitrobenzenesulfonate) to the extracellular solution was thought to inhibit chloride binding to both inner and outer surfaces of the membrane.[110] The authors state that DNDS is not interacting with two anion binding sites because the monovalent anion para-NBS causes the same effect. Yet, they do not rule out the distinct possibility that para-NBS could interact with the two interacting anion binding sites on band 3. As was seen in the careful kinetic studies of Dix and co-workers,[103] there are clearly two strongly interacting binding sites involved. This was also readily apparent in the interactions of PLP and the arylisothiocyanates, which are not that different in overall structure from para-NBS. Although it is not surprising that DNDS only inhibits from the outer membrane surface, it is surprising that para-NBS also only inhibits from the outside.[110]

Falke and co-workers[110] use the same argument to assert that the apparent simultaneous inhibition of outer and inner chloride binding by the exofacially acting agents is not due to an allosteric, or global conformational change since the inhibitor exhibits simple competition with the external substrate site. But the clear demonstration that DNDS produces a change in the global quaternary structure of band 3 has since been demonstrated (Chapter 2). Transport site ligands change the quaternary structure of band 3, and to assume they do not is invalid.

2. The Effect of Gradients on Probe Binding

If a chloride gradient is imposed across the membrane and if the single-site Ping-Pong model is used, then it has been shown[149] that a change in the ratio of inside facing to outside facing unloaded forms of the carrier will occur. The ratio of chloride in to chloride out is inversely proportional to the ratio of unloaded-inward to unloaded-outward forms ($Cl_i/Cl_o = E_o/E_i$). With an externally directed chloride gradient, there will be more outwardly facing sites and this change can be measured by studying K_i values for inhibitor binding. With more E_o forms, there will be more reactivity towards competitive inhibitors, and the inhibitory potency will actually increase. Knauf and co-workers have investigated the effect of gradients on the inhibitory potency of H_2DIDS,[182,183] NAP-taurine,[184] and niflumic acid.[185] Every one of these inhibitors, regardless of its mechanism of inhibition, shows stronger inhibitory potency when an outwardly directed chloride gradient is imposed. Salhany and Rauenbuehler[33] found a similar effect for reversible inhibition of dithionite transport by SITS consequent to the imposition of an external sulfate gradient. This effect once again questions the validity of making functional site assignments in an allosteric multisite protein like band 3. How can apparently competitive and truly noncompetitive inhibitors both respond to the extracellular gradient in the same way? Such a response is not consistent with the basic definition of a noncompetitive modifier site.

If both competitive and noncompetitive inhibitors are similarly affected by the conformation of the transporter, then addition of a noncompetitive inhibitor like NAP-taurine or niflumic acid or flufenamate should also affect substrate binding to the "transport site" on the other side of the membrane. We have not seen a direct test of this. However, addition of BS^3 to the DNDS binding site or addition of either DNDS or NAP-taurine seems to eliminate substrate inhibition. If the DNDS site is the external transport site, then we have the unusual situation that ligation of the external transport site has not only recruited all transport sites to the outside, but also in effect "recruited" the *trans* modifier site. If global conformational changes are occurring, then we must reconsider Ping-Pong arguments for site recruitment in terms of multiple allosterically linked sites on the protein.

It seems very clear from the kinetic studies of Dix and co-workers with chloride,[103] the findings of Salhany and co-workers with PLP,[122,128] and the additional studies cited above showing half-site reactivity, that more than one substrate binding site exists. One of these may be mutually exclusive with part of the stilbene-disulfonate site. There are intermonomeric allosteric interactions between the subdomains for interactions of small probes of the transport site, while stilbene disulfonates seem to uncouple those interactions under certain conditions.

C. ASYMMETRY

There are many examples of structural asymmetries in the red cell membrane. The very placement of the band 3 protein is the best example. Half of its mass is integral and half is water soluble and cytosolic. It is not surprising that this gross structural asymmetry extends to the level where kinetic constants for the transport process are also asymmetric. Asymmetries exist in transport kinetic constants, with exterior K_m values being smaller than interior values.[32,186] At equal chloride concentrations on both sides of the membrane, the Ping-Pong model would predict that there are 15 times as many inward-facing as outward-facing unloaded forms. The tighter binding of the substrate at the outside moves more sites in. The action of probes also reflects membrane asymmetry. Most of the important stilbene-disulfonate inhibitors which work at the outer surface have absolutely no effect at the inner surface. It is often suggested that the unusually large size of these molecules may be the reason. Yet, para-NBS also does not inhibit from the inner surface.[110]

In its simplest version, the Ping-Pong model is a mechanistically and kinetically symmetrical model. However, there is no obligation for kinetic symmetry. As pointed out, kinetic asymmetry simply means that the values of the various constants are not the same at comparable segments of the cycle. The source of the asymmetry has been investigated, and it seems to depend on the type of anion used. In the case of iodide, most of the asymmetry arises from different affinities of the two unloaded forms.[187] For chloride, on the other hand, the asymmetry seems to be due to differences in the intrinsic transport rate constants across the membrane, since, in experiments with niflumic acid, there was no difference in apparent chloride binding to either inward- or outward-facing forms.[185] Furthermore, there is evidence that the system is much more asymmetric at 38°C than at 0°C.[187,188] Keep in mind that many of these conclusions depend on several assumptions which in turn depend on the model used.

There are actually very few papers in the literature which have carefully compared the transport properties of the outside of the membrane with those of the inside. Few probes actually inhibit at both membrane surfaces. This comparison is important since it may offer a further test for the single-site Ping-Pong model. Although the model can easily accommodate kinetic asymmetry, it cannot explain mechanistic asymmetry. Consider the data of Schnell and Besl[62] on sulfate self-exchange. Variation in the external or internal anion concentration at constant *trans* anion concentration shows completely different Lineweaver-Burk patterns (see Figures 6 and 7). Negative cooperativity is seen for the out-to-in direction, while hyperbolic curves are seen for the in-to-out direction. If these differences are accepted, they directly suggest that the actual mechanism of transport is different at the two membrane surfaces. This is not easily accommodated by a single-site Ping-Pong model where mechanistic symmetry is the essence of the model.

D. KINETIC "ACID TESTS" FOR TRANSPORT CYCLE MODELS
1. Transient Kinetic Evidence

It is often said that kinetics can only disprove a given model. Disproofs can be powerful and even indispensable in situations where there are few structural correlates available. One simple test of the simultaneous model (i.e., the model in which the carrier always has sites facing opposite directions) is to see if the inward and outward movements of anions are coupled. Jennings[189,190] and Eidelman and Cabantchik[191,192] have studied this problem using transient kinetic approaches. Jennings[189] reasoned that sites could be recruited by placing the fast-moving chloride ion on the inside of the cell and mixing with sulfate. He measured the uptake of labeled sulfate in cells equilibrated in the absence of chloride and in the presence of a chloride-sulfate mixture. In the former case, the uptake was monophasic and linear, while with chloride present two phases were observed, both of which were linear, according to Jennings.[189] The fast phase was associated with chloride exit and proton entrance. According to the Ping-Pong model, the *trans* acceleration is a result of the recruitment of sites from inward- to outward-facing forms by internal chloride. With more transporters available, sulfate (with a proton) can enter faster. However, it is now known that sulfate can be transported both with and without a proton.[140,141,193]

Since both processes showed linear time courses, it seems possible that what Jennings was observing was not site recruitment, but rather two saturable forms of the carrier, each of which is capable of sulfate transport. The fast-exchanging form of the carrier is stabilized by proton and chloride binding. This form can even be stabilized in the absence of chloride and at constant pH by dansylation of band 3 in the absence, but especially in the presence, of APMB.[144,145] In this structure, anions are all "treated" like monovalent anions, and the rate of divalent transport is increased by up to three orders of magnitude.

If the fast phase in Jennings' experiments is a fast-exchanging state of the protein, then the rapid efflux of an internal counter anion should also be seen. Although Jennings did show the concomitant rapid efflux of chloride, Eidelman and Cabantchik,[191,192] studying the transient kinetic release of NBD-taurine (N(2-aminoethylsulfonate)-7-nitrobenz-2-oxa-1,3-diazole) from red cells under similar conditions (chloride in sulfate out), noted a lag period in NBD-taurine efflux. Conversely, with sulfate in and chloride out, the authors observed an apparent exponential "burst" of NBD-taurine release. The lag period for NBD-taurine exit could mean that initially there are more sites facing out (i.e., fewer sites facing "in" initially). Under the same general conditions as in Jennings' study cited above, sulfate and proton went in rapidly, consistent with the idea that the sites are indeed facing out under these conditions. If Jennings' results could be explained by the existence of a mixture of fast-exchanging and slow-exchanging states, then it would seem that NBD-taurine should have moved out of the cell rapidly when chloride was inside. Eidelman and Cabantchik[192] showed that increasing the chloride in the external medium progressively "killed" the lag. The half saturation for the effect was about 2.3 mM in chloride. This number is about the same as the half-saturation value for the porter at the outer surface.[32] Finally, Eidelman and Cabantchik[192] showed that with chloride in and sulfate out, the DNDS binding constant was about 0.8 μM, while for sulfate in and chloride out the constant was 22 μM.

Jennings[190] studied chloride half-cycle efflux into chloride-free phosphate medium and found that efflux was independent of internal chloride over a range between 20 and 170 mM, with K_m less than 2 mM. This contrasts with the K_m for internal chloride which is greater than 50 mM.[32] Jennings argues that the low apparent K_m is a result of the fact that the transporter is limited by the influx of the slower extracellular phosphate anion of which the K_m is in this range and therefore, that chloride efflux is uncoupled from phosphate influx. He also found that the inhibitory potency of H_2DIDS was increased, a result consistent with the Ping-Pong idea of outward facing site(s). Finally, he attempted to count the number of anions released in the half cycle and found a number consistent with the number of copies of band 3 porter in the membrane.

If there was some ambiguity about the results with probes concerning transmembrane site(s) alternation, there seems to be less difficulty in accepting these transient kinetic data. However, the results only disprove that type of two-site model in which the two sites face opposite bathing solutions, and the carrier conformational change occurs only when both sites are filled. The results do not rule out all two-site models. For example, two sites could be moving back and forth together.

2. Steady State Kinetic Evidence

There is a common tendency to equate apparent transmembrane site alternation with a single-site "Ping-Pong" kinetic model. It is true that all membrane Ping-Pong mechanisms have transmembrane site alternation. It is not true that all transmembrane site alternation mechanisms are Ping-Pong mechanisms. Fröhlich and Gunn[22] have given a detailed mathematical analysis of the single-site Ping-Pong mechanism. It is clear from this analysis that besides transmembrane site alternation the Ping-Pong model requires that once the site is facing one or the other side, the ion is released before another can add. This mechanism must occur on both sides of the membrane. If a second ion binds to a linked site somewhere in the cycle, the mechanism is not Ping-Pong despite transmembrane site alternation.

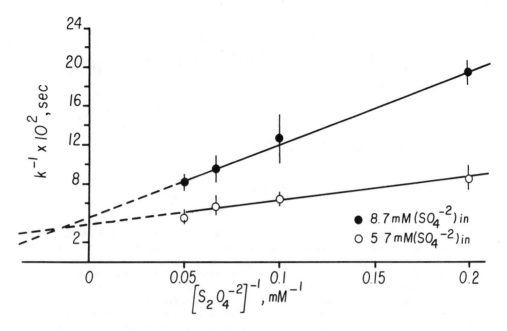

FIGURE 37. Dithionite-sulfate exchange kinetics at increasing *trans*-sulfate concentration. Temperature was 14°C. The two lines are not parallel. See original paper for experimental details. (From Salhany, J. M. and Rauenbuehler, P. B., *J. Biol. Chem.*, 258, 245, 1983. With permission.)

There is a kinetic experiment which can discriminate between Ping-Pong models and all other two-site models. It involves measuring anion saturation curves with respect to one side of the membrane at various constant *trans* anion concentrations. Intersecting lines in Lineweaver-Burk plots disprove the Ping-Pong mechanism. Parallel lines would support the mechanism.[22] This experiment has been performed by three groups. Gunn and Fröhlich (for chloride),[32] Salhany and Rauenbuehler (for dithionite-sulfate exchange),[33] and Hautmann and Schnell (for chloride).[34] The results of Gunn and Fröhlich[22] were scattered and difficult to interpret conclusively.[194] The same experimental question was approached using the spectrophotometrically based transport assay of Salhany and co-workers[58,59,63] and by Salhany and Rauenbuehler.[33] The results are shown in Figure 37. The authors measured dithionite-sulfate exchange at two different *trans* sulfate concentrations which were well below the range where the internal modifier site could be a problem. Their results show intersecting Lineweaver-Burk plots. To be sure that they were measuring a band 3-specific effect, they also showed that the inhibitory potency of SITS was greater in the high than in the low *trans* sulfate cells by a factor of 10.[33]

For several years, there was not a clear resolution to the question as to whether the Lineweaver-Burk plots were parallel or intersecting. However, Hautmann and Schnell[34] have recently repeated the work of Gunn and Fröhlich[32] with chloride. Their results are shown in Figure 9. There seems to be little question that the Lineweaver-Burk plots are *not parallel*. This aspect of the data confirms the findings of Salhany and Rauenbuehler.[33]

On the basis of the results just presented, we see that the kinetic "acid test" for the single-site Ping-Pong model fails to support the model. Does this mean that the Ping-Pong model is wrong? No! It simply means that this type of experiment does not support the model. There may be several technical reasons why the lines are not parallel. Perhaps even more effort should be put into this type of experiment, until all workers agree whether the lines are or are not parallel. As it currently stands, the lines are not parallel, and this would suggest the involvement of two sites in the transport mechanism. Furthermore, a two-site model seems strongly supported by the kinetic studies of chloride-stilbene disulfonate competition reported by Dix and co-workers.[103]

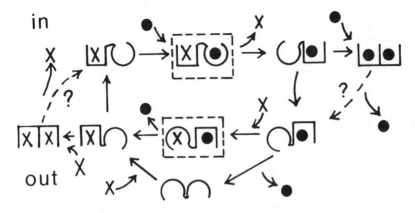

FIGURE 38.   Ordered sequential model for anion exchange by a band 3 dimer. In this model, each "site" is considered to be one band 3 monomer. The dashed box structure is shown to indicate the existence of some as-yet-unknown type of mechanism to distribute ligand between stable binary complexes at either membrane surface. Binary complexes are productive forms. A second type of productive form is the stable ternary complex. This form is populated at high anion concentration owing to the low affinity of the second monomer of the binary complex. The two monomers of the stable ternary complex are still considered to be conformationally coupled. The velocity through this low-affinity part of the cycle is considered to be slower than through the other productive part of the cycle involving binary complexes, and it can explain partial substrate inhibition.

VIII. WHAT IS THE ROLE OF SUBUNIT INTERACTIONS IN THE MECHANISM OF ANION TRANSPORT?

Allosteric coupling could serve to alternate the activity and affinity of each monomer so as to kinetically assist the binding and release of anions. At the membrane surface unstirred layer effects may be important. Providing a second low-affinity site for kinetic addition could facilitate the allosteric displacement of the bound anion. That is not to say that the bound anion could not dissociate or that there was not a dynamic and rapid equilibrium between bound and free anions. Coupling could provide a means of catalyzing release. This coupled pathway may dominate under most conditions.

Two coupled monomers of a dimeric unit could assist the anion binding and release steps of one another through an ordered sequential mechanism like that shown in Figure 38. In this model each monomer of the dimer has a separate channel, and the ligand induced change in the conformation at one channel affects the conformation of the other monomer. There are several conformational states: one outside facing, one intermediate state (not shown) and one inside facing. Both binary and ternary complexes can assume intermediate states, but they are short lived. The intermediate state of the binary complexes connects the two transmembrane binary forms, while the intermediate form of the ternary complex connects two *cis* binary complexes. All of these intermediate forms are in dashed boxes because they are not considered to be significantly populated during transport.

It will be noted that there is only one form of the unloaded porter dimer shown with all sites facing out. The actual direction that the unloaded form faces is arbitrarily chosen, but the mechanism requires that only one such form exist. This placement should yield mechanistic asymmetry as was suggested in certain kinetic experiments discussed above. Furthermore, since there is only one unloaded coupled dimer, there is an obligation to proceed through the transient ternary complex at the inner surface. This mechanistic obligation will produce intersecting Lineweaver-Burk plots when transport is measured as a function of the internal anion. When it is measured as a function of external anion, complex patterns may be seen depending on concentration.

Although the effect of inhibitors is not shown in this model for the sake of simplicity in presentation, transportable, coupled affinity probes such as PLP would trap the porter in one of the binary complexes of the cycle at half saturation. On the other hand, uncouplers would completely change the mechanism and allow each monomer to exchange anions independently. Assignment of the different structures implied by the BS^3 cross-linking patterns discussed in Chapter 2 to various states of the transport cycle is difficult at present since both PLP-half-labeled and DNDS-bound band 3 are cross-linkable to tetramers. It could be that the TC-state is a liganded quaternary state of the cycle, with the stilbene-bound substate being an outside-facing species on the cycle (because it is impermeant) and the PLP-bound substate being an inward-facing species (or an other intermediate state) because it is transportable.

If there are two substates of a single liganded quaternary structure, then what is the dimer cross-linkable state (the DC-state) identified in Chapter 2? It may be the unliganded quaternary structure of a transport cycle. The major mechanistically discriminating issue then becomes whether there is one substate to the unliganded quaternary DC-state (as suggested in Figure 38) or whether there are two unliganded substates of that quaternary structure, as expected in the Ping-Pong cycle.

IX. CONCLUDING REMARKS

An allosteric point of view was given for data in the band 3 porter literature. The basis for this view follows from the structural evidence that the porter monomeric structure seems to depend on the existence of the stable dimer. Alone this does not prove that there will or must be functionally significant interactions between monomers. Yet, an objective look at the kinetics reveals almost "textbook" allosteric patterns. These patterns are not artifacts since they show several consistencies. For example, if negative cooperativity were an artifact of the use of divalents, why is it only seen at the outer membrane surface and not the inner surface? Why does the degree of cooperativity depend on reversible stilbene-disulfonate binding, with cooperativity totally lost with partial covalent labeling of band 3? These changes speak of band 3-specific effects. Covalent BS^3 modification, which does not seem to alter arginine residues at the active site, also causes the pattern for monovalent anions to change from complex to hyperbolic. If arginines are independently functional at the active sites, then BS^3 modification has altered or eliminated superimposed interaction energies between these active sites. They now function independently by an as-yet-undetermined mechanism. Furthermore, it certainly looks as if the band 3 porter pH dependence is not solely a titration of active-site amino acids. Rather, the pH titration curve can convert between two characteristic forms through a variety of protein modifications. One can even modify an outside group and change the pH dependency at the inner surface, although this was interpreted as "thin barriers" rather than transmembrane allosterism. Finally, and perhaps most convincingly, porter ligands have been directly shown to change the porter quaternary structure between two identifiable states. Most, if not all, of these findings fit very well with what we expect to occur in Singer's homotropic dimer or tetramer model with multiple interacting active sites, each independently capable of functioning to exchange anions but performing that function within the coupled native state of an oligomer *in situ* so as to facilitate (i.e., catalyze) anion movement through the cycle.

X. ADDENDUM

Since submission of this manuscript a very important paper has been published by Legrum and Passow[195] which largely supports many of the points raised in this chapter about the significance of the stilbene disulfonate binding site with respect to the transport site. They found that chloride promotes dipyridamole binding to the stilbene site and that in the absence of monovalent anions (but with divalent anions present), dipyridamole is a totally ineffective

REFERENCES

1. **Jardetzky, O.,** Simple allosteric model for membrane pumps, *Nature (London),* 211, 969, 1966.
2. **Singer, S. J.,** Thermodynamics, the structure of integral membrane proteins and transport, *J. Supramol. Struct.,* 6, 313, 1977.
3. **Segel, I. H.,** *Enzyme Kinetics,* John Wiley & Sons, New York, 1975.
4. **Wieth, J. O. and Brahm, J.,** Cellular anion transport, in *The Kidney: Physiology and Pathophysiology,* Seldin, D. W. and Giebisch, G., Eds., Raven Press, New York, 1985, 49.
5. **Lowe, A. G. and Lambert, A.,** Chloride-bicarbonate exchange and related transport processes, *Biochim. Biophys. Acta,* 694, 353, 1983.
6. **Hoffmann, E. K.,** Anion transport systems in the plasma membrane of vertebrate cells, *Biochim. Biophys. Acta,* 864, 1, 1986.
7. **Shennan, D. B. and Boyd, C. A. R.,** Ion transport by the placenta: a review of membrane transport systems, *Biochim. Biophys. Acta,* 906, 437, 1987.
8. **Jennings, M. L.,** Oligomeric structure and the anion transport function of human erythrocyte band 3 protein, *J. Membr. Biol.,* 80, 105, 1984.
9. **Brahm, J.,** The physiology of anion transport in red cells, *Prog. Hematol.,* 14, 1, 1986.
10. **Passow, H. and Wood, P. G.,** Current concepts of the mechanism of anion permeability, in *Drugs and Transport Processes,* Callingham, B. A., Ed., University Park Press, Baltimore, 1974, 149.
11. **Dalmark, M.,** Chloride in the human erythrocyte. Distribution and transport between cellular and extracellular fluids and structural features of the cell membrane, *Prog. Biophys. Mol. Biol.,* 35, 145, 1976.
12. **Cabantchik, Z. I., Knauf, P. A., and Rothstein, A.,** The anion transport system of the red blood cell. The role of membrane protein evaluated by the use of "probes", *Biochim. Biophys. Acta,* 515, 239, 1978.
13. **Knauf, P. A.,** Erythrocyte anion exchange and the band 3 protein: transport kinetics and molecular structure, *Curr. Top. Membr. Transp.,* 12, 249, 1979.
14. **Gunn, R. B.,** Transport of anions across red cell membranes, in *Membrane Transport in Biology,* Vol. 2, Giebisch, G., Tosteson, D. C., and Ussing, H. H., Eds., Springer-Verlag, New York, 1979, 59.
15. **Deuticke, B.,** Properties and structural basis of simple diffusion pathways in the erythrocyte membrane, *Rev. Physiol. Biochem. Pharmacol.,* 78, 1, 1977.
16. **Gunn, R. B.,** Co- and Counter-transport mechanisms in cell membranes, *Annu. Rev. Physiol.,* 42, 249, 1980.
17. **Macara, I. G. and Cantley, L. C.,** The structure and function of band 3, in *Cell Membranes. Methods and Reviews,* Vol. 1, Elson, E., Frazier, W., and Glaser, L., Eds., Plenum Press, New York, 1983, 41.
18. **Jennings, M. L.,** Kinetics and mechanism of anion transport in red blood cells, *Annu. Rev. Physiol.,* 47, 519, 1985.
19. **Passow, H.,** Molecular aspects of band 3 protein-mediated anion transport across the red blood cell membrane, *Rev. Physiol. Biochem. Pharmacol.,* 103, 61, 1986.
20. **Jay, D. and Cantley, L.,** Structural aspects of the red cell anion exchange protein, *Annu. Rev. Biochem.,* 55, 511, 1986.
21. **Knauf, P. A.,** Anion transport in erythrocytes, in *Physiology of Membrane Disorders,* 2nd ed., Andreoli, T. E., Hoffman, J. F., Fanestil, D. D., and Schultz, S. G., Eds., Plenum Press, New York, 1986, 191.
22. **Fröhlich, O. and Gunn, R. B.,** Erythrocyte anion transport: the kinetics of a single-site obligatory exchange system, *Biochim. Biophys. Acta,* 864, 169, 1986.
23. **Stein, W. D.,** *Transport and Diffusion across Cell Membranes,* Academic Press, New York, 1986, 325.
24. **Chappell, J. B. and Crofts, A. R.,** Ion transport and reversible volume changes of isolated mitochondria, in *Regulation of Metabolic Processes in Mitochondria,* Tager, J. M., Papa, S., Quagliariello, E., and Slater, E. C., Eds., Elsevier, Amsterdam, 1966, 293.
25. **Harris, E. J. and Pressman, B. C.,** Obligate cation exchanges in red cells, *Nature (London),* 216, 918, 1967.
26. **Pressman, B. C. and Heeb, M. J.,** Effect of ionophorous antibiotics on the permeability of erythrocyte ghosts, *Biophys. J.,* 11, 310a, 1971.
27. **Scarpa, A., Cecchetto, A., and Azzone, G. F.,** Permeability of erythrocytes to anions and the regulation of cell volume, *Nature (London),* 219, 529, 1968.
28. **Scarpa, A., Cecchetto, A., and Azzone, G. F.,** The mechanism of anion translocation and pH equilibration in erythrocytes, *Biochim. Biophys. Acta,* 219, 179, 1970.
29. **Hunter, M. J.,** A quantitative estimate of the non-exchange-restricted chloride permeability of the human red cell, *J. Physiol. (London),* 218, 49P, 1971.
30. **Hunter, M. J.,** Human erythrocyte anion permeabilities measured under conditions of net charge transfer, *J. Physiol. (London),* 268, 35, 1977.
31. **Brahm, J.,** Temperature-dependent changes of chloride transport kinetics in human red cells, *J. Gen. Physiol.,* 70, 283, 1977.

32. **Gunn, R. B. and Fröhlich, O.,** Asymmetry in the mechanism for anion exchange in human red blood cell membranes. Evidence for reciprocating sites that react with one transported anion at a time, *J. Gen. Physiol.,* 74, 351, 1979.

33. **Salhany, J. M. and Rauenbuehler, P. B.,** Kinetics and Mechanism of erythrocyte anion exchange, *J. Biol. Chem.,* 258, 245, 1983.

34. **Hautmann, E. K. and Schnell, K. F.,** Concentration dependence of the chloride selfexchange and homoexchange fluxes in human red cell ghosts, *Pfluegers Arch.,* 405, 193, 1985.

35. **Lassen, U. V., Pape, L., and Vestergaard-Bogind, B.,** Chloride conductance of the Amphiuma red cell membrane, *J. Membr. Biol.,* 39, 27, 1978.

36. **Hoffman, J. F. and Laris, P. C.,** Determination of membrane potentials in human and Amphiuma red blood cells by means of a fluorescent probe, *J. Physiol. (London),* 239, 519, 1974.

37. **Freedman, J. C. and Hoffman, J. F.,** Ionic and osmotic equilibrium of human red blood cells treated with nystatin, *J. Gen. Physiol.,* 74, 157, 1979.

38. **Knauf, P. A., Fuhrmann, G. F., Rothstein, S., and Rothstein, A.,** The relationship between anion exchange and net anion flow across the human red blood cell membrane, *J. Gen. Physiol.,* 69, 363, 1977.

39. **Kaplan, J. H., Pring, M., and Passow, H.,** Band-3 protein-mediated anion conductance of the red cell membrane, *FEBS Lett.,* 156, 175, 1983.

40. **Fröhlich, O., Leibson, C., and Gunn, R. B.,** Chloride net efflux from intact erythrocytes under slippage conditions. Evidence for a positive charge on the anion binding/transport site, *J. Gen. Physiol.,* 81, 127, 1983.

41. **Knauf, P. A., Law, F.-Y., and Marchant, P. J.,** Relationship of net chloride flow across the human erythrocyte membrane to the anion exchange mechanism, *J. Gen. Physiol.,* 81, 95, 1983.

42. **Falke, J. J. and Chan, S. I.,** Molecular mechanisms of band 3 inhibitors. I. Transport site inhibitors, *Biochemistry,* 25, 7888, 1986.

43. **Tosteson, D. C.,** Halide transport in red blood cells, *Acta Physiol. Scand.,* 46, 19, 1959.

44. **Fröhlich, O.,** Relative contributions of the slippage and tunneling mechanisms to anion net efflux from human erythrocytes, *J. Gen. Physiol.,* 84, 877, 1984.

45. **Fröhlich, O.,** How channel-like is a biological carrier. Studies with the erythrocyte anion transporter, *Biophys. J.,* 45, 93, 1984.

46. **Fröhlich, O.,** The "tunneling" mode of biological carrier-mediated transport, *J. Membr. Biol.,* 101, 189, 1988.

47. **Aronson, P. S.,** Kinetic properties of the plasma membrane Na^+-H^+ exchanger, *Annu. Rev. Physiol.,* 47, 545, 1985.

48. **Gottipaty, V. K. and Fröhlich, O.,** Effects of extracellular sulfonates on chloride net efflux, *Biophys. J.,* 53, 531a, 1988.

49. **Bardsley, W. G. and Childs, R. E.,** Sigmoid curves, non-linear double-reciprocal plots and allosterism, *Biochem. J.,* 149, 313, 1975.

50. **Bardsley, W. G., Leff, P., Kavanagh, J., and Waight, R. D.,** Deviations from Michaelis-Menten kinetics, *Biochem. J.,* 187, 739, 1980.

51. **Dalmark, M.,** Effects of halides and bicarbonate on chloride transport in human red blood cells, *J. Gen. Physiol.,* 67, 223, 1976.

52. **Gunn, R. B., Dalmark, M., Tosteson, D. C., and Wieth, J. O.,** Characteristics of chloride transport in human red blood cells, *J. Gen. Physiol.,* 61, 185, 1973.

53. **Cass, A. and Dalmark, M.,** Equilibrium dialysis of ions in nystatin-treated red cells, *Nature (London) New Biol.,* 244, 47, 1973.

54. **Schnell, K. F., Gerhardt, S., and Schöppe-Fredenburg, A.,** Kinetic characteristics of the sulfate selfexchange in human red blood cells and red blood cell ghosts, *J. Membr. Biol.,* 30, 319, 1977.

55. **Tanford, C.,** Simple model can explain self-inhibition of red cell anion exchange, *Biophys. J.,* 47, 15, 1985.

56. **Falke, J. J., Pace, R. J., and Chan, S. I.,** Chloride binding to the anion transport binding sites of band 3. A ^{35}Cl NMR study, *J. Biol. Chem.,* 259, 6472, 1984.

57. **Knauf, P. A. and Mann, N. A.,** Location of the chloride self-inhibitory site of the human erythrocyte anion exchange system, *Am. J. Physiol.,* 251, C1, 1986.

58. **Salhany, J. M. and Swanson, J. C.,** Kinetics of passive anion transport across the human erythrocyte membrane, *Biochemistry,* 17, 3354, 1978.

59. **Salhany, J. M., Cordes, K. A., and Gaines, E. D.,** Light-scattering measurements of hemoglobin binding to the erythrocyte membrane. Evidence for transmembrane effects related to a disulfonic stilbene binding to band 3, *Biochemistry,* 19, 1447, 1980.

60. **Salhany, J. M., Rauenbuehler, P. B., and Sloan, R. L.,** Alterations in pyridoxal 5′-phosphate inhibition of human erythrocyte anion transport associated with osmotic hemolysis and resealing, *J. Biol. Chem.,* 262, 15974, 1987.

61. **Shoemaker, D. G., Bender, C. A., and Gunn, R. B.,** Sodium-phosphate cotransport in human red blood cells. Kinetics and role in membrane metabolism, *J. Gen. Physiol.,* 92, 449, 1988.

62. **Schnell, K. F. and Besl, E.,** Concentration dependence of the unidirectional sulfate and phosphate flux in human red cell ghosts under selfexchange and under homoexchange conditions, *Pfluegers Arch.,* 402, 197, 1984.
63. **Salhany, J. M. and Gaines, E. D.,** Steady state kinetics of erythrocyte anion exchange. Evidence for site-site interactions, *J. Biol. Chem.,* 256, 11080, 1981.
64. **Salhany, J. M., Gaines, E. D., and Sullivan, R.,** Steady and transient state kinetics of erythrocyte anion exchange. Evidence for cooperativity in substrate and inhibitor binding suggesting site-site interactions within the band 3 protein dimer, *J. Supramol. Struct. Cell. Biochem. Suppl.,* 5, 125, 1981.
65. **Ku, C. P., Jennings, M. L., and Passow, H.,** A comparison of the inhibitory potency of reversibly acting inhibitors of anion transport on chloride and sulfate movements across the human red cell membrane, *Biochim. Biophys. Acta,* 553, 132, 1979.
66. **Barzilay, M., Ship, S., and Cabantchik, Z. I.,** Anion transport in red blood cells. I. Chemical properties of anion recognition sites as revealed by structure-activity relationships of aromatic sulfonic acids, *Membr. Biochem.,* 2, 227, 1979.
67. **Barzilay, M. and Cabantchik, Z. I.,** Anion transport in red blood cells. II. Kinetics of reversible inhibition by nitroaromatic sulfonic acids, *Membr. Biochem.,* 2, 255, 1979.
68. **Macara, I. G. and Cantley, L. C.,** Interactions between transport inhibitors at the anion binding sites of the band 3 dimer, *Biochemistry,* 20, 5095, 1981.
69. **Staros, J. V. and Kakkad, B. P.,** Cross-linking and chymotryptic digestion of the extracytoplasmic domain of the anion exchange channel in intact human erythrocytes, *J. Membr. Biol.,* 74, 247, 1983.
70. **Jennings, M. L. and Nicknish, J. S.,** Localization of a site of intermolecular cross-linking in human red blood cell band 3 protein, *J. Biol. Chem.,* 260, 5472, 1985.
71. **Jennings, M. L., Monaghan, R., Douglas, S. M., and Nicknish, J. S.,** Functions of extracellular lysine residues in the human erythrocyte anion transport protein, *J. Gen. Physiol.,* 86, 653, 1985.
72. **Passow, H.,** Effects of pronase on passive ion permeability of the human red blood cell, *J. Membr. Biol.,* 6, 233, 1971.
73. **Cabantchik, Z. I. and Rothstein, A.,** Membrane proteins related to anion permeability of human red blood cells. II. Effects of proteolytic enzymes on disulfonic stilbene sites of surface proteins, *J. Membr. Biol.,* 15, 227, 1974.
74. **Jennings, M. L. and Passow, H.,** Anion transport across the erythrocyte membrane, in situ proteolysis of band 3 protein, and cross-linking of proteolytic fragments by 4,4′-diisothiocyano dihydrostilbene-2,2′-disulfonate, *Biochim. Biophys. Acta,* 554, 498, 1979.
75. **Jennings, M. L. and Adams, M. F.,** Modification by papain of the structure and function of band 3, the erythrocyte anion transport protein, *Biochemistry,* 20, 7118, 1981.
76. **Grinstein, S., Ship, S., and Rothstein, A.,** Anion transport in relation to proteolytic dissection of band 3 protein, *Biochim. Biophys. Acta,* 507, 294, 1978.
77. **Cousin, J. L. and Motais, R.,** Inhibition of anion transport in the red blood cell by anionic amphiphilic compounds. I. Determination of the flufenamate-binding site by proteolytic dissection of the band 3 protein, *Biochim. Biophys. Acta,* 687, 147, 1982.
78. **Cousin, J. L. and Motais, R.,** Inhibition of anion transport in the red blood cell by anionic amphiphilic compounds. II. Chemical properties of the flufenamate-binding site on the band 3 protein, *Biochim. Biophys. Acta,* 687, 156, 1982.
79. **Falke, J. J., Kanes, K. J., and Chan, S. I.,** The minimal structure containing the band 3 anion transport site. A ^{35}Cl NMR study, *J. Biol. Chem.,* 260, 13294, 1985.
80. **Lepke, S. and Passow, H.,** Effects of incorporated trypsin on anion exchange and membrane proteins in human red blood cell ghosts, *Biochim. Biophys. Acta,* 455, 353, 1976.
81. **Garcia, A. M., Kopito, R., and Lodish, H. F.,** Expression of band 3 in Xenopus Laevis oocytes microinjected with in vitro prepared mRNA, *Biophys. J.,* 51, 567a, 1987.
82. **Jennings, M. L., Adams-Lackey, M., and Denney, G. H.,** Peptides of human erythrocyte band 3 protein produced by extracellular papain cleavage, *J. Biol. Chem.,* 259, 4652, 1984.
83. **Matsuyama, H., Kawano, Y., and Hamasaki, N.,** Anion transport activity in the human erythrocyte membrane modulated by proteolytic digestion of the 38,000-dalton fragment in band 3, *J. Biol. Chem.,* 258, 15376, 1983.
84. **Jennings, M. L.,** Reductive methylation of the two 4,4′-diisothiocyanodihydrostilbene-2,2′-disulfonate-binding lysine residues of band 3, the human erythrocyte anion transport protein, *J. Biol. Chem.,* 257, 7554, 1982.
85. **Wieth, J. O., Bjerrum, P. J., and Borders, C. L., Jr.,** Irreversible inactivation of red cell chloride exchange with phenylglyoxal, an arginine-specific reagent, *J. Gen. Physiol.,* 79, 283, 1982.
86. **Bjerrum, P. J., Wieth, J. O., and Borders, C. L., Jr.,** Selective phenylglyoxalation of functionally essential arginyl residues in the erythrocyte anion transport protein, *J. Gen. Physiol.,* 81, 453, 1983.

143

87. **Bjerrum, P. J.,** Identification and location of amino acid residues essential for anion transport in red cell membranes, in *Structure and Function of Membrane Proteins,* Quagliariello, E. and Palmieri, F., Eds., Elsevier, Amsterdam, 1983, 107.

88. **Zaki, L.,** Inhibition of anion transport across red blood cells with 1,2-cyclohexanedione, *Biochem. Biophys. Res. Commun.,* 99, 243, 1981.

89. **Zaki, L.,** The effect of arginine specific reagents on anion transport across red blood cells, in *Protides of the Biological Fluids,* 29th Colloq., 1981, Peeters, H., Ed., Pergamon Press, New York, 1982, 279.

90. **Zaki, L.,** Anion transport in red blood cells and arginine specific reagents. I. Effect of chloride and sulfate ions on phenylglyoxal sensitive sites in the red blood cell membrane, *Biochem. Biophys. Res. Commun.,* 110, 616, 1983.

91. **Zaki, L.,** Anion transport in red blood cells and arginine-specific reagents. The location of [^{14}C] phenylglyoxal binding sites in the anion transport protein in the membrane of human red cells, *FEBS Lett.,* 169, 234, 1984.

92. **Zaki, L. and Julien, T.,** Anion transport in red blood cells and arginine-specific reagents. Interaction between the substrate-binding site and the binding site of arginine-specific reagents, *Biochim. Biophys. Acta,* 818, 325, 1985.

93. **Julien, T. and Zaki, L.,** New evidence for the essential role of arginine residues in anion transport across the red blood cell membrane, *Biochim. Biophys. Acta,* 900, 169, 1987.

94. **Julien, T. and Zaki, L.,** Studies on inactivation of anion transport in human red blood cell membrane by reversibly and irreversibly acting arginine-specific reagents, *J. Membr. Biol.,* 102, 217, 1988.

95. **Takahashi, K.,** The reaction of phenylglyoxal with arginine residues in proteins, *J. Biol. Chem.,* 243, 6171, 1968.

96. **Fröhlich, O.,** The external anion binding site of the human erythrocyte anion transporter: DNDS binding and competition with chloride, *J. Membr. Biol.,* 65, 111, 1982.

97. **Kaufmann, E., Eberl, G., and Schnell, K. F.,** Characterization of the band 3 substrate site in human red cell ghosts by NDS-TEMPO, a disulfonatostilbene spin probe: the function of protons in NDS-TEMPO and substrate-anion binding in relation to anion transport, *J. Membr. Biol.,* 91, 129, 1986.

98. **Macara, I. G. and Cantley, L. C.,** Mechanism of anion exchange across the red cell membrane by band 3: interactions between stilbenedisulfonate and NAP-taurine binding sites, *Biochemistry,* 20, 5695, 1981.

99. **Rao, A., Martin, P., Reithmeier, R. A. F., and Cantley, L. C.,** Location of the stilbene disulfonate binding site of the human erythrocyte anion-exchange system by resonance energy transfer, *Biochemistry,* 18, 4505, 1979.

100. **Dix, J. A., Verkman, A. S., Solomon, A. K., and Cantley, L. C.,** Human erythrocyte anion exchange site characterized using a fluorescent probe, *Nature (London),* 282, 520, 1979.

101. **Schnell, K. F., Elbe, W., Käsbauer, J., and Kaufmann, E.,** Electron spin resonance studies on the inorganic-anion-transport system of the human red blood cell. Binding of a disulfonatostilbene spin label (NDS-TEMPO) and inhibition of anion transport, *Biochim. Biophys. Acta,* 732, 266, 1983.

102. **Verkman, A. S., Dix, J. A., and Solomon, A. K.,** Anion transport inhibitor binding to band 3 in red blood cell membranes, *J. Gen. Physiol.,* 81, 421, 1983.

103. **Dix, J. A., Verkman, A. S., and Solomon, A. K.,** Binding of chloride and a disulfonic stilbene transport inhibitor to red cell band 3, *J. Membr. Biol.,* 89, 211, 1986.

104. **Lieberman, D. M. and Reithmeier, R. A. F.,** Characterization of the stilbenedisulfonate binding site of the band 3 polypeptide of human erythrocyte membranes, *Biochemistry,* 22, 4028, 1983.

105. **Anjaneyulu, P. S. R., Beth, A. H., Sweetman, B. J., Faulkner, L. A., and Staros, J. V.,** Bis(sulfo-*N*-succinimidyl)[^{15}N, ^{2}H$_{16}$] Doxyl-2-spiro-4'-pimelate, a stable isotope-substituted, membrane-impermeant bifunctional spin label for studies of the dynamics of membrane proteins: application to the anion-exchange channel in intact human erythrocytes, *Biochemistry,* 27, 6844, 1988.

106. **Falke, J. J. and Chan, S. I.,** Molecular mechanisms of band 3 inhibitors. II. Channel blockers, *Biochemistry,* 25, 7895, 1986.

107. **Falke, J. J. and Chan, S. I.,** Molecular mechanisms of band 3 inhibitors. III. Translocation inhibitors, *Biochemistry,* 25, 7899, 1986.

108. **Falke, J. J. and Chan, S. I.,** Evidence that anion transport by band 3 proceeds via a ping-pong mechanism involving a single transport site. A ^{35}Cl NMR study, *J. Biol. Chem.,* 260, 9537, 1985.

109. **Shami, Y., Carver, J., Ship, S., and Rothstein, A.,** Inhibition of Cl$^-$ binding to anion transport protein of the red blood cell by DIDS (4,4'-diisothiocyano-2,2'-stilbene disulfonic acid) measured by [^{35}CL] NMR, *Biochem. Biophys. Res. Commun.,* 76, 429, 1977.

110. **Falke, J. J., Pace, R. J., and Chan, S. I.,** Direct observation of the transmembrane recruitment of band 3 transport sites by competitive inhibitors. A ^{35}Cl NMR study, *J. Biol. Chem.,* 259, 6481, 1984.

111. **Jacobs, M. H., Stewart, D. R., and Butler, M. K.,** Some effects of tannic acid on the cell surface, *Am. J. Med. Sci.,* 205, 154, 1943.

112. **Passow, H.,** Passive ion permeability of the erythrocyte membrane. An assessment of scope and limitations of the fixed charge hypothesis, *Prog. Biophys. Mol. Biol.,* 19, 424, 1969.

113. **Passow, H. and Schnell, K. F.,** Chemical modifiers of passive ion permeability of the erythrocyte membrane, *Experientia,* 25, 460, 1969.

114. **Knauf, P. A. and Rothstein, A.,** Chemical modification of membranes. I. Effects of sulfhydryl and amino reactive reagents on anion and cation permeability of the human red blood cell, *J. Gen. Physiol.,* 58, 190, 1971.

115. **Obaid, A. L., Rega, A. F., and Garrahan, P. J.,** The effect of maleic anhydride on the ionic permeability of red cells, *J. Membr. Biol.,* 9, 385, 1972.

116. **Maddy, A. H.,** A fluorescent label for the outer components of the plasma membrane, *Biochim. Biophys. Acta,* 88, 390, 1964.

117. **Cabantchik, Z. I. and Rothstein, A.,** Membrane proteins related to anion permeability of human red blood cells. I. Localization of disulfonic stilbene binding sites in proteins involved in permeation, *J. Membr. Biol.,* 15, 207, 1974.

118. **Steck, T. L.,** Cross-linking the major proteins of the isolated erythrocyte membrane, *J. Mol. Biol.,* 66, 295, 1972.

119. **Ship, S., Shami, Y., Breuer, W., and Rothstein, A.,** Synthesis of tritiated 4,4'-diisothiocyano-2,2'-stilbene disulfonic acid ([³H]DIDS) and its covalent reaction with sites related to anion transport in human red blood cells, *J. Membr. Biol.,* 33, 311, 1977.

120. **Lepke, S., Fasold, H., Pring, M., and Passow, H.,** A study of the relationship between inhibition of anion exchange and binding to the red blood cell membrane of 4,4'-diisothiocyano stilbene-2,2'-disulfonic acid (DIDS) and its dihydro derivative (H₂DIDS), *J. Membr. Biol.,* 29, 147, 1976.

121. **Kampmann, L., Lepke, S., Fasold, H., Fritzsch, G., and Passow, H.,** The kinetics of intramolecular cross-linking of the band 3 protein in the red blood cell membrane by 4,4'-diisothiocyano dihydrostilbene-2,2'-disulfonic acid (H₂DIDS), *J. Membr. Biol.,* 70, 199, 1982.

122. **Salhany, J. M., Rauenbuehler, P. B., and Sloan, R. L.,** .Characterization of pyridoxal 5'-phosphate affinity labeling of band 3 protein. Evidence for allosterically interacting transport inhibitory subdomains, *J. Biol. Chem.,* 262, 15965, 1987.

123. **Cabantchik, Z. I., Balshin, M., Breuer, W., Markus, H., and Rothstein, A.,** A comparison of intact human red blood cells and resealed and leaky ghosts with respect to their interactions with surface labeling agents and proteolytic enzymes, *Biochim. Biophys. Acta,* 382, 621, 1975.

124. **Cabantchik, Z. I., Balshin, M., Breuer, W., and Rothstein, A.,** Pyridoxal phosphate. An anionic probe for protein amino groups exposed on the outer and inner surfaces of intact human red blood cells, *J. Biol. Chem.,* 250, 5130, 1975.

125. **Nanri, H., Hamasaki, N., and Minakami, S.,** Affinity labeling of erythrocyte band 3 protein with pyridoxal 5-phosphate. Involvement of the 35,000-dalton fragment in anion transport, *J. Biol. Chem.,* 258, 5985, 1983.

126. **Salhany, J. M., Rauenbuehler, P. B., and Sloan, R. L.,** Evidence for multisite allosteric interactions on the band 3 monomer, *Biochem. Biophys. Res. Commun.,* 143, 959, 1987.

127. **Kawano, Y. and Hamasaki, N.,** Isolation of a 5,300-dalton peptide containing a pyridoxal phosphate binding site from the 38,000-dalton domain of band 3 of human erythrocyte membranes, *J. Biochem. (Tokyo),* 100, 191, 1986.

128. **Salhany, J. M., Rauenbuehler, P. B., and Sloan, R. L.,** Direct evidence for intermonomeric cooperativity in substrate binding to the band 3 dimer in intact red cells. A ligand distribution study, submitted.

129. **Kawano, Y., Okubo, K., Tokunaga, F., Miyata, T., Iwanaga, S., and Hamasaki, N.,** Localization of the pyridoxal phosphate binding site at the COOH-terminal region of erythrocyte band 3 protein, *J. Biol. Chem.,* 263, 8232, 1988.

130. **Dockham, P. A. and Vidaver, G. A.,** Comparison of human and pigeon erythrocyte membrane proteins by one- and two-dimensional gel electrophoresis, *Comp. Biochem. Physiol.,* 87B, 171, 1987.

131. **Dockham, P. A., Steinfeld, R. C., Stryker, C. J., Jones, S. W., and Vidaver, G. A.,** An isoelectric focusing procedure for erythrocyte membrane proteins and its use for two-dimensional electrophoresis, *Anal. Biochem.,* 153, 102, 1986.

132. **Cornish-Bowden, A. and Koshland, D. E., Jr.,** Diagnostic uses of the Hill (Logit and Nernst plots), *J. Mol. Biol.,* 95, 201, 1975.

133. **Cuppoletti, J., Goldinger, J., Kang, B., Jo, I., Berenski, C., and Jung, C. Y.,** Anion carrier in the human erythrocyte exists as a dimer, *J. Biol. Chem.,* 260, 15714, 1985.

134. **Verkman, A. S., Skorecki, K. L., Jung, C. Y., and Ausiello, D. A.,** Target molecular weights for red cell band 3 stilbene and mercurial binding sites, *Am. J. Physiol.,* 251, C541, 1986.

135. **Mond, R.,** Umkehr der Anionenpermeabilität der roten Blutkörperchen in eine elektive Durchlässigkeit für Kationen, *Pfluegers Arch. Gesamte Physiol. Menschen Tiere,* 217, 618, 1927.

136. **Rummel, W., Pfleger, K., and Seifen, E.,** Die pH-Abhangigkeit der Aufnahme und Abgabe von anorganischem Phosphat am Erythrocyten, *Biochem. Z.,* 330, 310, 1958.

137. **Schnell, K. F.,** On the mechanism of inhibition of the sulfate transfer across the human erythrocyte membrane, *Biochim. Biophys. Acta,* 282, 265, 1972.

138. **Funder, J. and Wieth, J. O.,** Chloride transport in human erythrocytes and ghosts: a quantitative comparison, *J. Physiol. (London),* 262, 679, 1976.

139. **Lepke, S. and Passow, H.,** Inverse effects of dansylation of red blood cell membrane on band 3 protein-mediated transport of sulphate and chloride, *J. Physiol. (London),* 328, 27, 1982.

140. **Milanick, M. A. and Gunn, R. B.,** Proton-sulfate co-transport. Mechanism of H⁺ and sulfate addition to the chloride transporter of human red blood cells, *J. Gen. Physiol.,* 79, 87, 1982.

141. **Milanick, M. A. and Gunn, R. B.,** Proton inhibition of chloride exchange: asynchrony of band 3 proton and anion transport sites, *Am. J. Physiol.,* 250, C955, 1986.

142. **Obaid, A. L. and Crandall, E. D.,** HCO₃⁻/Cl⁻ exchange across the human erythrocyte membrane: effects of pH and temperature, *J. Membr. Biol.,* 50, 23, 1979.

143. **Wieth, J. O. and Bjerrum, P. J.,** Titration of transport and modifier sites in the red cell anion transport system, *J. Gen. Physiol.,* 79, 253, 1982.

144. **Legrum, B., Fasold, H., and Passow, H.,** Enhancement of anion equilibrium exchange by dansylation of the red blood cell membrane, *Hoppe Seyler's Z. Physiol. Chem.,* 361, 1573, 1980.

145. **Berghout, A., Raida, M., Romano, L., and Passow, H.,** pH dependence of phosphate transport across the red blood cell membrane after modification by dansyl chloride, *Biochim. Biophys. Acta,* 815, 281, 1985.

146. **Wood, P. G. and Passow, H.,** Iodide transport in the human red blood cell, *Int. Congr. Physiol. Sci. Proc.,* 608, 1071, 1974.

147. **Gunn, R. B.,** A titratable carrier model for both mono- and di-valent anion transport in human red blood cells, in *Oxygen Affinity of Hemoglobin and Red Cell Acid Base Status,* Rorth, M. and Astrup, P., Eds., Munksgaard, Copenhagen, 1972, 823.

148. **Deuticke, B., Dierkesmann, R., and Bach, D.,** Neuere Studien zur Anionen-Permeabilität menschlicher Erythrocyten, in *1st Int. Symp. on Metabolism and Membrane Permeability of Erythrocytes and Thrombocytes,* Deutsch, E., Gerlach, E., and Moser, K., Eds., Georg Thieme Verlag, Stuttgart, 1968, 430.

149. **Dalmark, M.,** Chloride transport in human red cells, *J. Physiol. (London),* 250, 39, 1975.

150. **Labotka, R. J. and Omachi, A.,** The pH dependence of red cell membrane transport of titratable anions studied by NMR spectroscopy, *J. Biol. Chem.,* 263, 1166, 1988.

151. **Matsuyama, H., Kawano, Y., and Hamasaki, N.,** Involvement of a histidine residue in inorganic phosphate and phosphoenol-pyruvate transport across the human erythrocyte membrane, *J. Biochem. (Tokyo),* 99, 495, 1986.

152. **Hamasaki, N., Kawano, Y., and Inoue, H.,** The active center of transport for phosphoenolpyruvate and inorganic phosphate in the human erythrocyte membrane, *Biomed. Biochim. Acta,* 46, S51, 1987.

153. **Romano, L. and Passow, H.,** Characterization of anion transport system in trout red blood cell, *Am. J. Physiol.,* 246, C330, 1984.

154. **Jennings, M. L.,** Proton fluxes associated with erythrocyte membrane anion exchange, *J. Membr. Biol.,* 28, 187, 1976.

155. **Jennings, M. L.,** Characteristics of CO₂-independent pH equilibration in human red blood cells, *J. Membr. Biol.,* 40, 365, 1978.

156. **Passow, H.,** The molecular basis of ion discrimination in the erythrocyte membrane, in *The Molecular Basis of Membrane Function,* Tosteson, D. C., Ed., Prentice-Hall, Englewood Cliffs, NJ, 1969, 319.

157. **Wieth, J. O., Andersen, O. S., Brahm, J., Bjerrum, P. J., and Borders, C. L., Jr.,** Chloride-bicarbonate exchange in red blood cells: physiology of transport and chemical modification of binding sites, *Philos. Trans. R. Soc. London Ser. B,* 299, 383, 1982.

158. **Raida, M. and Passow, H.,** Enhancement of divalent anion transport across the human red blood cell membrane by the water-soluble dansyl chloride derivative 2-(*N*-piperidine) ethyl-amine-1-naphthyl-5-sulfonylchloride (PENS-Cl), *Biochim. Biophys. Acta,* 812, 624, 1985.

159. **Jennings, M. L. and Al-Rhaiyel, S.,** Modification of a carboxyl group that appears to cross the permeability barrier in the red blood cell anion transporter, *J. Gen. Physiol.,* 92, 161, 1988.

160. **Zaki, L., Fasold, H., Schuhmann, B., and Passow, H.,** Chemical modification of membrane proteins in relation to inhibition of anion exchange in human red blood cells, *J. Cell. Physiol.,* 86, 471, 1975.

161. **Ho, M. K. and Guidotti, G.,** A membrane protein from human erythrocytes involved in anion exchange, *J. Biol. Chem.,* 250, 675, 1975.

162. **Drickamer, L. K.,** Fragmentation of the 95,000-dalton transmembrane polypeptide in human erythrocyte membranes. Arrangement of the fragments in the lipid bilayer. *J. Biol. Chem.,* 251, 5115, 1976.

163. **Rakitzis, E. T., Gilligan, P. J., and Hoffman, J. F.,** Kinetic analysis of the inhibition of sulfate transport in human red blood cells by isothiocyanates, *J. Membr. Biol.,* 41, 101, 1978.

164. **Sigrist, H., Kempf, C., and Zahler, P.,** Interaction of phenylisothiocyanate with human erythrocyte band 3 protein. I. Covalent modification and inhibition of phosphate transport, *Biochim. Biophys. Acta,* 597, 137, 1980.

165. **Kempf, C., Brock, C., Sigrist, H., Tanner, M. J. A., and Zahler, P.,** Interaction of phenylisothiocyanate with human erythrocyte band 3 protein. II. Topology of phenylisothiocyanate binding sites and influence of *p*-sulfophenylisothiocyanate on phenylisothiocyanate modification, *Biochim. Biophys. Acta,* 641, 88, 1981.

166. **Cacciola, S. O., Sigrist, H., Reist, M., Cabantchik, Z. I., and Zahler, P.,** Functional evidence for distinct interaction of hydrophobic arylisothiocyanates with the erythrocyte anion transport protein, *J. Membr. Biol.,* 81, 139, 1984.

167. **Sigrist, H. and Zahler, P.,** Selective covalent modification of membrane components, in *The Enzymes of Biological Membranes,* Vol. 1, Martonosi, A. N., Ed., Plenum Press, New York, 1985, 333.

168. **Poensgen, J. and Passow, H.,** Action of 1-fluoro-2,4-dinitrobenzene on passive ion permeability of the human red blood cell, *J. Membr. Biol.,* 6, 210, 1971.

169. **Rudloff, V., Lepke, S., and Passow, H.,** Inhibition of anion transport across the red cell membrane by dinitrophenylation of a specific lysine residue at the H_2DIDS binding site of the band 3 protein, *FEBS Lett.,* 163, 14, 1983.

170. **Andersen, O. S., Bjerrum, P. J., Borders., C. L., Jr., Broda, T., and Wieth, J. O.,** Essential carboxyl groups in the anion exchange protein of human red blood cell membranes, *Biophys. J.,* 41, 164a, 1983.

171. **Craik, J. D. and Reithmeier, R. A. F.,** Reversible and irreversible inhibition of phosphate transport in human erythrocytes by a membrane impermeant carbodiimide, *J. Biol. Chem.,* 260, 2404, 1985.

172. **Jennings, M. L., and Anderson, M. P.,** Chemical modification and labeling of glutamate residues at the stilbene-disulfonate site of human red blood cell band 3 protein, *J. Biol. Chem.,* 262, 1691, 1987.

173. **Werner, P. K. and Reithmeier, R. A. F.,** The mechanisms of inhibition of anion exchange in human erythrocytes by 1-ethyl-3-[3-(trimethylammonio)propyl]carbodiimide, *Biochim. Biophys. Acta,* 942, 19, 1988.

174. **Renner, M., Dietl, M., and Schnell, K. F.,** Chloride mediated inhibition of the phosphate and the sulfate transport by dipyridamole in human erythrocyte ghosts, *FEBS Lett.,* 238, 77, 1988.

175. **Macara, I. G., Kuo, S., and Cantley, L. C.,** Evidence that inhibitors of anion exchange induce a transmembrane conformational change in band 3, *J. Biol. Chem.,* 258, 1785, 1983.

176. **Rothstein, A., Cabantchik, Z. I., and Knauf, P.,** Mechanism of anion transport in red blood cells: role of membrane proteins, *Fed. Proc.,* 35, 3, 1976.

177. **Passow, H., Fasold, H., Gärtner, E. M., Legrum, B., Ruffing, W., and Zaki, L.,** Anion transport across the red blood cell membrane and the conformation of the protein in band 3, *Ann. N.Y. Acad. Sci.,* 341, 361, 1980.

178. **Grinstein, S., McCulloch, L., and Rothstein, A.,** Transmembrane effects of irreversible inhibitors of anion transport in red blood cells. Evidence for mobile transport sites, *J. Gen. Physiol.,* 73, 493, 1979.

179. **Hsu, L. and Morrison, M.,** The interaction of human erythrocyte band 3 with cytoskeletal components, *Arch. Biochem. Biophys.,* 227, 31, 1983.

180. **Deuticke, B.,** Transformation and restoration of biconcave shape of human erythrocytes induced by amphiphilic agents and changes of ionic environment, *Biochim. Biophys. Acta,* 163, 494, 1968.

181. **Fujii, T., Sato, T., Tamura, A., Wakatsuki, M., and Kanaho, Y.,** Shape changes of human erythrocytes induced by various amphipathic drugs acting on the membrane of the intact cells, *Biochem. Pharmacol.,* 28, 613, 1979.

182. **Furuya, W., Tarshis, T., Law, F.-Y., and Knauf, P. A.,** Transmembrane effects of intracellular chloride on the inhibitory potency of extracellular H_2DIDS. Evidence for two conformations of the transport site of the human erythrocyte anion exchange protein, *J. Gen. Physiol.,* 83, 657, 1984.

183. **Knauf, P. A., Tarshis, T., Grinstein, S., and Furuya, W.,** Spontaneous and induced asymmetry of the human erythrocyte anion exchange system as detected by chemical probes, in *Membrane Transport in Erythrocytes,* Alfred Benzon Symp. 14, Lassen, U. V., Ussing, H. H., and Wieth, J. O., Eds., Munksgaard, Copenhagen, 1980, 389.

184. **Knauf, P. A., Law, F.-Y., Tarshis, T., and Furuya, W.,** Effects of the transport site conformation on the binding of external NAP-taurine to the human erythrocyte anion exchange system. Evidence for intrinsic asymmetry, *J. Gen. Physiol.,* 83, 683, 1984.

185. **Knauf, P. A. and Mann, N. A.,** Use of niflumic acid to determine the nature of the asymmetry of the human erythrocyte anion exchange system, *J. Gen. Physiol.,* 83, 703, 1984.

186. **Schnell, K. F., Besl, E., and Manz, A.,** Asymmetry of the chloride transport system in human erythrocyte ghosts, *Pfluegers Arch.,* 375, 87, 1978.

187. **Knauf, P. A., Brahm, J., Bjerrum, P., and Mann, N.,** Kinetic asymmetry of the human erythrocyte anion exchange system, in *8th School on Biophysics of Membrane Transport. School Proc.,* Poland, May 4—13, 1986, 158.

188. **Knauf, P. A. and Brahm, J.,** Asymmetry of the human red blood cell anion transport system at 38°C., *Biophys. J.,* 49, 579a, 1986.

189. **Jennings, M. L.,** Apparent "recruitment" of SO_4 transport sites by the Cl gradient across the human erythrocyte membrane, in *Membrane Transport in Erythrocytes, Alfred Benzon Symp. 14,* Lassen, U. V., Ussing, H. H., and Wieth, J. O., Eds., Munksgaard, Copenhagen, 1980, 450.

190. **Jennings, M. L.,** Stoichiometry of a half-turnover of band 3, the chloride transport protein of human erythrocytes, *J. Gen. Physiol.,* 79, 169, 1982.

191. **Eidelman, O. and Cabantchik, Z. I.,** The mechanism of anion transport across human red blood cell membranes as revealed with a fluorescent substrate. I. Kinetic properties of NBD-taurine transfer in symmetric conditions, *J. Membr. Biol.,* 71, 141, 1983.

192. **Eidelman, O. and Cabantchik, Z. I.,** The mechanism of anion transport across human red blood cell membranes as revealed with a fluorescent substrate. II. Kinetic properties of NBD-taurine transfer in asymmetric conditions, *J. Membr. Biol.,* 71, 149, 1983.

193. **Milanick, M. A. and Gunn, R. B.,** Proton-sulfate co-transport: external proton activation of sulfate influx into human red blood cells, *Am. J. Physiol.,* 247, C247, 1984.

194. **Gunn, R. B. and Fröhlich, O.,** Arguments in support of a single transport site on each anion transporter in human red cells, in *Chloride Transport in Biological Membranes,* Zadunaisky, J. A., Ed., Academic Press, New York, 1982, 33.

195. **Legrum, B. and Passow, H.,** Inhibition of inorganic anion transport across the human red blood cell membrane by chloride-dependent association of dipyridamole with a stilbene disulfonate binding site on the band 3 protein, *Biochim. Biophys. Acta,* 979, 193, 1989.

Chapter 4

CYTOSOLIC ASSOCIATIONS OF BAND 3 PROTEIN AND THE POTENTIAL FOR HETEROTROPIC ALLOSTERIC CONTROL OF ANION EXCHANGE

I. INTRODUCTION

To keep pace in a setting of severe exercise, band 3 anion exchange must be sufficiently fast to prevent any rate limitation from occurring in the evolution of CO_2 at the lung. Yet the papers discussed in Chapter 1 suggested that at least based on the measured exchange rate for oxygenated red cells, band 3 anion exchange may be too slow to provide sufficient CO_2 clearance from blood at the lung. A compensatory mechanism involving band 3 could exist to increase the rate of anion exchange during severe exercise. Compensatory mechanisms are commonplace in respiratory physiology. The discovery that 2,3-diphosphoglycerate (DPG) facilitates oxygen release from hemoglobin is a classic example.[1,2] A similar "fine-tuning" of the rate of anion exchange would require that band 3 be an allosteric porter with both homotropic and heterotropic interactions. The heterotropic effect should involve oxygen-linked hemoglobin binding to a cytosolic porter extension which could increase the rate of anion exchange at the two homotropic transport sites through a conformationally based connection. In this way the anion exchange rate could keep pace with the demands of exercise. The structure and function of band 3 would seem to favor heterotropic allosteric modulation of anion transport. Band 3 appears to function as a homotropic porter dimer, while fully half of its mass extends into the cytosol and forms a dimeric association with a neighboring monomer, cytoplasmic domain of band 3 (CDB3). The conformation of this dimeric extension seems poised to change in response to cytosolic interactions (Chapter 2).

In this chapter evidence will be presented that hemoglobin binds to the dimeric extension on human band 3 in an oxygen-linked fashion under conditions which closely approximate the physiological. We will show that the hemoglobin binding site and the anion transport sites are linked. Inhibitor binding to the transport domain of the porter alters hemoglobin binding to CDB3 while hemoglobin binding increases the rate of anion exchange, thus supporting the linkage hypothesis. Other functions for the cytosolic extension will also be discussed. One of these is the finding that glycolytic enzymes bind to the porter extension. Although binding inactivates glycolytic enzymes, persuasive circumstantial evidence is presented that the amino acid repeat at the enzyme binding site on band 3 (Chapter 2) may serve to bind two glycolytic enzymes. While the binary enzyme-band 3 complex may be catalytically inactive, we propose that a ternary 2-enzyme-band 3 complex may be catalytically active. Finally, this proposed "action" at the cytosolic extension of band 3 must be integrated with the structural role for the porter extension. Band 3 functions as a "docking site" for the cytoskeleton by providing a binding site for a connecting protein known as ankyrin (Chapter 2). The ankyrin-band 3 interaction is often viewed statically, which is not conducive to the dynamic purposes of transport control. Yet, (1) too few ankyrin molecules exist to form a stoichiometric complex with each band 3 monomer present, (2) new evidence exists showing that ankyrin-free band 3 can rapidly exchange with ankyrin-bound band 3, and (3) evidence discussed in Chapter 2 showed that transport site ligands can modulate the global quaternary structure of band 3. These facts all speak strongly in favor of the potential for heterotropic allosteric modulation of porter transport sites by agents which bind to the cytosolic extension of the porter.

II. CYTOSKELETAL ASSOCIATIONS

A. ANKYRIN
1. Introduction

Solubilization of the red cell membrane bilayer in a nonionic detergent reveals a network of proteins in a sub-bilayer array (Chapter 2). Attachment of this protein superstructure to the bilayer is essential to the maintenance of membrane integrity. Several groups of workers in a long series of studies[3-17] led most notably by Bennett and Stenbuck[10] and Branton and co-workers[14] showed that the spectrin component of the superstructure is attached to the cytoplasmic extension of band 3 through a connecting protein known as ankyrin (band 2.1) (Chapter 2). Band 3 participates in a high-affinity association with ankyrin under physiological conditions. The aspect of the interaction which seems relevant to a cytosolic modulation theory is lack of stoichiometry.[3] This raises two issues. The first is whether there might be an isoform of band 3 designed to uniquely interact with ankyrin. However, this possibility was disproven by Bennett.[16] The second issue concerns the mechanism of association.

2. Mode and Dynamics of the Band 3-Ankyrin Interaction

Several studies suggest that the predominant factor controlling rotational diffusion of integral membrane proteins is the association with other membrane proteins.[18,19] In unsealed ghosts, band 3 rotational diffusion can be resolved into two components with different degrees of mobility.[20] About 40% (4×10^5/cell) of the band 3 is immobile.[20] If this immobile component is connected to ankyrin, the stoichiometry would be consistent with an ankyrin linkage with 10^5 band 3 tetramers.[3] Cleavage of the cytosolic extension causes a substantial increase in the rapidly rotating component,[20] consistent with the severing of the connection of band 3 to the cytoskeleton. In support of this effect of the cytoskeletal connection, several authors have shown that addition of exogenous ankyrin and other cytoskeletal proteins to band 3 in reconstituted systems or to unsealed ghosts decreases translational and rotational diffusion.[21-26]

One model for these interactions which seems consistent with the data was proposed by Tsuji and Ohnishi[25] which they call the "cytoskeletal fence" model.[26] It has the following features: (1) ankyrin-bound band 3 which is associated to the cytoskeleton is translationally restricted; (2) ankyrin-free band 3 is not bound to the cytoskeleton, but these molecules are considered to be trapped in the superstructure, freely able to diffuse within boundaries defined by the spectrin tetramers of the network; (3) dissociation of the spectrin tetramers to dimers allows wider diffusional freedom.[26] Thus, polymerization states of spectrin can influence the long-range translational movement of ankyrin-free band 3 dimers. Tsuji and co-workers[26] conclude that the translationally immobile component is also rotationally immobile when cytoskeleton-bound.

If 40 to 60% of the band 3 is both directly and indirectly associated to ankyrin as an imobile band 3 tetramer while the remaining band 3 dimers are translationally and rotationally mobile, is there a rapid communion between these two states? Are the transport properties of the two states different in either gross or subtly discernible ways? The answer to the first question was recently given in a potentially important paper by Ueno and co-workers.[27] They studied the factors which influence the rate of exchange between ankyrin-free band 3 and ankyrin-bound band 3 in Triton X-100 "shells". The study involved labeling CDB3 with ^{125}I in intact cells using the lactoperoxidase method. The exchange between band 3 states at 37°C and physiological salt was remarkably fast ($t_{1/2} < 1$ min). The exchange process was inhibitable by addition of isolated CDB3, showing the specificity of the process. The questions which remain unresolved are do such rapid exchanges occur *in situ;* what factors modulate the rate of exchange and are the two states of band 3 functionally distinct.

3. Circumstantial Evidence That the Ankyrin-Band 3 Interactions May Be Modulatable and May Alter the Anion-Exchange Function

It is always difficult to extrapolate conclusions based on work with ghosts or detergent solutions, to the *in situ* condition. Still, the evidence discussed above gives a working hypothesis for further consideration. The picture suggests that band 3 has different association states within the membrane plane. The ankyrin-bound state consists of an immobile porter tetramer which does not rotate. The ankyrin-free porter rotates around an axis perpendicular to the membrane plane and undergoes translational movement nonspecifically restricted by the encumbrance of the underlying spectrin superstructure. However, these two states may be in relatively rapid exchange depending on, at least, temperature. This situation potentially lends itself to other types of modulation which may determine the equilibrium position between ankyrin-free and ankyrin-bound band 3 dimers.

Does ligation of band 3 with transport site ligands significantly shift the equilibrium between ankyrin-free and ankyrin-bound forms of band 3? It was seen in Chapter 2 that both PLP (pyridoxal 5'-phosphate) covalent binding and DNDS (4,4'-dinitrostilbene-2,2'-disulfonate) reversible binding convert the BS[3] (bis[sulfosuccinimidyl]suberate) cross-linking pattern from mostly dimer-cross-linkable to entirely tetramer-cross-linkable states. Other evidence suggesting that the cytosolic and transport domains of band 3 may be in communication was also discussed. Any of these changes could represent shifts between ankyrin-free and ankyrin-bound states.

Additional evidence that there is a band 3-mediated connection between the integral transport domain and the cytoskeleton is seen in the demonstration by Hsu and Morrison[28] that spectrin and ankyrin were less easily extractable from membranes isolated from 4,4'-diisothiocyanostilbene-2,2'-disulfonate (DIDS)-labeled red cells compared to control cells. Very recently, Mosior and co-workers[29] found that there is a significant increase in osmotic fragility with DIDS treatment. The change correlated with DIDS inhibition of anion transport, suggesting an involvement of band 3. This change was not related to changes in the water transport properties of the cell. The authors relate the increase in osmotic fragility to an alteration of the conformation of band 3. Later in this chapter, we will offer a possible unified model to explain these and the other DIDS-induced changes still to be discussed. It seems clear that the structure of band 3, because of its pivotal role in ankyrin binding, can have a widespread and major influence on the physical properties of the red cell.

In Chapter 2, the literature was discussed showing that band 3 can be phosphorylated at tyrosine 8 and perhaps at tyrosine 21 of the extreme N terminus of CDB3 (Figure 6 of Chapter 2). Phosphorylation of either ankyrin or band 3 may also influence the states of association and the transport function of the porter. Tao and co-workers[30] studied the effect of CDB3 phosphorylation on the association with ankyrin. Although band 3 phosphorylation did not affect ankyrin binding, ankyrin phosphorylation reduced the binding stoichiometry with CDB3.[30] One complex observed by Tao and co-workers[30] contained 2 mol of band 3 fragment per mole of ankyrin, while another had a binding stoichiometry of 0.5 mol of fragment per mole of ankyrin, yet the proportion of both complexes was reduced with phosphorylation of ankyrin. The phosphorylation sites on ankyrin are thought to be located in the spectrin binding domain[3] even though phosphorylation of ankyrin does not alter spectrin binding.[3] Rather it seems to alter the mode of binding to the cytoplasmic fragment of band 3.[30]

The interaction of ankyrin with band 3 and the role of phosphorylation in that interaction may have been clarified by the recent studies of Hall and Bennett[31] and Pontremoli and associates.[32] The latter authors had shown that activation of the calpain system resulted in an increase in the phosphorylation of band 3. Hall and Bennett[31] report that calpain releases a 20-kDa domain from ankyrin (band 2.1) leading to the formation of band 2.2 as a proteolytic product. Significantly, this domain of ankyrin is involved in the binding to band 3.[31,33-35]

If phosphorylation of ankyrin or the calpain activity effects the state of association with band 3, it becomes interesting to note work of Bursaux and co-workers[36] suggesting that phosphorylation of red cell membranes increases the rate of anion exchange. Since band 3 is the major phosphorylation site on the membrane (see Section VIII. A.2 of Chapter 2), it would be interesting if phosphorylation modulated different states of band 3-ankyrin associations which have significantly different transport properties. Some evidence with a mutant band 3 supports such a connection. Kay and co-workers[37] found a mutation of human band 3 with an insertion of between 2 and 4 kDa in the CH17 subdomain of the transport site. The cells showed faster anion transport, and there was evidence for lower ankyrin binding. The differences could be related to different states of band 3-ankyrin association.

B. BANDS 4.1 AND 4.2

Yu and Steck,[38] working with band 3 in Triton extracts, discovered its associations with band 4.2. The reason they did not detect the even stronger association with ankyrin is that the small fraction of band 3 which was tightly bound to ankyrin sedimented with the Triton shells upon centrifugation, while the bulk of the band 3 remained in the supernatant. There are about 200,000 copies of band 4.2 in the red cell (Chapter 2). Korsgren and Cohen[39] have presented electron microscopic studies showing that band 4.2 ranges in size from about 80 to 150 Å in diameter and hydrodynamic studies in which it behaves as a heterogeneous mixture. However there is also evidence that it exists as a tetramer.[40,41] Band 4.2 binds to the cytoplasmic domain of band 3 at a different site from that of ankyrin and can even bind with low affinity to ankyrin and band 4.1.[42] Band 4.2 is also associated with those band 3 molecules bound to ankyrin in Triton shells.[13,16,17] Yet, band 4.2 can be found in the component of band 3 present in the Triton supernate.[38,43] This apparent paradox may be explained by the studies of Ueno and co-workers,[27] which show that ankyrin-free band 3 and ankyrin-bound band 3 can rapidly exchange, depending on temperature. Perhaps the band 4.2-associated band 3 molecules seen in solution were all originally associated with ankyrin-bound band 3. This point has been discussed in the literature by Bennett,[16] who favors an exchange hypothesis, and by Lange and co-workers.[44] The rapid exchange between free and ankyrin-bound band 3 means that the observed differences may only be due to experimental conditions and to the factors which modulate the exchange. The work of Korsgren and Cohen[39,42] has nevertheless established the interaction of band 4.2 with the cytoplasmic domain of band 3 on the red cell membrane. Binding was eliminated by proteolytic removal of the cytoplasmic domain of band 3 or by the addition of isolated band 3 cytoplasmic fragment. Very recently, Rybicki and co-workers[45] have identified a patient with a deficiency in band 4.2 protein. They presented evidence suggesting that the patient's band 4.2 associates normally with the membrane, but that ion depletion leads to an excessive release of ankyrin. In normal cells virtually no ankyrin is released. The authors suggest that band 4.2 may play some role in stabilizing ankyrin binding to band 3. This seems to be a complex effect since band 4.2 was shown not to influence the binding of ankyrin to band 3 in reassociation studies.[14]

The band 4.1 molecule has a similar (slightly higher) molecular weight as compared with band 4.2 and is also present at about 200,000 copies per cell.[3] It is a bipolar, monomeric protein which mediates the interaction between spectrin and actin.[46-49] Band 4.1 is primarily attached to an integral periodic acid Schiff (PAS) staining protein (either glycophorin or glycoconnectin, Chapter 2). A weaker *in vitro* association with the cytoplasmic domain of band 3 has been proposed.[50] Pasternack and co-workers[50] showed that about 65% of band 4.1 was associated with band 3, while 35% was bound to a PAS-staining protein. However, since the PAS staining protein site has a higher affinity, it should bind band 4.1 preferentially.

C. SUMMARY

From the perspective of a heterotropic allosteric theory, it is significant that all copies of band 3 porter are not rigidly held. There is a population which has rotational freedom and some translational freedom within confines nonspecifically defined by the underlying spectrin network. Finally, there is at least the potential for an exchange between the ankyrin-bound and the ankyrin-free band 3 dimer. Transport-site ligands may alter the distribution of band 3 between states. Another factor which may affect that exchange is ankyrin phosphorylation.

Membrane phosphorylation affects anion transport and there is a mutant which has an altered transport function and interacts with ankyrin abnormally. This supports a connection between ankyrin binding and the anion-exchange rate function of band 3. What needs to be demonstrated is a clear difference in transport activity between ankyrin-free and ankyrin-bound band 3. Other factors which may shift the equilibrium between states need to be defined.

III. CYTOSOLIC ASSOCIATIONS : GENERAL CONSIDERATIONS

A. INTRODUCTION

The study of the red cell may be divided conceptually into four broad categories. They are hemoglobin, carbonic anhydrase, cell metabolism, and the membrane. For many years each of these systems was studied as if the others did not exist. Indeed, hemoglobin researchers were discarding membranes to prepare isolated hemoglobin while membrane molecular biologists were discarding hemoglobin, taking pains to prepare hemoglobin-free isolated ghosts for study.[51-58] This was the predominant approach until recently, when two major turning points were reached which necessitated a more integrated molecular view of the respiratory function of the red cell. The first was the demonstration by Benesch and Benesch[1] and by Chanutin and Curnish[2] that DPG is a regulator of hemoglobin function. This discovery connects red cell metabolism with hemoglobin oxygenation. The second turning point is coming into view only now. It involves the evidence that certain glycolytic enzymes and hemoglobin of the cytoplasm make specific protein-protein associations with band 3 porter.

Although the discussion of these associations will be largely confined to the specifics of the red blood cell, there is a more general context within which the interactions should be viewed. This has to do with the role of enzyme organization in cellular metabolic regulation.[59-70] Biochemists have been characterizing the structure and function of soluble enzymes and other proteins for many years, clarifying the relationships of structure and activity. This classic legacy does not provide knowledge as to how the various enzymes are assembled within the cell and whether systems which are functionally connected are, in fact, in spatial proximity. Furthermore, since membranes are selective barriers to solutes, it is reasonable to consider a possible link between solute transport and enzyme action on the transported solute if it is a substrate of the enzyme. Ligand-linked enzyme binding to integral membrane transport proteins may be involved in the regulation of substrate transport. For a general review of glycolytic enzyme associations and binding to cellular structures, the reader should consult the monograph by Friedrich.[71]

Some of the earliest evidence of glycolytic enzyme association with supramolecular structures came from work with the red cell membrane.[56,72-74] These studies appeared simultaneously with a very large literature on the association of hemoglobin with the red cell membrane.[51-56,75-79] Indeed, Bürker[80] first proposed as early as 1922 the idea that the hemoglobin of the red cell was "held by union with the membrane". Several studies followed showing that there was indeed a tight association of glyceraldehyde-3-phosphate dehydrogenase (G3PD) and other glycolytic enzymes with isolated red cell ghosts,[81-87] while other workers were demonstrating the ability of hemoglobin to reassociate with the membrane.[58,88-92]

B. GLYCOLYTIC ENZYME ASSOCIATION WITH THE RED CELL MEMBRANE
1. Introduction

The association of ankyrin with band 3 was determined under physiological conditions of ionic strength and pH, and therefore can be expected to exist *in situ*. By contrast, the association of glycolytic enzymes with cellular structures *in situ* is weaker and until recently, most reassociation studies have been performed under conditions of low ionic strength. Nevertheless, the interactions with cellular structures have been shown to involve specific sites of association with specific consequences of enzyme binding to activity.[71] The specificity of the various interactions continues to stimulate much discussion on the physiological relevance of these interactions.[67-70] One of the first exciting advances in this field was the demonstration in some laboratories that incorporation of labeled extracellular inorganic phosphate into ATP and other glycolytic intermediates was more rapid than the appearance of labeled intracellular phosphate. Such preferential incorporation of extracellular inorganic phosphate into the glycolytic pathway suggested a close proximity of G3PD to the membrane.[93-95] The idea of a connection between phosphate uptake and glycolysis was not immediately accepted;[96-98] but the effect was later confirmed by Niehaus and Hammerstedt[99] in both HeLa cells and erythrocytes at lower extracellular phosphate levels. Also, a compartmental kinetic analysis of inorganic phosphate uptake into red cells showed that it required a membrane-bound ATP synthesizing unit.[100] Shoemaker and co-workers[101] have recently suggested that there is no difference in the rate of incorporation of extracellular orthophosphate between the cytosolic pools of orthophosphate and nucleotide phosphate. Despite these controversies, it may be significant that Green and co-workers[74] and Schrier[72,102,103] and others[73,104] showed that G3PD and other glycolytic enzyme activities are associated with the isolated red cell membrane fraction.

2. Glyceraldehyde-3-Phosphate Dehydrogenase Binding to the Red Cell Membrane

With the development of modern methods in membrane molecular biology, the protein components of the isolated erythrocyte membrane were soon characterized (Chapter 2).[105] One of the Coomassie blue-staining protein bands found on SDS gels was identified as G3PD.[83,105,106] Several groups of workers then demonstrated that G3PD is a reversible binding membrane-associated protein,[84-86,107] while Yu and Steck[38] found it tightly associated with band 3 in the supernatant of Triton extracts of white ghosts. McDaniel and co-workers[86] observed the reassociation of G3PD with "stripped" membranes under a wide variety of conditions. They confirmed the earlier results of Kant and Steck84 concerning the general binding characteristics, except that under their conditions, biphasic Scatchard plots were obtained. Analysis of the plots revealed that 2×10^5 molecules of G3PD bind with high affinity ($K_d = 2.6 \ \mu M$) while 6×10^5 molecules bind with relatively lower affinity ($K_d = 9 \ \mu M$). McDaniel and co-workers[86] also showed the salt dependence of binding. The enzyme is only partially salt-elutable over the physiological range. It is interesting to note that the authors found that the binding characteristics of rabbit muscle G3PD, although qualitatively similar, were quantitatively different from human erythrocyte G3PD. This contrasts with the reassociation results of Yu and Steck[38] with rabbit muscle G3PD, where positive cooperativity in G3PD binding was noted. Although the pH values used in the two types of experiments were slightly different (7.5 vs. 8), it is not clear why one group finds negative cooperativity while the other group finds positive cooperative isotherms.

3. Aldolase Binding to the Red Cell Membrane

Aldolase was one of the first glycolytic enzymes found associated with the red cell membrane fraction in early studies.[56,72,74,81,82] Strapazon and Steck[108,109] studied the reassociation of both rabbit muscle aldolase[108] and human erythrocyte membrane aldolase[109] and found quite different binding isotherms. Those of the rabbit muscle form were biphasic, while those of the human erythrocyte version were hyperbolic. The differences suggest that the specific properties of glycolytic enzyme binding are, to a very large degree, the main factor determining the shape of the binding isotherm. Strapazon and Steck[109] showed the effect of ionic strength and metabolites on the binding of aldolase to the membrane. The effect of the various metabolites in eluting aldolase corresponded to their potency as substrates and competitive inhibitors of catalytic activity.[109]

4. Phosphofructokinase Binding to the Red Cell Membrane

Uyeda and co-workers[110,111] have extensively characterized the interaction of phosphofructokinase (PFK) with the red cell membrane. Their data on the reassociation of the enzyme showed some evidence for the existence of positive cooperativity. Like G3PD and aldolase, the binding was both pH and ionic strength dependent. Later Jenkins and co-workers[112] studied the reassociation of human PFK with inside-out vesicles and found the same association constant as Uyeda and co-workers,[111] but did not find evidence for positive cooperativity. They also showed that the order of potency in the ability of anions to displace PFK from the membrane was ADP > ATP > NADH > fructose-6-P > fructose $1,6-P_2$ > DPG > sulfate.

5. Other Membrane Associations of Glycolytic Enzymes

The inner surface of the red cell membrane is sufficiently heterogeneous, containing both charged lipids and proteins, to provide additional binding sites for proteins. Glycolytic enzyme binding can show biphasic Scatchard plots.[86,108] Complex binding isotherms can mean that there are multiple binding sites or that there are interactions in enzyme binding to several sites on a specific protein. Unfortunately, there is little evidence in the enzyme binding literature which might settle this issue. Since binding studies are performed at low ionic strength, why search for low-affinity binding sites under those conditions? Nevertheless, information of mechanistic or pathophysiological significance may still be uncovered. Some possible sites of membrane association aside from band 3 would be charged phospholipids and F-actin.

Michalak and co-workers[113] have recently demonstrated that G3PD can bind to phosphatidylinositol liposomes. The availability of phosphatidylinositol binding sites on the inner surface of the membrane was not studied. Although glycolytic enzymes may bind to other sites, there is evidence that chicken erythrocyte membranes do not bind G3PD and that this is due to the absence of acidic N-terminal residues on chicken band 3.[114] Unless there are also major differences in phospholipid and other integral membrane proteins, the absence of nonspecific G3PD binding to chicken membranes at low ionic strength and low pH suggests that such interactions do not occur with an intact membrane.

6. Functional Properties of Membrane-Associated Glycolytic Enzymes

Some of the earlier work on the association of glycolytic enzymes with the membrane fraction seemed to indicate that the membrane-bound form of the enzyme was active. Several studies on the activity of G3PD upon binding to phospholipid vesicles gave varying results, depending on the type of vesicle preparation used.[115,116] Addition of G3PD to erythrocyte membranes caused an increase in both V_{max} and K_m.[116] Eby and Kirtley[117] found that both the specific activity and the stability of human erythrocyte G3PD were increased by washing of the cell membranes. In more recent detailed studies it has been unequivocally established that the activity of the bound form of G3PD is completely inhibited.[107,118] Aldolase, like G3PD, also loses activity when bound to the membrane.[107,109]

PFK activity is functional both on and off of the red cell membrane, unlike the other glycolytic enzymes studied. PFK has traditionally been viewed as the regulatory enzyme in the glycolytic pathway. However, new nuclear magnetic resonance (NMR) studies have suggested that the glycolytic rate is controlled at a step in glycolysis above PFK.[119] The allosteric nature of PFK is evident in the sigmoidal dependence of its activity curve on the substrate fructose-6-P in the presence of ATP. Significantly, Karadsheh and Uyeda[110] found that in the presence of ATP and Mg^{2+} PFK binding to the erythrocyte membrane caused loss of the sigmoidal nature of the catalytic curve and led to an insensitivity toward ATP and DPG as if binding blocked those allosteric sites on the enzyme.

C. HEMOGLOBIN ASSOCIATION WITH THE RED CELL MEMBRANE
1. Introduction

There is approximately 5 mM hemoglobin tetramer present in the red blood cell. At this relatively enormous concentration compared with other cellular proteins, it would be surprising not to find some association of hemoglobin with the membrane. Difficulty in completely removing hemoglobin from membranes led Hanahan and co-workers[55,56] to better define the conditions necessary for the complete removal of membrane-associated hemoglobin. The authors systematically studied the pH and ionic strength dependence of hemoglobin removal, and because of this apparently weak association, suggested that it was nonspecific. Still, questions of the possible specific pathophysiological if not physiological association stimulated a continued interest in this subject.[58,76,88,89] Fischer and associates[88] published a study on the reassociation of various hemoglobins with hemoglobin-free red cell membranes. They clearly demonstrated the electrostatic nature of the interaction by studying the pH dependence and by showing that Hb A_2, which is more positively charged then Hb A, is more avidly bound to the membrane. Furthermore, the hemoglobin-free membranes had a large binding capacity, saturating at about 5×10^2 heme-bound membrane protein. This suggests the involvement of multiple membrane sites of association.

The inner surface phospholipid could account for the bulk of hemoglobin binding since it is the most abundant membrane component. There is a large literature to support the idea that such interactions do indeed occur at least in phospholipid liposome preparations.[120-126] Yet, the available evidence suggests that interactions with such artificial preparations cause irreversible denaturation of hemoglobin,[126] while the interaction of hemoglobin with the natural red cell membrane is fully structurally and functionally reversible under most routine conditions. In a recent study it was demonstrated that the presence of membrane cholesterol prevents hemoglobin intercalation into the lipid and subsequent denaturation.[127] Because the normal red cell membrane retains its cholesterol content when isolated,[104] hemoglobin penetration of the bilayer of unsealed ghosts seems unlikely.

2. Sites of Hemoglobin Association with the Red Cell Membrane

Titration of the salt-stripped (i.e., Hb- and G3PD-depleted) white, unsealed ghosts with oxyhemoglobin (oxyHb) in 5 mM phosphate buffer, pH6, reveals the presence of two distinct classes of sites.[128-130] The existence of two classes of sites was also demonstrated in hemoglobin binding kinetic studies.[131] There are about 1×10^6 high-affinity binding sites per ghost and between 4 and 6×10^6 low-affinity sites present. Hemoglobin binding to all sites is completely reversible over reasonable periods of time upon addition of high salt or upon raising the pH. Shaklai and co-workers[129] presented the first evidence for the possible involvement of band 3 as the high-affinity hemoglobin binding site. They showed that G3PD addition could displace hemoglobin from its association with that class of binding sites. Salhany and co-workers[130] extended this work by showing (1) that G3PD and hemoglobin showed competitive binding under affinity conditions; (2) that selective proteolysis of the inner surface sites (which removes the cytoplasmic aspect of band 3) significantly reduced the number of high affinity sites; and (3) that titration of the extracellular surface of band 3 with DIDS caused a reduction in hemoglobin binding. This reduction correlated with DIDS inhibition of anion transport (after subtracting a nonspecific DIDS site) and changed the mechanism of hemoglobin binding to the membrane inner surface. The DIDS effect is particularly important to our discussion and will be considered in detail later. It is interesting and also potentially important that the lowering of hemoglobin affinity by DIDS is opposite to the effect of DIDS on the extractability of spectrin and ankyrin.[28] The DIDS-induced decrease in extractability suggests tighter ankyrin binding to DIDS-bound band 3.

Direct evidence for a competition of hemoglobin for band 3 sites was given by Salhany and co-workers[130] using isolated CDB3. They showed that formation of a stoichiometric complex of oxyHb and CDB3 in solution altered the functional properties of hemoglobin in a manner identical to that seen earlier by Salhany and Shaklai[132] when they added hemoglobin to the high-affinity sites on isolated white ghosts. Another indication of the specificity of the interaction was the demonstration by Cordes and Salhany[133] that myoglobin only showed low affinity binding to unsealed ghosts under the low pH and ionic strength conditions where hemoglobin binding was tight and stoichiometric. In addition, phosphorylation of the tyrosines on CDB3 blocks hemoglobin and glycolytic enzyme binding under conditions of low pH and ionic strength, despite the incorporation of one or more additional negative charges into the protein.[134] There is clearly a specific interaction between hemoglobin and CDB3.

Rauenbuehler and his co-workers[135] have attempted to identify the low-affinity binding sites on the inner surface of the erythrocyte membrane. Proteolytically insensitive sites on the inner surface of the membrane were shown to account for about 25% of the sites, in agreement with the static titrations and the known number of band 3 protomers. Phospholipid cleavage released only about 38% of the bound hemoglobin. The authors demonstrated that the other approximately 40 to 60% of the low-affinity sites was located on the cytoplasmic portion of glycophorin. Glycophorin is known to have a very acidic but smaller cytoplasmic extension than band 3 (see Chapter 2). Titration of hemoglobin binding sites on rabbit red cell membranes showed fewer sites due to the lack of glycophorin.[135] Rauenbuehler and co-workers[135] also reconstituted human glycophorin into phospholipid liposomes and saw an increase in hemoglobin binding.

Other hemoglobin binding sites may exist on the membrane. It has been proposed that hemoglobin binds to spectrin.[136] However, Cassoly[137] was not able to demonstrate binding under his conditions. There may be a nonspecific effect of any protein, including cellular hemoglobin, on the self-association properties of spectrin, stabilizing it in the tetrameric form.[138] This effect of proteins on the state of spectrin association may explain the findings of Wiedenmann and Elbaum[139] of the effect of hemoglobin on the echinocyte-discocyte transition of ghosts and other effects. However, Cordes and Salhany[133] showed that under conditions of specific binding of hemoglobin or G3PD to band 3 (but not myoglobin), the ability of ghosts to decompose to inside-out vesicles after ion depletion was greatly reduced. Thus, specific protein binding to band 3 biases the factors involved in membrane vesicle formation toward the formation of right-side-out vesicles.

Another potentially important interaction of hemoglobin with the membrane which could have pathological significance is the specific interaction of deoxyhemoglobin with G-actin.[140] Although the actin of the cytoskeleton is in the F form, it is possible that deoxyhemoglobin, like DNase I[141] could bind to the pointed end of the short F-actin microfilaments of the red cell cytoskeleton.

It has been known for many years that divalent cations can have a profound effect on the binding of hemoglobin to the membrane,[55,82,88] some of which may be related to cation-stimulated resealing and trapping of hemoglobin.[104] As little as 10 μM calcium markedly increases Hb retention to ghosts.[82] Prasanna-Murthy and co-workers[142] have studied the effects of Mg^{2+} on hemoglobin and glycolytic enzyme binding to the isolated cytoplasmic domain of band 3. Their results indicate that although Mg^{2+} significantly reduces the binding of glycolytic enzymes, it has no effect on hemoglobin binding. Calcium was not studied. Eaton and co-workers[143] have confirmed the earlier work on the potentiation of hemoglobin binding by calcium and showed, in addition, that DIDS labeling of band 3 greatly reduces the calcium-mediated hemoglobin binding effect.

3. Functional Properties of Membrane-Bound Hemoglobin
a. Addition of Oxyhemoglobin

Salhany and Shaklai[132] measured the oxygen release and carbon monoxide (CO) binding properties of hemoglobin bound to salt-stripped unsealed ghosts under conditions in which the high-affinity site on band 3 was saturated. They performed CO binding studies under conditions where the rate of CO binding (after oxygen release) was rate limiting. The oxygenated form of hemoglobin almost always contains a significant fraction of alpha-beta dimer which reacts with CO about ten times faster than does the deoxyhemoglobin tetramer. The fraction of dimer present can be quite large in dilute hemoglobin solutions. Figure 1 shows the CO binding results

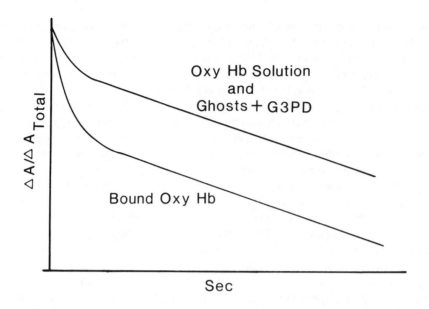

FIGURE 1.   Carbon monoxide (CO) binding to hemoglobin in solution (top curve) and bound to band 3 on unsealed red cell ghosts (lower curve). The top curve is also the condition where G3PD is added after formation of the hemoglobin-band 3 complex on the membrane. G3PD and hemoglobin compete for the same site with G3PD having a higher affinity. When hemoglobin is membrane bound, CO binding after rapidly removing oxygen shows a predominance of rapid reacting phase characteristic of membrane-bound hemoglobin dimers. Addition of G3PD displaces hemoglobin from band 3, and the time course is indistinguishable from that in solution. (Redrawn from Salhany, J. M. and Shaklai, N., *Biochemistry,* 18, 893, 1979. With permission.)

of Salhany and Shaklai.[132] Saturation of the band 3 high-affinity sites on the inner surface of the membrane led to a substantial increase in the fraction of fast-reacting, dimeric hemoglobin. Furthermore, addition of G3PD, which displaces hemoglobin from band 3, caused the amount of fast reacting form to revert back to that seen in solutions free of membranes under otherwise identical conditions. These results were interpreted as indicating that band 3 bound oxyhemoglobin is stabilized in the hemoglobin dimeric state. The authors also measured oxygen release rates of band 3-bound oxyhemoglobin and were able to demonstrate a 20-times slower rate of oxygen release from the beta-chain of bound oxyhemoglobin dimer. This was demonstrated by studying the wavelength dependence of the oxygen-CO replacement reaction.[144] The wavelength dependence is a consequence of a difference in the spectral-kinetic properties of the beta vs. the alpha-chain of hemoglobin.[144]

b. Deoxyhemoglobin

Unlike oxyhemoglobin, the tetramer to dimer dissociation constant for deoxyhemoglobin is such that there will be no dimer present under most solution conditions. Salhany and Shaklai[132] showed that deoxyhemoglobin could bind to the membrane and that there was no fast CO-reacting component present. This result, and those for oxyhemoglobin, indicates that there must be multiple modes of hemoglobin binding. Yet it was not possible to tell, in those studies, if there was a difference in affinity between oxy- and deoxyhemoglobin.

D. OTHER CYTOSOLIC ASSOCIATIONS WITH THE RED CELL MEMBRANE
1. Catalase

Catalase is an important red cell component which serves to rid the cell of hydrogen peroxide generated from superoxide production consequent to hemoglobin oxidation. Although catalase is predominantly a cytosolic protein, there have been reports of its association with the membrane.[145-148] Aviram and Shaklai[148] studied the reassociation of catalase with the red cell membrane and were able to demonstrate a specific interaction. There was a single class of sites (10^6 per ghost) with tight binding under the low ionic strength and pH conditions used. However, unlike the case of hemoglobin and the glycolytic enzymes, there was no change in the functional properties of membrane-bound catalase. Competition studies with proteins which bind to band 3 suggested that band 3 was the site of association.[148] The authors proposed that maintenance of catalytic activity for membrane-bound catalase may serve to protect the membrane lipids from daily oxidative stress if the enzyme is associated *in situ.*.

2. Association of Tyrosine Kinase with Band 3

In Chapter 2, the evidence that band 3 is variably phosphorylated was discussed. The phosphorylation sites are located on the cytoplasmic domain of band 3 at tyrosine 8, and perhaps at tyrosine 21 in the repeat sequence.[134] Protein phosphorylation of tyrosine residues within nucleated cells has been connected with the regulation of normal cell growth as well as with the onset of cell transformation. Thus band 3 phosphorylation may provide an experimentally approachable model system for this problem. In order for the cytoplasmic fragment of band 3 to be phosphorylated, tyrosine kinase must be located in close proximity and be able to bind to the cytoplasmic domain.

Habib-Mohamed and Steck[149] studied the topographic relationship of band 3 tyrosine kinase with the other proteins on the erythrocyte membrane. They found that band 3 tyrosine kinase was associated with the Triton X-100 insoluble membrane skeleton, but not with spectrin or actin. The kinase activity could be reversibly dissociated from the skeleton by elevation of the ionic strength. The membrane binding capacity for the kinase exceeded the native complement of the enzyme by a factor of 60, and inside-out, peripheral protein-depleted vesicles had a strong binding capacity for the enzyme. Addition of excess G3PD was found both to inhibit phosphorylation of tyrosine 8 on band 3 and to cause the release of the tyrosine kinase activity into solution. The isolated cytoplasmic fragment of band 3 was an equally good substrate for the enzyme and caused the release of the enzyme from Triton-extracted skeletons. Thus, erythrocyte tyrosine kinase may be viewed as being preferentially associated with the cytoplasmic end of those few band 3 molecules which remain tightly associated with the Triton-extracted cytoskeleton, although it can bind to and phosphorylate the remaining band 3 population just as well.

3. Hemichrome Binding to Band 3

Low and co-workers[150-154] have shown that the oxidative product of hemoglobin known as hemichrome binds tightly to band 3. This binding has been proposed to cause an in-plane co-polymerization of band 3-hemichrome complexes. The clumped band 3 is thought to be recognized at the outer surface as the IgG binding site, and this may be part of the cell aging process. The difference in the structure of hemichromes and hemoglobin is subtle. Hemichrome formation leads to increased dimerization of the protein. This form of the hemichrome seems not only to bind very tightly to band 3, but also to cross-link band 3 dimers to higher oligomeric states.[151]

The evidence that the complexes of band 3 and hemichrome actually form *in situ* and *in vivo* and contain IgG is now becoming fairly clear.[153-155] The sickle cell is a good model system in which to look for these complexes.[153,154] The complex is so stable that it can be isolated from solubilized, extracted vesicles under isotonic conditions.[154] It is remarkable that the complex contains not only band 3 and hemichrome, but also autologous IgG, glycophorins A and B, ankyrin, and bands 4.1 and 4.9. The fact that band 4.1 is included may be related to the age-dependent changes in the ratio of band 4.1a vs. band 4.1b, noted by Mueller and co-workers.[156]

Although the accumulating evidence favors hemichrome-induced band 3 clustering as an explanation of red cell aging, efforts to demonstrate clustering in high-density adult erythrocytes (i.e. "old cells") through electron-microscope studies have not been successful to date.[157] There is indirect evidence with bovine erythrocyte cross-linking which could be interpreted as supporting a clustering hypothesis.[158] Problems in identifying clusters may be related to membrane loss.

Owing to the apparently substantial change in band 3 structure with hemichrome binding, one may ask if there are major associated changes in the anion exchange rate. There is no clear answer to this question in the literature. There have been transport studies on old vs. young cells but with conflicting findings.[159-161] Considering that the mechanism of red cell aging is controversial,[162,163] direct evidence is needed concerning the effect of hemichrome binding to band 3 on the anion-exchange rate.

Lelkes and co-workers[164] have very recently published a paper which challenges the hemichrome-band 3 clumping hypothesis. They found a random distribution of band 3-intramembrane particles both over phenylhydrazine-induced, membrane-bound Heinz bodies and in the intervening areas in a freeze-fracture electron-microscopic study. This specific finding is at variance with the data published by Low and co-workers.[152] Lelkes and co-workers[164] also showed that acridine orange-induced band 3 aggregation was not prevented by preformation of membrane-bound Heinz bodies, further supporting the idea that there may be no significant interaction between the Heinz body and band 3 *in situ*. If the procedures used by the two groups are indeed identical, then this discrepancy needs to be resolved. If band 3 is not the site of Heinz body association, other candidates include the acidic phospholipids[120-127] or the acidic C terminus of glycophorin, which binds hemoglobin weakly.[135] Since rabbits[135] and certain humans[165] lack glycophorin, one may wonder if Heinz bodies can be attached to the membranes of those cells under physiological conditions.

4. Evidence for Direct Calcium Binding to Band 3

Because there is an ATP-driven pump in the red cell membrane, free intracellular calcium is kept very low. With age and in certain hemoglobinopathies, substantial concentrations of calcium accumulate. There is good evidence that calcium activates certain proteases to cleave band 3.[166,167] However, relatively little attention has been given to direct effects of calcium on band 3 structure and function. Direct calcium interactions with the amino-terminal end seem likely for several reasons. Addition of cytosolic, but not extracellular calcium causes a conformational change in band 3 such that a CH17 integral lysine becomes unreactive towards dinitrophenylation,[168] and there is also a potent, but partial inhibition of anion transport.[169]

The inhibition constant is about 3 μM, suggesting the involvement of a specific calcium binding site on band 3, rather than a non-specific interaction with lipid. It would seem very worthwhile to understand how calcium can exert such a potent inhibitory force from the inner surface.

One way to understand the effects of calcium is to know just where it is binding. Salhany and co-workers[211] have recently proposed that the N-terminal end of band 3 has a homology of charge comparable to loop regions of EF-hand segments of calcium binding proteins (unpublished observations). This is illustrated in Figure 2. Comparison of the sequence of human band 3, starting with amino acid 2, shows that negative charge exists at the putative calcium coordinate x, z, −x, and −z positions. The charge homology for band 3 compared to domain 3 of calmodulin and TN-C3 from rabbit muscle seems striking. Interestingly, tyrosine 8, the tyrosine which can be phosphorylated on band 3, is at coordination position-y. One hypothesis is that calcium binding to the acidic N terminus could lead to a conformational change in CDB3, dislodging the ankyrin connection and simultaneously attenuating anion transport. This could cause a significant osmotic effect. The result may well be calcium-mediated membrane exocytotic events. Preliminary experiments indicate that isolated CDB3 can specifically bind calcium.

	X		Y		Z		−Y		−X			−Z	
Domain 3 of Calmodulin	Asp	Lys	Asp	Gly	Asn	Gly	Tyr	Iso	Ser	Ala	Ala	Gly	Leu
TN-C3 (Rabbit Skel. Musc.)	Asp	Arg	Asn	Ala	Asp	Gly	Tyr	Iso	Asp	Ala	Glu	Gly	Leu
Human Band 3 (Starting at amino acid #2)	Glu	Glu	Leu	Gln	Asp	Asp	Tyr	Glu	Asp	Asp	Met	Glu	Glu
	2	3	4	5	6	7	8	9	10	11	12	13	14

FIGURE 2. Amino acid sequence of domain 3 of calmodulin, TN-C3 protein from rabbit skeletal muscle, and the first acidic segment of the 23 amino acid N-terminal repeat of human erythrocyte band 3 beginning at amino acid 2. Note the charge homology at the putative calcium coordinate sites x, y, z, −y, −x, and −z. All three proteins have a phosphorylatable tyrosine at the −y position. This charge homology suggests that the first repeat of the acidic N terminus of band 3 is a calcium binding site.

IV. MODE OF ASSOCIATION OF CYTOSOLIC PROTEINS WITH THE CYTOPLASMIC FRAGMENT OF BAND 3

A. DO GLYCOLYTIC ENZYMES FORM AN ACTIVE MULTIENZYME COMPLEX ON BAND 3?

Many of the experiments just described support the view that the glycolytic enzymes, especially G3PD, as well as hemoglobin, bind to a mutually exclusive site on the cytoplasmic surface of the membrane; and that site is believed to be band 3. However, there are some studies published which have suggested that enzyme and hemoglobin binding may not be completely mutually exclusive.[111,118,170-172] Higashi and co-workers[111] showed that PFK may bind to band 3, by demonstrating that aldolase and G3PD are competitive. However, they found that hemoglobin is not able to displace PFK and concluded that hemoglobin and PFK must be binding to different sites. Unfortunately, this conclusion may not be totally supportable since later work showed that hemoglobin,[142] aldolase,[171,172] G3PD,[118,173] and PFK[112] all bind to the acidic, first 23 amino acids of the N terminus of band 3. The reason aldolase and G3PD could prevent PFK binding while hemoglobin could not[111] is that the competition studies were performed at pH 7, where the enzymes bind tightly to band 3 but where low concentrations of oxyhemoglobin (like the conditions used by Higashi and co-workers[111]) bind weakly. Hemoglobin competition studies with PFK need to be performed under conditions where there is significant hemoglobin binding.

Although the protection studies of Higashi and co-workers[111] suggest a mutually exclusive binding site for PFK and the other glycolytic enzymes, stoichiometric replacement of bound PFK was only seen with aldolase. Very high levels of G3PD were required to release PFK despite the apparent sharing of the same site. Other questions about the location of the enzyme binding sites on the membrane have been raised.[170,172] Wilson and co-workers[170] showed that the membrane site for aldolase binding can be denatured with little effect on G3PD binding. This result may be related to the finding of Steck and co-workers[118,171] who showed that band 3 fragments containing residues 1 to 13, displace both aldolase and G3PD from the membrane, while a fragment containing residues 13 to 23 only displaces aldolase. Yet, one segment is nearly (but not exactly) a perfect repeat of the other (Figure 6 of Chapter 2).[174] If the 13 to 23 segment were the aldolase binding site and the 1 to 13 the G3PD binding site, then we might have an explanation for the results of Wilson and co-workers.[170] Such differences would explain why Higashi and co-workers[111] could not easily displace bound PFK with G3PD, while aldolase was

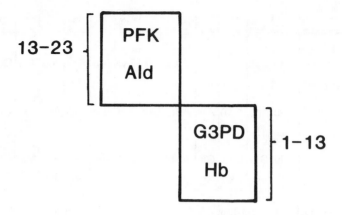

FIGURE 3. Protein binding site assignments on the two repeating subdomains of the acidic N terminus of human erythrocyte band 3. The first 13 amino acids are assigned as the binding sites for G3PD and hemoglobin, while the second series of amino acids are assigned to PFK and aldolase (ald). See text for further details.

found to be a good eluent. If PFK binds to the putative aldolase binding residues at 13 to 23, then aldolase, but not G3PD would be expected to displace PFK. Furthermore, even if favorable hemoglobin binding conditions were used, hemoglobin may still not be able to displace PFK if it binds to the G3PD site consisting of residues 1 to 13. Indeed, if aldolase and PFK are accepted as being mutually exclusive at residues 13 to 23, it then is quite interesting to note that Kirschner-Zilber and Shaklai[172] found that aldolase does not compete with hemoglobin for band 3 sites.[175]

The findings of Wilson and co-workers,[170] Steck and co-workers,[118,171] Prasanna-Murthy and co-workers,[142] Kirschner-Zilber and Shaklai,[172,175] and Higashi and co-workers[111] may be summarized by the schematic model given in Figure 3. The model indicates that the repeated segments of the N terminus of band 3 provide binding sites for two enzymes, or one enzyme and deoxy-hemoglobin. The structural difference between the two segments is subtle, and the various enzymes may be forced onto one or the other segment, but this is not the natural order according to the model. The idea of multiple enzyme binding to band 3 dimers (or tetramers) is important since many of the theories on these interactions involve multienzyme complexes.[71] Furthermore, although binding of a given glycolytic enzyme may turn off substrate catalysis, there is no clear evidence as to whether binding of a second type of enzyme to one subdomain might "restart" catalysis of the first enzyme bound to the other subdomain (even though it is still bound as a ternary band 3-double enzyme complex). Deoxyhemoglobin binding may perform a similar function, and this would further link glycolysis to the oxygen transport function of the cell. These views are certainly speculative. Yet, the competition studies quoted above inevitably lead to such speculations. In this regard, it may be very misleading to perform competitive binding studies based on enzyme activity alone. Direct experimental tests of the model in Figure 3 seem possible.

If there are two classes of enzyme binding sites formed by the amino acid repeat at the N terminus of band 3, then the mode of glycolytic enzyme binding should reflect such complex interactions. Jenkins and co-workers[112] studied the activity of PFK and its binding to inside-out vesicles. They observed strictly hyperbolic binding but also noticed a slow inactivation of the enzyme with time. It will be recalled that the earlier studies with this enzyme suggested that band 3 was binding to the allosteric site since sigmoidal behavior in catalysis was lost despite the presence of ATP.[110] The loss of PFK activity has been attributed to the dissociation to dimers of PFK on band 3.[112] Jenkins and co-workers[112] show the time course of inactivation when PFK is bound to inside-out vesicles or to the 23-kDa proteolytic subdomain of the cytoplasmic fragment of band 3. The dimerization of PFK on band 3 strongly resembles what happens to hemoglobin when it binds to band 3 in the oxygenated form.[132] Perhaps dimerization reflects the presence of two binding sites on the repeat sequence. To test this, one needs to see if the first 11 amino acids of the repeat do not cause dimerization in contrast to a 23-amino acid peptide where dimerization should be observed.

Aldolase activity is nearly completely inhibited by binding to band 3.[171] The near total inhibition of enzyme activity is remarkable since the enzyme has four identical, catalytically active subunits, yet it binds to band 3 with a 1:1 tetramer-to-band 3 monomer stoichiometry.[171] This result does not support a simple competitive model for inhibition of enzyme activity. Careful inspection of the inhibition patterns by Steck and co-workers[171] demonstrated that complete inhibition was never achieved, even at saturating concentrations of band 3. The authors surmised that although band 3 and the substrate of aldolase can displace each other from the enzyme, a partially catalytically active ternary complex of band 3, substrate and enzyme must form.[171] It would appear that the binding of a single band 3 to one subunit of aldolase reduces the affinity of the remaining subunits for substrate, suggesting strong negative cooperativity. If aldolase participates in a glycolytic enzyme complex on the cytoplasmic domain of band 3, the ability of the unbound subunits to react with substrate may be important to the mechanism by which substrate fluxes can reactivate the enzyme and/or release it from band 3.

When G3PD is bound to the cytoplasmic fragment of band 3, its catalytic activity, unlike that of aldolase, seems to be totally inhibited.[118,173] Although the catalytic activity of membrane-bound G3PD is hyperbolically inhibited, the isolated 23-kDa subdomain inhibits activity completely but with a slight sigmoid dependence.[118] This behavior suggests that multiple band 3 fragments bind to the enzyme with positive cooperative interactions between subunits. It is curious that while the 23-kDa subdomain can inhibit enzyme activity as completely as was seen for the membrane bound enzyme, its ability to elute the enzyme from the membrane was 30-fold lower than band 3.[118]

In summary, we have seen that there may, indeed, be two classes of enzyme binding sites at the acidic N terminus of band 3, due to the repeated sequence (Chapter 2). This could allow formation of at least ternary complexes which may have different catalytic properties compared to systems in which enzymes add singularly to CDB3. Inhibition studies suggest that the bound enzymes are usually allosterically inhibited, which would favor the hypothetical restoration of that activity with ternary complex formation suggested above. However, if active multienzyme complexes do not form on the cytoplasmic N terminus of band 3, then other hypotheses for a functional role of enzyme binding are needed. The central fact to consider is that the addition of single enzymes to band 3 has been found to inactivate them. The loss of activity is associated with stable enzyme structures, and binding to band 3 may be a mechanism of enzyme storage.[65] Another possibility is that substrate control of the concentration of active enzyme forms may allow rapid establishment of new steady states with swings in substrate concentration.[65]

B. EVIDENCE FOR LINKAGES BETWEEN THE HEMOGLOBIN BINDING SITE AND THE ANION TRANSPORT SITE ON HUMAN BAND 3

1. Introduction

The predominant linkage between the two fundamental respiratory gas transport processes is today known to be through the binding and release of the Bohr proton to hemoglobin. In light of this linkage, should we expect there also to be a linkage between hemoglobin oxygenation and chloride-bicarbonate exchange through band 3? If there could be a direct linkage, it would be to satisfy an apparent need which occurs during exercise when the band 3-mediated chloride-bicarbonate exchange rate may be too slow to keep pace with the other demands of the system (Chapter 1).

The factors needed to establish a linkage between hemoglobin deoxygenation and bicarbonate transport include the following. Band 3 would need to be an allosteric porter with homotropic interactions between two independently active domains. A fixed and rigid channel with a small internal site of limited flexibility would seem difficult to modulate. The porter would need a heterotropic cytosolic extension to bind hemoglobin in an oxygen-linked fashion. Since the model proposes linked functions between heterotropic and homotropic sites, hemoglobin binding to the heterotropic porter affector site should alter the binding and activity of the transport site, while ligand binding to the transport site should alter hemoglobin binding to the porter affector site. In what follows we will discuss some key facts which suggest at least the plausibility of heterotropic allosteric linkage between the hemoglobin binding site and the anion transport sites on the band 3.

2. Mode of Interaction of Hemoglobin With Band 3: Evidence That the Acidic N Terminus of Band 3 Binds to the 2,3-Diphosphoglycerate Binding Site of Deoxyhemoglobin

There is much evidence on the mode of the specific interaction between hemoglobin and band 3. Prasanna-Murthy and co-workers[142] showed that the dissected domain of the cytoplasmic fragment of band 3 containing the first 23 amino acids could bind to hemoglobin. It is significant that the remaining C-terminal portion of CDB3, which very probably contains the ankyrin binding site, does not bind hemoglobin. This latter subdomain of CDB3 contains an interfacial pocket holding the only two sulfhydryl groups on the fragment (Chapter 2). These sulfhydryl groups are over 100 Å from the N-terminal hemoglobin binding site (Chapter 2), thus precluding disulfide formation between hemoglobin and the same band 3 monomer to which it is bound. This was confirmed by Cassoly and Salhany,[176] who reported an inability to cross-link a stoichiometric complex of CDB3 and hemoglobin using the Cu^{2+}-orthophenanthroline method. However, either nonspecific interactions occur when hemoglobin is membrane bound or the structural setting is different, since in unsealed ghosts hemoglobin can be cross-linked to band 3.[177,178]

While the hemoglobin binding site on CDB3 seems quite considerably distant from the C-terminal anion transport domain, to what extent are they structurally connected? CDB3 is a dimeric structure, and hemoglobin binding could change its conformation. Such conformational changes could then be transmitted in any number of ways to the transport domain. However, saturation transfer electron spin resonance (ESR) data of spin-labeled hemoglobin and G3PD binding to band 3 in membranes do not seem to support this view. The integral domain and the CDB3 dimer seem to rotate independently.[179,180] On the other hand, one may ask if the two domains are also motionally independent when the probe proteins are not bound. Perhaps there are protein-induced transitions in motional freedom which have functional consequence, as was discussed above.

The rationale for the interaction of hemoglobin with the acidic N terminus of band 3 was given by Walder and co-workers.[181] They showed that a synthetic peptide containing amino acids 1 to 11, could bind to deoxyhemoglobin. Since the first 11 amino acids of the N terminus of band 3 are extremely acidic, it is reasonable to suppose that the binding site on hemoglobin is the well-characterized DPG binding site between the beta-chains. Walder and co-workers[181] were able to cocrystallize a peptide consisting of the first 11 amino acids, and they confirmed that it binds to the DPG binding site along the molecular dyad axis of symmetry. Their X-ray difference maps are shown in Figure 4A-4D. Figures 4A and B are views looking down the molecular dyad axis, while Figures 4C and D are perpendicular views. The "finger" of positive difference density extends inside the central cavity to the level of the beta-heme groups.

Although electrostatic effects are important to binding, they cannot be the sole determinant. Low and co-workers[134] have recently demonstrated that phosphorylation of tyrosine 8 and possibly tyrosine 21 of the 23-amino acid fragment causes a substantial inhibition of both hemoglobin and glycolytic enzyme binding despite the fact that the degree of negative charge of the fragment had increased significantly. Apparently, phosphorylation of the fragment

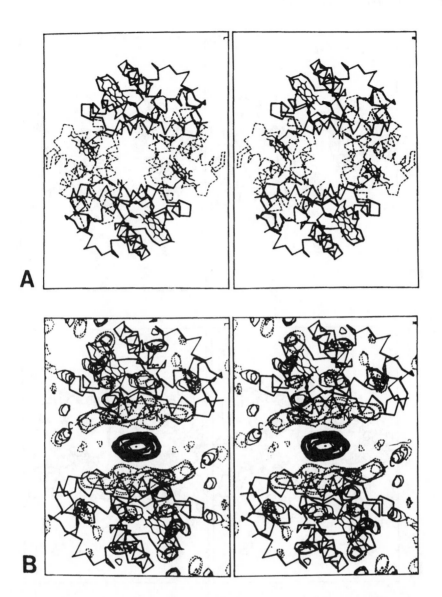

FIGURE 4. Difference electron density maps of the deoxyhemoglobin-peptide complex minus deoxyhemoglobin, superimposed on alpha-carbon plots of the hemoglobin subunits. The difference in electron density is contoured in two-dimensional sections spaced 1 Å apart with contours starting at ±2 sigma, where sigma is defined as the root mean square density over the entire map. Dashed (negative) contours show decreases in electron density; solid (positive) contours show increases in electron density. (A) Stereo drawing of the alpha-carbon plot of deoxyhemoglobin viewed down the molecular dyad. Beta-subunits are shown as *thick solid lines,* alpha-subunits as *dashed lines,* and the heme groups are drawn with *thin solid lines*. (B) 13 sections of the difference in electron density map superimposed on the alpha-carbon tracing of the beta-subunits shown in A. The position of the 11-amino acid peptide is clearly revealed by the intense positive peak along the molecular dyad. The largest negative features show that peptide binding causes disordering of 12 residues of the COOH-terminus of the beta-chains as well as the 3 NH_2-terminal residues before the alpha helix. (C) Stereo drawing of the alpha-carbon tracing of deoxyhemoglobin viewed perpendicular to the molecular dyad. One alpha-subunit has been omitted for clarity. (D) Seven sections of the difference in electron density map superimposed on the alpha-carbon tracing shown in C. The "finger" of positive difference density along the molecular dyad shows that the peptide ligand extends inside the central cavity to the level of the beta-heme groups. (From Walder, J. A. Chatterjee, R., Steck, T. L., Low, P. S., Musso, G. F., Kaiser, E. T., Rogers, P. H., and Arnone, A., *J. Biol. Chem.,* 259, 10238, 1984. With permission.)

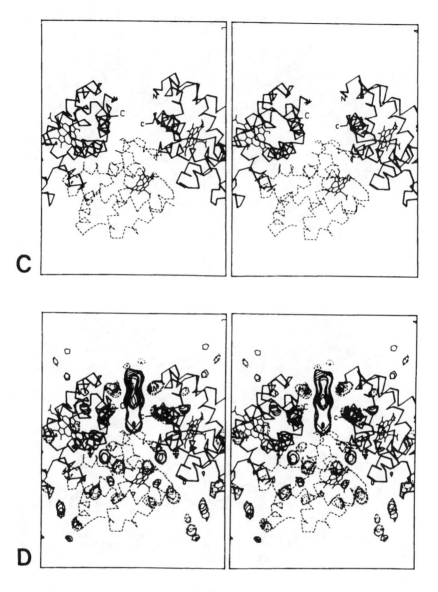

FIGURE 4 (continued)

changes its conformation such that it no longer can bind. However, the physiological implications of the phosphorylation effects are unclear, since phosphotyrosine has been difficult to demonstrate on band 3 *in vivo*.[182]

Since the N-terminal end of band 3 binds to the DPG binding site on hemoglobin, one might expect binding to cause a reduction in oxygen affinity. There is indeed a significant increase in P_{50}.[181,183] The effect of band 3 on log P_{50} is shown in Figure 5, from the paper by Tsuneshige and co-workers.[183] Yet, we saw above that addition of oxyhemoglobin to membranes[132] or to isolated cytoplasmic fragment[130,176,184] stabilizes the oxyhemoglobin dimer (Figure 1). Cassoly has clarified the situation by studying the flash photolysis of carboxyhemoglobin (HbCO) as a function of increasing ratios of HbCO to CDB3 (Figure 6).[184] As the stoichiometric ratio increases, there is an increase in the rapid CO binding component, indicating stabilization of the "R-state" dimer in agreement with the membrane study.[132] The curves in Figure 6B are computer simulations of the dependence of the fraction of fast phase on the concentration of band 3

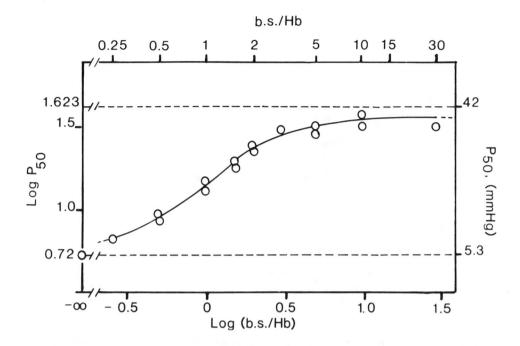

FIGURE 5. Dependence of P_{50} (the oxygen half-saturation of hemoglobin [Hb]) on Hb-membrane mixing ratio expressed by the number of binding sites on the membrane per Hb tetramer (b.s./Hb), and corresponding P_{50} values. The upper limit was calculated by extrapolation of a log P_{50} vs. 1/(b.s./Hb) plot. The point on the curve at the lower left corresponds to a measurement of Hb alone. Hb concentration, 3 μM on a tetramer basis; in 5 mM sodium phosphate buffer, pH 6.5; at 25°C. (From Tsuneshige, A., Imai, K. and Tyuma, I., *J. Biochem. (Tokyo)*, 101, 695, 1987. With permission.)

fragment, according to the mechanism shown in Figure 7. The best fit was that in which two dimers of hemoglobin could bind to one band 3 fragment, or one hemoglobin tetramer could bind and the bound forms interconvert, with the tetramer affinity being higher than that of the dimer. This behavior is a consequence of the thermodynamics of the scheme. If the tetramer and dimer binding constants were the same or if the tetramer had a lower affinity, then there should have been 100% fast phase, and this was not observed.

One structural explanation for stabilization of the oxy dimer on band 3 is that there are only two ways for band 3 to bind to the DPG binding site. Either the hemoglobin molecule must be split to form two alpha-beta dimers, which could then bind, or the hemoglobin "T-state" tetramer (liganded or unliganded) would have to bind at the open DPG pocket. There is some evidence that the ligand-bound hemoglobin tetramer on band 3 may be in the liganded T-state.[184]

In summary, we see that the extremely acidic N terminus of band 3 can stabilize either the oxyhemoglobin dimer or the T-state tetramer. But clearly T-state tetramers must bind with a higher affinity, and this is what would be required if deoxyhemoglobin binding is to affect the anion transport rate in response to severe exercise, where the steady-state level of deoxyhemoglobin may increase within the cell.

3. Evidence for Linkages Between the Hemoglobin Binding Site and the Anion Transport Site on Band 3

If oxygen-linked hemoglobin binding to band 3 is to modulate anion transport, then there should be evidence for a linkage between the hemoglobin binding site and the anion transport site. Salhany and co-workers[130] established such a transmembrane linkage by showing that titration of exofacial transport domain on band 3 with DIDS lowered the hemoglobin affinity at

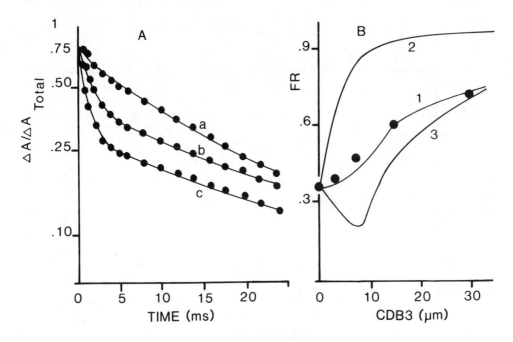

FIGURE 6. Flash photolysis experiments on carboxyhemoglobin in the presence of increasing amounts of CDB3.(A) Curves a, b and c represent the time course for the recombination of CO with photodissociated hemoglobin. Concentrations were carboxyhemoglobin, 30 μM (per heme); [CO], 280 μM; CDB3, curve a, 0; curve b, 15 μM per monomer; curve c, 30 μM. (B) FR represents the fraction of the fast reacting material measured from the time courses of the reaction as a function of CDB3 concentration. In the absence of CDB3, the value found for FR indicates that the dimer-tetramer equilibrium is governed by a dissociation constant $K_{4,2}$ of 6 μM. The points are experimental. Curve 1 corresponds with $K_D = 1.5 \times 10^{-7} M$ and $K_T = 2 \times 10^{-9} M$. Curve 2 corresponds with $K_D = 1.5 \times 10^{-7} M$ and $K_T = 2 \times 10^{-8} M$. Curve 3 was computed for a simpler scheme with only 1 hemoglobin dimer binding site/B$_3$F monomer with $K_D = 1.5 \times 10^{-7} M$ and $K_T = 10^{-8} M$. (Cassoly, R., *J. Biol. Chem.*, 258, 3859, 1983. With permission.)

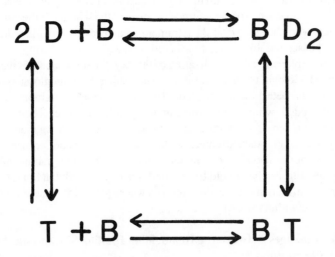

FIGURE 7.   Mechanism of hemoglobin dimers (D) and tetramer (T) binding to CDB3 (B).

its cytoplasmic site in a manner which correlated with the inhibition of anion transport by DIDS. Their findings are shown in Figure 8. Figure 8A shows DIDS inhibition of anion transport in intact red cells. Figure 8B shows the corresponding reduction in hemoglobin binding to unsealed ghosts derived from the same cells, determined using a light-scattering method.[130] In the control, the reduction of hemoglobin affinity was not stoichiometric with DIDS coverage because of a complicating secondary DIDS site. This component was subtracted through an involved mathematical analysis which is fully detailed in the paper.[130] Figure 9 shows plots of the components extracted from the fit. One component correlated strongly with transport inhibition, while the other did not. The secondary component could be experimentally removed by chymotrypsin treatment of cells after DIDS labeling. As seen in Figures 8B and 9 (open circles), this component shows a strong correlation with anion transport inhibition by DIDS. DIDS binding to the exofacial site on band 3 also changes the mechanism of hemoglobin binding (Figure 10). The control panel shows hyperbolic binding of oxyhemoglobin, while the DIDS-labeled cells showed negative cooperative hemoglobin binding. Taken together, it seems that hemoglobin binds with greater difficulty to CDB3 when DIDS is bound to the transport domain.

For many years the effect of DIDS on hemoglobin binding was not considered significant despite the publication of evidence that DIDS binding altered cytoskeletal protein extractability.[28] It was argued that anion transport could occur even when CDB3 was cleaved from the membrane-bound domain of the porter.[185] However, this argument seems to miss an important point. If hemoglobin is a heterotropic allosteric affector of the band 3 anion-transport function, one would not expect anion transport to be absolutely dependent on the presence of hemoglobin. As an example, it is clear that oxygen binds very well to hemoglobin in the absence of hemoglobin allosteric affectors (but with different constants). Would one use the above logic to propose that DPG is physiologically irrelevant because hemoglobin can work in its absence? Similarly, chicken band 3 lacks the acidic N terminus and probably does not bind hemoglobin. But because several hemoglobins from various species do not bind DPG, does this mean that DPG is physiologically irrelevant to human physiology?

If there is any validity to the hypothesis linking hemoglobin binding to the anion-transport function of band 3, then one must demonstrate that hemoglobin does indeed alter anion transport. Hemoglobin binding should also alter reversible inhibitor binding to the transport domain. Several recent papers have been published which provide the needed evidence to support this part of the linkage hypothesis. The most notable is the recent study by Racker and co-workers[186] using a reconstituted band 3 system. They found that the addition of hemoglobin significantly increases the rate of phosphate transport and that the effect is markedly potentiated by the presence of Mg^{2+}. They also were able to confirm that addition of DIDS to the transport domain lowered affinity of hemoglobin to the cytoplasmic domain. These results offer the evidence to complete the allosteric linkage argument begun earlier.[130] However, more work is still needed since the role of Mg^{2+} is unclear. Recall that Prasanna-Murthy and co-workers[142] found that Mg^{2+} reduced G3PD binding but had no effect on hemoglobin binding. Perhaps the Mg^{2+} effect in Racker's study[186] clears residual G3PD, making more hemoglobin binding sites available.

Does hemoglobin binding to CDB3 lower the affinity of reversible stilbene binding to the transport domain? Static binding measurements suggest that reversible stilbene binding to band 3 in intact red cells is the same as in isolated band 3.[187] On the other hand, Solomon and co-workers[188] have recently applied their more-sensitive kinetic method[189] to measure DBDS (4,4'-dibenzamido-2,2'-stilbene disulfonate) binding kinetics and have observed significant differences in the kinetic parameters for red cells vs. "pink" ghosts and white ghosts.[188] They conclude that the conformation at the stilbene-disulfonate binding site is progressively altered as red cells become "pink" ghosts and then white ghosts. Since hemoglobin is being progressively eluted in these transitions, it seems possible that the changes are related to differential hemoglobin binding, but this must be directly tested in reassociation studies.

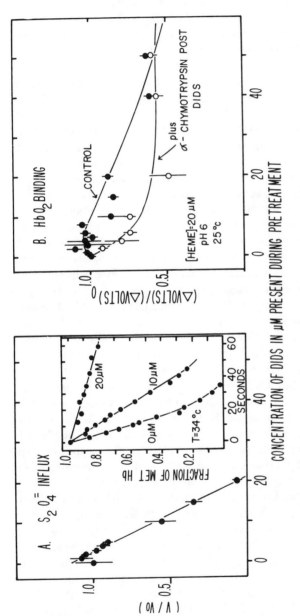

FIGURE 8. Effect of DIDS reaction with intact erythrocytes (A) on the velocity of dithionite–sulfate heteroexchange and (B) on the light-scattering change due to hemoglobin binding to membranes isolated from similarly treated cells. (A) Dithionite flux. Methemoglobin-containing erythrocytes were prepared and reacted with DIDS at 50% hematocrit. Dithionite–sulfate heteroexchange for intact cells was measured at 34°C for a 1% hematocrit after mixing. The concentration of dithionite was constant at 50 mM after mixing. The data are plotted as the ratio of the measured velocities over the velocity at zero DIDS. Mean and standard deviations are shown. The intercept at the DIDS axis was 21.2 μM, which corresponds to ~1.8 × 10⁶ DIDS binding sites per cell. The insert shows a plot of typical time courses for 0, 10, and 20 μM DIDS. (B) Light scattering due to hemoglobin binding to membranes from DIDS- reacted erythrocytes and DIDS-reacted alpha-chymotrypsin-treated erythrocytes. Cells were reacted with various DIDS concentrations and membranes were isolated or they were reacted with DIDS and then with alpha-chymotrypsin, following which membranes were isolated. Total protein present after mixing in each case was 36 μg/ml. Hemoglobin was constant at 20 μM after the mixing. Binding was studied in 5 mM phosphate, pH 6 at 25°C, and is presented as the normalized voltage change relative to zero DIDS control or alpha-chymotrypsin predigested. (Note: predigestion with alphachymotrypsin had no significant effect on light scattering.) The data are presented as mean values ± SE from three separate determinations on different days with different samples of blood. The curves shown are best-fitting curves from weighted nonlinear curve-fitting procedures discussed in the original paper. (From Salhany, J. M., Cordes, K. A., and Gaines, E. D., *Biochemistry, 19*, 1447, 1980. With permission.)

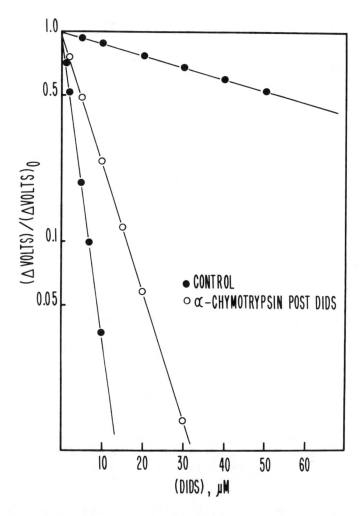

FIGURE 9. Theoretical plot of the individual exponential terms from the fit to the data in Figure 8 describing the effect of externally reacted DIDS on hemoglobin affinity for the cytoplasmic portion of the membrane. The symbols have the same meaning as those in Figure 8. (From Salhany, J. M., Cordes, K. A. and Gaines, E. D., *Biochemistry,* 19, 1447, 1980. With permission.)

4. Mechanism of the Linkage Between the Hemoglobin Binding Site and the Anion Transport Domain

Although there seems to be clear evidence for the existence of transmembrane effects involving band 3,[28,130,143,186] it is not clear by what mechanism these changes can occur. Both the integral and the cytoplasmic domains of band 3 can exist independently as at least stable dimers. Allosteric interactions between sites on each monomer of the cytoplasmic domain could be transmitted to the integral domain, despite the evidence for the apparent independence of the two domains in some instances.[179,180,185,190] One mechanism may involve interactions between monomers of a band 3 dimer or higher-order state of association. Evidence for interactions at the cytoplasmic domain indicates cooperativity in hemoglobin binding.[130,191] Premachandra[191] demonstrated the presence of apparent positive cooperativity in "deoxy" hemoglobin binding to isolated band 3. Shaklai and Abrahami[192] did not see complex binding of deoxyhemoglobin. Salhany and co-workers[130] attributed the appearance of positive cooperativity to the presence of multiple binding sites on the membrane. However, the experiments of Premachandra[191] and

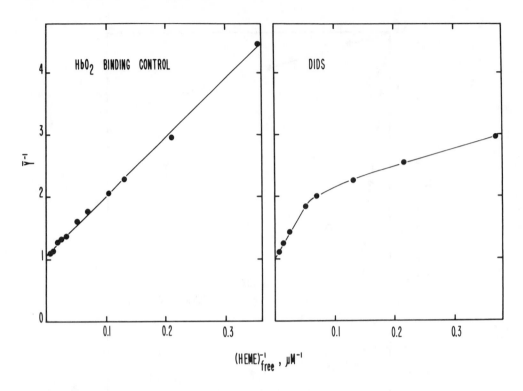

FIGURE 10.   Effect of DIDS pretreatment on the mechanism of hemoglobin binding. The conditions were 5 mM phosphate pH 6 and 25°C, with all ghost concentrations at 36 μg/ml after the mixing. Double-reciprocal plots of the fraction of hemoglobin saturation of membrane sites vs. the concentration of free heme are shown for control (A) and DIDS-reacted (B) membranes. The concentration of DIDS during pretreatment of cells was 50 μM. The value of K_d for the control was 2 μM (tetramer). K_d values were estimated for the two components of the DIDS-treated membranes and found to be 0.4 μM for the high-affinity component and 4.3 μM for the low-affinity component. (From Salhany, J. M., Cordes, K. A., and Gaines, E. D., *Biochemistry,* 19, 1447, 1980. With permission.)

Salhany and co-workers[130] are not directly comparable (one study uses oxyhemoglobin[130] and membranes, while the other uses isolated band 3 and "deoxy" hemoglobin[191]).

Salhany and Cassoly[193] have recently hypothesized that hemoglobin binding to the acidic N terminus should produce long-range conformational changes in CDB3 which could potentially affect higher-order interactions. These conformational changes could link the band 3 transport site to the hemoglobin binding site. To demonstrate long-range conformational changes the authors used the fact that the cluster of sulfhydryl groups on CDB3 is over 100 Å from the hemoglobin site (Chapter 2). The rate of *p*-chloromercuribenzoate (PMB) binding to those sulfhydryl groups was then used to see if stoichiometric addition of hemoglobin could change sulfhydryl reactivity over such great distances. Figure 11 shows the effect of formation of a 1:1 stoichiometric hemoglobin tetramer/CDB3 monomer complex on the reactivity of PMB with CDB3 sulfhydryls. Both reaction phases were drastically slowed. Investigation of the mechanism showed that the initial PMB affinity step (Chapter 2) was lowered by hemoglobin binding (Figure 12). The authors proposed a mechanism involving a long-range hemoglobin-induced "closure" of the "pocket of sulfhydryls" at the C-terminal end of CDB3. A schematic structural model for this effect is given in Figure 13.

Such long-range conformational changes have the potential to explain functional communication between the hemoglobin binding site and the anion transport site on band 3. Suppose, for the sake of discussion that band 3 exists as a tetramer which can take two quaternary conformational states (Chapter 2). These states are shown in Figure 14. One state will be called

173

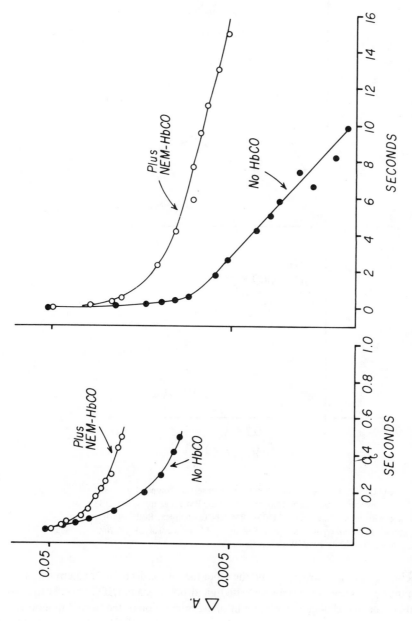

FIGURE 11. Reaction time courses of PMB with CDB3 and with the stoichiometric CDB3/NEM-HbCO complex. The left-hand panel shows the early phase of the time course to illustrate that formation of a stoichiometric complex with NEM-HbCO decreases the apparent rate of reaction. The right-hand panel shows the time course over longer periods to illustrate that the slow phase is also diminished in apparent rate. The final concentration of PMB was 5 μM. (From Salhany, J. M. and Cassoly, R., *J. Biol. Chem.*, 264, 1399, 1989. With permission.)

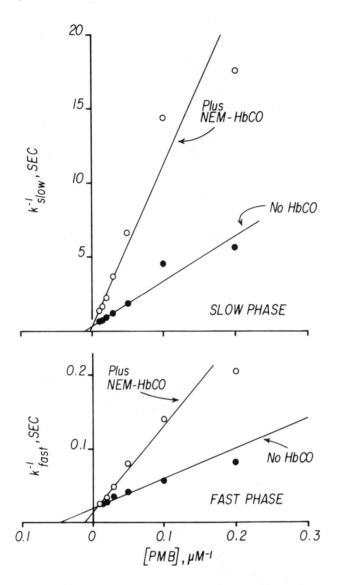

FIGURE 12. Double reciprocal plots of the observed, computer-extracted rate constants for the fast and slow phases of the PMB reaction with CDB3 and with the stoichiometric CDB3/NEM-HbCO complex. Both data sets follow hyperbolic patterns. (From Salhany, J. M. and Cassoly, R., *J. Biol. Chem.*, 264, 1399, 1989. With permission.)

an "outward-facing" quaternary structure, and the other the "inward-facing" quaternary structure. We assign the "out" state as the transport-site ligand-bound state. DIDS or other ligands would bind to that state and change the relative in-plane orientation of the band 3 monomers. This change in quaternary structure would then be transmitted to CDB3, causing a tighter association with ankyrin. Such an effect could explain the greater difficulty in extracting cytoskeletal proteins from DIDS-labeled membranes[28] while at the same time explaining the weaker binding of hemoglobin.[130,143,186] In contrast, the "in" quaternary state would have a different CDB3 conformation allowing those band 3 dimers not directly bound to ankyrin to bind hemoglobin (Figure 14). Hemoglobin binding may drive the in-plane dimerization reaction of the "in" quaternary structure (not shown in Figure 14). Keep in mind that these "in" and "out"

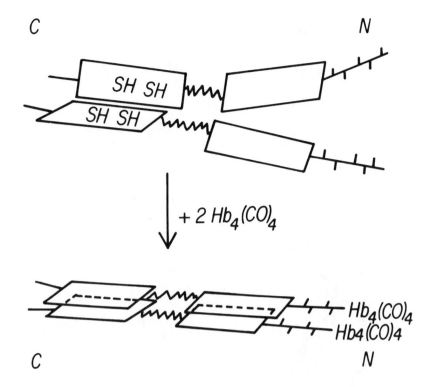

FIGURE 13.   Schematic drawing showing the effect of hemoglobin on the global conformation of the CDB3 dimer to account for the reduction in the reactivity of the pocket of sulfhydryls over 100 Å from the hemoglobin binding site. (From Salhany, J. M. and Cassoly, R, *J. Biol. Chem.* 264,1399, 1989. With permission.)

states may be equivalently called fast anion-exchange ("in") and slow anion-exchange ("out") states.This is one example of the type of heterotropic allosteric modulation which might follow from a tetramer of homotropic dimers. There surely may be other possible scenarios, but Figure 14 offers some unifying quality for the data, especially the differential effect of DIDS binding on cytoskeletal protein extractability and hemoglobin binding.

V. EVIDENCE FOR CYTOSOLIC PROTEIN BINDING UNDER PHYSIOLOGICAL CONDITIONS AND *IN SITU*

The question of the physiological relevance of cytosolic protein binding has been an issue since Bürker first proposed in 1922 that hemoglobin may be "held by union with the membrane".[80] By contrast, the probable physiological binding of ankyrin to band 3 has not been questioned since tight binding is observed under conditions of physiological pH and ionic strength.

Solti and co-workers[194] presented some of the first evidence for the membrane association of G3PD *in situ*. Human erythrocytes were treated with highly tritiated iodoacetate under conditions such that half of the label became attached to G3PD. They quantitated the autoradiographs using a computer and found that the distribution of the grains was heaviest near the membrane. Yeltman and Harris[195] and Keokitichai and Wrigglesworth[196] added glutaraldehyde to intact cells and were able to show that up to 90% of the total cellular enzyme remained associated with the membrane residue. There was some evidence that one site of interaction of aldolase *in situ* consists of erythrocyte actin microfilaments.[195]

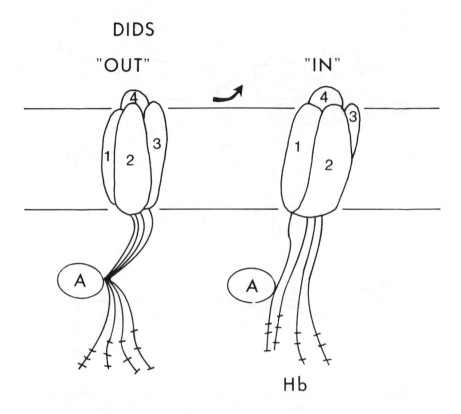

FIGURE 14.   Different conformations of a band 3 tetramer. The DIDS-bound conformational state
has CDB3 more tightly associated with ankyrin (A). The DIDS-free state can take a different
conformation in which the association with ankyrin of one band 3 dimer is looser and deoxyhemoglobin
can bind.

Steck and students[197,198] have made a kinetic analysis of the release of glycolytic enzymes
from the cell consequent to rapid hemolysis with saponin. They examined the activity of the
enzyme in the filtrate as a function of time and extrapolated the data back to the zero-time axis
to determine the amount bound in the intact cell. They found that 40% of the aldolase is bound,
50% of the PFK is bound, and 65% of the G3PD is bound.[197,198] The percentages bound were
independent of the ionic strength of the hemolyzing solution. Szabolcsi and Cseke[199] used a
similar approach, and their results would also support the hypothesis that G3PD may be located
near the membrane. However, others have criticized the filtration technique.[200] Also, use of an
NMR method with intact cells has shown that the G3PD step is not rate limiting *in situ*.[201] If
multiple enzyme complexes are active (an untested hypothesis), the determination of enzyme
binding on the basis of activity alone may be misleading. Steck and co-workers[212] have used
fluorescence immunocytochemical labeling of G3PD on sections of fixed, intact red cells and
were able to demonstrate a membrane localization.

Although the existence of functional, band 3-bound multiple enzyme complexes *in situ* has
not been directly established, there is evidence for its existence. Fossel and Solomon[202-205] have
presented functional evidence for the existence of a membrane-bound glycolytic complex on
band 3 which is in direct contact with the $(Na^+ + K^+)$-ATPase. It is interesting to note that the
authors were able to isolate a 10^6-Da particle from erythrocyte hemolysates containing G3PD,
aldolase, and phosphoglycerate kinase.[203] Whether this complex is attached to band 3 *in situ* or
not remains to be firmly established. Friedrich and co-workers have also presented functional
evidence favoring a red cell glycolytic enzyme complex.[206]

There may be several reasons to organize glycolytic enzymes into complexes on the membrane. Maintenance of membrane integrity through provision of ATP for pumps is one reason for membrane proximity. Yet, one of the longest standing controversies has centered around data suggesting that extracellular orthophosphate is more rapidly incorporated into cell metabolites than into the cytosolic orthophosphate pool.[93-103] Clearly, if an active glycolytic complex exists on some of the copies of band 3, this possibility becomes even more plausible. However, recent studies by Shoemaker and co-workers[101] suggest that there is no difference between the rate of incorporation of extracellular orthophosphate into the cytosolic orthophosphate pool and the rate of incorporation into cytosolic nucleotide phosphate. There was evidence that the membrane component of the nucleotide pool reached steady state with extracellular orthophosphate much more rapidly than the cytosolic pool of nucleotides. Interestingly, DNDS had no effect on the rate of incorporation into the membrane nucleotide pool. However, removal of sodium from the extracellular medium decreased the level of incorporation by 90%. The authors suggest that a separate Na-phosphate cotransport system exists, perhaps distinct from band 3, which is in direct contact with the membrane nucleotide synthetic system. Perhaps a class of band 3 exists which is refractory to DNDS inhibition. It would be interesting to know if this sodium-phosphate cotransport pathway was also insensitive to covalent DIDS binding. Furthermore, since DNDS changes the quaternary structure of band 3 (Chapter 2) it becomes possible that glycolytic enzyme binding to the cytosolic sites of the porter is also dependent on quaternary structure.

The interaction of hemoglobin and band 3 under physiological conditions seems relatively well established. Eisinger and co-workers[207] used fluorescence energy transfer to show that as the intracellular pH was lowered, hemoglobin caused more quenching of both lipid-placed and band 3-bound fluorophores. Their results are shown in Figure 15. The top portion of the figure shows the pH-dependent quenching of various x-AS (i.e., x-(9-anthroyloxy)stearic acid) derivatives, while the bottom shows the quenching of DIDS.[207] It is clear from the x-AS data that intracellular hemoglobin is the acceptor of the fluorescence since placement of the fluorophore deeper in the bilayer caused relatively more quenching by hemoglobin. DIDS fluorescence was also reduced as the pH was lowered. Since lower pH favors hemoglobin binding, a closer approach of hemoglobin to band 3 was suggested based on calculations. However, the interpretation of the data in terms of the presence of specific binding was not made by the authors and distances are only as good as the model used as was discussed by Eisinger and co-workers.[207,208]

Studies have been published indicating hemoglobin binding at physiological pH.[209] Chétrite and Cassoly[210] have recently presented direct measurements of CDB3-hemoglobin association constants as a function of ionic strength over the physiological range. Their results are shown in Figure 16. They demonstrate that deoxyhemoglobin has a much higher affinity for CDB3 than does oxyhemoglobin and that binding is sensitive to the presence of phosphate buffer and 2,3-DPG (data not shown here). The dissociation constant is on the order of $10^{-4} M$ at 120 mM NaCl. On the basis of this value they estimated that about 50% of the band 3 may interact with deoxyhemoglobin *in situ*. Nonidealities at the membrane surface may be expected to further promote binding.

VI. CONCLUSIONS

In this chapter much data have been summarized to show that although band 3 functions as an anion porter, it also has a structural role in the cell. Yet it seems equally clear that that role should not be viewed in static terms. The connection of band 3 with ankyrin is not stoichiometric. Several other ligand binding sites are available on CDB3, and the conformation of the CDB3 dimer is sensitive to protein binding over extraordinarily long ranges. These facts may offer at least the beginning of a rational basis from the demonstration of linkages between the

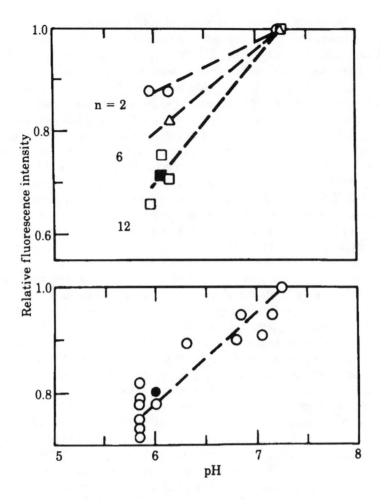

FIGURE 15.   Front-face fluorescence intensity ratios for x-AS- (upper) and DIDS-(lower) labeled intact cells as a function of internal pH, normalized to the intensity at pH 7.25. DIDS is bound to band 3 protein, while x-AS probes are in the phospholipid bilayer regions of the cell. [■], intensity ratio derived from comparison of the decay functions; [●], intensity ratio for deoxygenated cells. These data were used to estimate donor-acceptor distances. (From Eisinger, J., Flores, J., and Salhany, J. M., *Proc. Natl. Acad. Sci. U.S.A.,* 79, 408, 1982. With permission.)

hemoglobin binding site and the anion transport domain of band 3. Such linkages, if established *in situ,* offer a way to further integrate the two major functions of the human red blood cell: oxygen and carbon dioxide transport.

VII. ADDENDUM

Since submission of this manuscript a paper by Davis and co-workers[213] has appeared showing that the ankyrin binding site on CDB3 is not defined by a short continuous sequence but invovles more complex interactions. In addition Cherry and co-workers[214] have published new transient dichroism studies on band 3 rotation suggesting that ankyrin linkage to band 3 may in fact not act as a restraint on band 3 rotation.

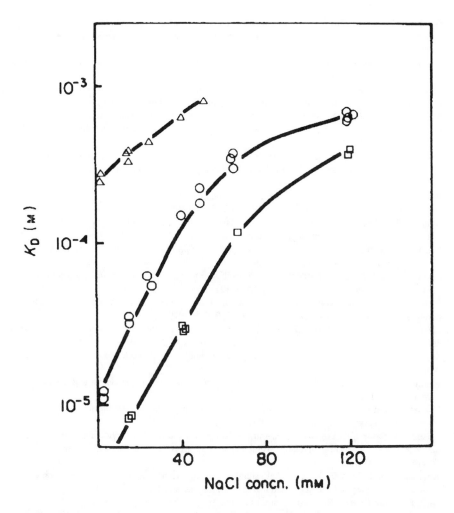

FIGURE 16. Equilibrium dissociation constant of oxy- and deoxyhemoglobin for immobilized CDB3 as a function of NaCl concentration. (Δ) Oxyhemoglobin in 10 mM phosphate buffer (pH 7.2); (m) deoxyhemoglobin in 10 mM phosphate buffer (pH 7.2); (q) deoxyhemoglobin in 10 mM bisTris buffer (pH 7.2). The ordinate for K_D is logarithmic. According to the amounts of immobilized CDB3 that could be used practically, $K_D = 10^{-3} \, M$ represents an upper limit in the measurement of the dissociation constant. Consequently, the association of oxyhemoglobin with CDB3 at pH 7.2 could be estimated only below 50 mM salt. The concentration of hemoglobin was varied between 2×10^{-5} M and $9 \times 10^{-5} \, M$. In the presence of a large excess of DPG (3 mM), the association of deoxyhemoglobin to immobilized CDB3 was too low to be measurable. For salt concentrations below 40 mM NaCl, the concentration of matrix-bound CDB3 was varied between $3 \times 10^{-5} \, M$ and $10^{-4} \, M$. (From Chétrite, G. and Cassoly, R., *J. Mol. Biol.*, 185, 639, 1985. With permission.)

REFERENCES

1. **Benesch, R. and Benesch, R. E.,** The effect of organic phosphates from the human erythrocyte on the allosteric properties of hemoglobin, *Biochem. Biophys. Res. Commun.*, 26, 162, 1967.
2. **Chanutin, A. and Curnish, R. R.,** Effect of organic and inorganic phosphates on the oxygen equilibrium of human erythrocytes, *Arch. Biochem. Biophys.*, 121, 96, 1967.
3. **Bennett, V.,** The membrane skeleton of human erythrocytes and its implications for more complex cells, *Annu. Rev. Biochem.*, 54, 273, 1985.

4. **Nicolson, G. L. and Painter, R. G.,** Anionic sites of human erythrocyte membranes. II. Antispectrin-induced transmembrane aggregation of the binding sites for positively charged colloidal particles, *J. Cell Biol.,* 59, 395, 1973.

5. **Elgsaeter, A. and Branton, D.,** Intramembrane particle aggregation in erythrocyte ghosts. I. The effects of protein removal, *J. Cell Biol.,* 63, 1018, 1974.

6. **Elgsaeter, A., Shotton, D. M., and Branton, D.,** Intramembrane particle aggregation in erythrocyte ghosts. II. The influence of spectrin aggregation, *Biochim. Biophys. Acta,* 426, 101, 1976.

7. **Shotton, D., Thompson, K., Wofsy, L., and Branton, D.,** Appearance and distribution of surface proteins of the human erythrocyte membrane. An electron microscope and immuno-chemical labeling study, *J. Cell Biol.,* 76, 512, 1978.

8. **Bennett, V. and Branton, D.,** Selective association of spectrin with the cytoplasmic surface of human erythrocyte plasma membranes. Quantitative determination with purified [^{32}P] spectrin, *J. Biol. Chem.,* 252, 2753, 1977.

9. **Bennett, V.,** Purification of an active proteolytic fragment of the membrane attachment site for human erythrocyte spectrin, *J. Biol. Chem.,* 253, 2292, 1978.

10. **Bennett, V. and Stenbuck, P. J.,** Identification and partial purification of ankyrin, the high affinity membrane attachment site for human erythrocyte spectrin, *J. Biol. Chem.,* 254, 2533, 1979.

11. **Yu, J. and Goodman, S. R.,** Syndeins: the spectrin-binding protein(s) of the human erythrocyte membrane, *Proc. Natl. Acad. Sci. U.S.A.,* 76, 2340, 1979.

12. **Luna, E. J., Kidd, G. H., and Branton, D.,** Identification by peptide analysis of the spectrin-binding protein in human erythrocytes, *J. Biol. Chem.,* 254, 2526, 1979.

13. **Bennett, V. and Stenbuck, P. J.,** The membrane attachment protein for spectrin is associated with band 3 in human erythrocyte membranes, *Nature (London),* 280, 468, 1979.

14. **Hargreaves, W. R., Giedd, K. N., Verkleij, A., and Branton, D.,** Reassociation of ankyrin with band 3 in erythrocyte membranes and in lipid vesicles, *J. Biol. Chem.,* 255, 11965, 1980.

15. **Sheetz, M. P.,** Integral membrane protein interaction with triton cytoskeletons of erythrocytes, *Biochim. Biophys. Acta,* 557, 122, 1979.

16. **Bennett, V.,** Isolation of an ankyrin-band 3 oligomer from human erythrocyte membranes, *Biochim. Biophys. Acta,* 689, 475, 1982.

17. **Bennett, V. and Stenbuck, P. J.,** Association between ankyrin and the cytoplasmic domain of band 3 isolated from the human erythrocyte membrane, *J. Biol. Chem.,* 255, 6424, 1980.

18. **Kusumi, A., Sakaki, T., Yoshizawa, T., and Ohnishi, S.,** Protein-lipid interaction in rhodopsin recombinant membranes as studied by protein rotational mobility and lipid alkyl chain flexibility measurements, *J. Biochem. (Tokyo),* 88, 1103, 1980.

19. **Kusumi, A. and Hyde, J. S.,** Spin-label saturation-transfer electron spin resonance detection of transient association of rhodopsin in reconstituted membranes, *Biochemistry,* 21, 5978, 1982.

20. **Nigg, E. A. and Cherry, R. J.,** Anchorage of a band 3 population at the erythrocyte cytoplasmic membrane surface: protein rotational diffusion measurements, *Proc. Natl. Acad. Sci. U.S.A.,* 77, 4702, 1980.

21. **Chang, C.-H., Takeuchi, H., Ito, T., Machida, K., and Ohnishi, S.,** Lateral mobility of erythrocyte membrane proteins studied by the fluorescence photobleaching recovery technique, *J. Biochem. (Tokyo),* 90, 997, 1981.

22. **Sakaki, T., Tsuji, A., Chang, C.-H., and Ohnishi, S.,** Rotational mobility of an erythrocyte membrane integral protein band 3 in dimyristoylphosphatidylcholine reconstituted vesicles and effect of binding of cytoskeletal peripheral proteins, *Biochemistry,* 21, 2366, 1982.

23. **Sheetz, M. P., Schindler, M., and Koppel, D. E.,** Lateral mobility of integral membrane proteins is increased in spherocytic erythrocytes, *Nature (London)* 285, 510, 1980.

24. **Golan, D. E. and Veatch, W.,** Lateral mobility of band 3 in the human erythrocyte membrane studied by fluorescence photobleaching recovery: evidence for control by cytoskeletal interactions, *Proc. Natl. Acad. Sci. U.S.A.,* 77, 2537, 1980.

25. **Tsuji, A. and Ohnishi, S.,** Restriction of the lateral motion of band 3 in the erythrocyte membrane by the cytoskeletal network: dependence on spectrin association state, *Biochemistry,* 25, 6133, 1986.

26. **Tsuji, A., Kawasaki, K., Ohnishi, S., Merkle, H., and Kusumi, A.,** Regulation of band 3 mobilities in erythrocyte ghost membranes by protein association and cytoskeletal meshwork, *Biochemistry,* 27, 7447, 1988.

27. **Ueno, E., Sato, S., Jinbu, Y., and Nakao, M.,** Dynamic association of band 3 with Triton shells in human erythrocyte ghosts, *Biochim. Biophys. Acta* 915, 77, 1987.

28. **Hsu, L. and Morrison, M.,** The interaction of human erythrocyte band 3 with cytoskeletal components, Arch. *Biochem. Biophys.,* 227, 31, 1983.

29. **Mosior, M., Bialas, W. A., and Gomulkiewicz, J.,** Effect of DIDS on osmotic properties of bovine erythrocytes, *Biochim. Biophys. Acta,* 945, 51, 1988.

30. **Soong, C.-J., Lu, P.-W., and Tao, M.,** Analysis of band 3 cytoplasmic domain phosphorylation and association with ankyrin, *Arch. Biochem. Biophys.,* 254, 509, 1987.
31. **Hall, T. G. and Bennett, V.,** Regulatory domains of erythrocyte ankyrin, *J. Biol. Chem.,* 262, 10537, 1987.
32. **Pontremoli, S., Sparatore, B., Salamino, F., De Tullio, R., Pontremoli, R., and Melloni, E.,** The role of calpain in the selective increased phosphorylation of the anion-transport protein in red cell of hypertensive subjects, *Biochem. Biophys. Res. Commun.,* 151, 590, 1988.
33. **Wallin, R., Culp, E. N., Coleman, D. B., and Goodman, S. R.,** A structural model of human erythrocyte band 2.1: alignment of chemical and functional domains, *Proc. Natl. Acad. Sci. U.S.A.,* 81, 4095, 1984.
34. **Weaver, D. C. and Marchesi, V. T.,** The structural basis of ankyrin function. I. Identification of two structural domains, *J. Biol. Chem.,* 259, 6165, 1984.
35. **Weaver, D. C., Pasternack, G. R., and Marchesi, V. T.,** The structural basis of ankyrin function. II. Identification of two functional domains, *J. Biol. Chem.,* 259, 6170, 1984.
36. **Bursaux, E., Hilly, M., Bluze, A., and Poyart, C.,** Organic phosphates modulate anion self-exchange across the human erythrocyte membrane, *Biochim. Biophys. Acta,* 777, 253, 1984.
37. **Kay, M. M. B., Bosman, G. J. C. G. M., and Lawrence, C.,** Functional topography of band 3: specific structural alteration linked to functional aberrations in human erythrocytes, *Proc. Natl. Acad. Sci. U.S.A.,* 85, 492, 1988.
38. **Yu, J. and Steck, T. L.,** Associations of band 3, the predominant polypeptide of the human erythrocyte membrane, *J. Biol. Chem.,* 250, 9176, 1975.
39. **Korsgren, C. and Cohen, C. M.,** Purification and properties of human erythrocyte band 4.2. Association with the cytoplasmic domain of band 3, *J. Biol. Chem.,* 261, 5536, 1986.
40. **Steck, T. L.,** Cross-linking the major proteins of the isolated erythrocyte membrane, *J. Mol. Biol.,* 66, 295, 1972.
41. **Wang, K. and Richards, F. M.,** An approach to nearest neighbor analysis of membrane proteins. Application to the human erythrocyte membrane of a method employing cleavable cross-linkages, *J. Biol. Chem.,* 249, 8005, 1974.
42. **Korsgren, C. and Cohen, C. M.,** Associations of human erythrocyte band 4.2 binding to ankyrin and to the cytoplasmic domain of band 3, *J. Biol. Chem.,* 263, 10212, 1988.
43. **Lukacovic, M. F., Feinstein, M. B., Sha'afi, R. I., and Perrie, S.,** Purification of stabilized band 3 protein of the human erythrocyte membrane and its reconstitution into liposomes, *Biochemistry,* 20, 3145, 1981.
44. **Lange, Y., Hadesman, R. A., and Steck, T. L.,** Role of the reticulum in the stability and shape of the isolated human erythrocyte membrane, *J. Cell Biol.,* 92, 714, 1982.
45. **Rybicki, A. C., Heath, R., Wolf, J. L., Lubin, B., and Schwartz, R. S.,** Deficiency of protein 4.2 in erythrocytes from a patient with a Coombs negative hemolytic anemia. Evidence for a role of protein 4.2 in stabilizing ankyrin on the membrane, *J. Clin. Invest.,* 81, 893, 1988.
46. **Leto, T. L. and Marchesi, V. T.,** A structural model of human erythrocyte protein 4.1, *J. Biol. Chem.,* 259, 4603, 1984.
47. **Ohanian, V. and Gratzer, W.,** Preparation of red-cell-membrane cytoskeletal constituents and characterization of protein 4.1, *Eur. J. Biochem.,* 144, 375, 1984.
48. **Tyler, J. M., Reinhardt, B. N., and Branton, D.,** Associations of erythrocyte membrane proteins. Binding of purified bands 2.1 and 4.1 to spectrin, *J. Biol. Chem.,* 255, 7034, 1980.
49. **Ungewickell, E., Bennett, P. M., Calvert, R., Ohanian, V., and Gratzer, W. B.,** *In vitro* formation of a complex between cytoskeletal proteins of the human erythrocyte, *Nature (London),* 280, 811, 1979.
50. **Pasternack, G. R., Anderson, R. A., Leto, T. L., and Marchesi, V. T.,** Interactions between protein 4.1 and band 3. An alternative binding site for an element of the membrane skeleton, *J. Biol. Chem.,* 260, 3676, 1985.
51. **Jorpes, E.,** The protein component of the erythrocyte membrane or stroma, *Biochem. J.,* 26, 1488, 1932.
52. **Adams, G. A.,** The nature of haemoglobin in the red blood corpuscle, *Biochem. J.,* 32, 646, 1938.
53. **Anderson, H. M. and Turner, J. C.,** Preparation and the haemoglobin content of red cell 'ghosts', *Nature (London),* 183, 112, 1959.
54. **Anderson, H. M. and Turner, J. C.,** Relation of hemoglobin to the red cell membrane, *J. Clin. Invest.,* 39, 1, 1960.
55. **Dodge, J. T., Mitchell, C., and Hanahan, D. J.,** The preparation and chemical characteristics of hemoglobin-free ghosts of human erythrocytes, *Arch. Biochem. Biophys.,* 100, 119, 1963.
56. **Mitchell, C. D., Mitchell, W. B., and Hanahan, D. J.,** Enzyme and hemoglobin retention in human erythrocyte stroma, *Biochim. Biophys. Acta,* 104, 348, 1965.
57. **Weed, R. I., LaCelle, P. L., and Merrill, E. W.,** Metabolic dependence of red cell deformability, *J. Clin. Invest.,* 48, 795, 1969.
58. **Hanahan, D. J., Ekholm, J., and Hildenbrandt, G.,** Biochemical variability of human erythrocyte membrane preparations, as demonstrated by sodium-potassium-magnesium and calcium adenosine triphosphatase activities, *Biochemistry,* 12, 1374, 1973.

59. **Oparin, A. I.,** Richtungseinstellung der Invertasewirkung in der lebenden Pflanzenzelle, *Enzymologia,* 4, 13, 1937.

60. **Siekevitz, P.,** On the meaning of intracellular structure for metabolic regulation, in *CIBA Foundation Symposium on the Regulation of Cell Metabolism,* Wolstenholme, G. E. W. and O'Connor, C. M., Eds., Little, Brown, Boston, 1958, 17.

61. **Keleti, T., Batke, J., Ovádi, J., Jancsik, V., and Bartha, F.,** Macromolecular interactions in enzyme regulation, *Adv. Enzyme Regul.,* 15, 233, 1977.

62. **Masters, C. J.,** Metabolic control and the microenvironment, *Curr. Top. Cell. Regul.,* 12, 75, 1977.

63. **Masters, C. J.,** Interactions between soluble enzymes and subcellular structure, *Trends Biochem. Sci.,* 3, 206, 1978.

64. **Welch, G. R.,** On the role of organized multienzyme systems in cellular metabolism: a general synthesis. *Prog. Biophys. Mol. Biol.,* 32, 103, 1977.

65. **Wilson, J. E.,** Ambiquitous enzymes: variation in intracellular distribution as a regulatory mechanism, *Trends Biochem. Sci.,* 3, 124, 1978.

66. **Masters, C. J.,** Interactions between soluble enzymes and subcellular structure, *CRC Crit. Rev. Biochem.,* 11, 105, 1981.

67. **Clarke, F., Stephan, P., Morton, D., and Weidemann, J.,** Glycolytic enzyme organization via the cytoskeleton and its role in metabolic regulation, in *Regulation of Carbohydrate Metabolism,* Vol. 2, Beitner, R., Ed., CRC Press, Boca Raton FL, 1985, 1.

68. **Friedrich, P. and Hajdu, J.,** The structure, mechanism, control and organization of glycolytic enzymes in relation to their function in muscle. An overview of supramolecular enzyme organization, *Biochem. Soc. Trans.,* 15, 973, 1987.

69. **Bernhard, S. A. and Srivastava, D. K.,** Functional consequences of the direct transfer of metabolites in muscle glycolysis, *Biochem. Soc. Trans.,* 15, 977, 1987

70. **Masters, C. J., Reid, S., and Don, M.,** Glycolysis — new concepts in an old pathway, *Mol. Cell. Biochem.,* 76, 3, 1987.

71. **Friedrich, P.,** *Supramolecular Enzymes Organization: Quaternary Structure and Beyond,* Pergamon Press, New York, 1985.

72. **Schrier, S. L.,** Studies of the metabolism of human erythrocyte membranes, *J. Clin. Invest.,* 42, 756, 1963.

73. **Salmon, B., Murer, E., and Brierley, G. P.,** Association of glycolytic enzymes with membranes of the red blood corpuscle, *J. Cell Biol.,* 23, 81A, 1964.

74. **Green, D. E., Murer, E., Hultin, H. O., Richardson, S. H., Salmon, B., Brierley, G. P., and Baum, H.,** Association of integrated metabolic pathways with membranes. I. Glycolytic enzymes of the red blood corpuscle and yeast, *Arch. Biochem. Biophys.,* 112, 635, 1965.

75. **Hoffman, J. F.,** Physiological characteristics of human red blood cell ghosts, *J. Gen. Physiol.,* 42, 9, 1958.

76. **Klipstein, F. A. and Ranney, H. M.,** Electrophoretic components of the hemoglobin of red cell membranes, *J. Clin. Invest.,* 39, 1894, 1960.

77. **Zittle, C. A., DellaMonica, E. S., and Custer, J. H.,** Purification of human red cell acetylcholinesterase, *Arch. Biochem. Biophys.,* 48, 43, 1954.

78. **Weed, R. I., Reed, C. F, and Berg, G.,** Is hemoglobin an essential structural component of human erythrocyte membranes? *J. Clin. Invest.,* 42, 581, 1963.

79. **Rifkind, R. A. and Danon, D.,** Heinz body anemia — an ultra-structural study. I. Heinz body formation, *Blood,* 25, 885, 1965.

80. **Bürker, K.,** Das Gesetz der Verteilung des Hämoglobins auf die Oberfläche der Erythrocyten, *Pfluegers Arch. Gesamte Physiol. Menschen Tiere,* 195, 516, 1922.

81. **Nilsson, O. and Ronquist, G.,** Enzyme activities and ultra-structure of a membrane fraction from human erythrocytes, *Biochim. Biophys. Acta,* 183, 1, 1969.

82. **Duchon, G. and Collier, H. B.,** Enzyme activities of human erythrocyte ghosts: effects of various treatments, *J. Membr. Biol.,* 6, 138, 1971.

83. **Tanner, M. J. A. and Gray, W. R.,** The isolation and functional identification of a protein from the human erythrocyte 'ghost', *Biochem. J.,* 125, 1109, 1971.

84. **Kant, J. A. and Steck, T. L.,** Specificity in the association of glyceraldehyde 3-phosphate dehydrogenase with isolated human erythrocyte membranes, *J. Biol. Chem.,* 248, 8457, 1973.

85. **Shin, B. C. and Carraway, K. L.,** Association of glyceraldehyde 3-phosphate dehydrogenase with the human erythrocyte membrane, *J. Biol. Chem.,* 248, 1436, 1973.

86. **McDaniel, C. F., Kirtley, M. E., and Tanner, M. J. A.,** The interaction of glyceraldehyde 3-phosphate dehydrogenase with human erythrocyte membranes, *J. Biol. Chem.,* 249, 6478, 1974.

87. **Arese, P., Bosia, A., Pescarmona, G. P., and Till, U.,** 2,3-diphosphoglycerate synthesis by human white ghosts, *FEBS Lett.,* 49, 33, 1974.

88. **Fischer, S., Nagel, R. L., Bookchin, R. M., Roth, E. F., Jr., and Tellez-Nagel, I.,** The binding of hemoglobin to membranes of normal and sickle erythrocytes, *Biochim. Biophys. Acta,* 375, 422, 1975.

89. **Bank, A., Mears, G., Weiss, R., O'Donnell, J. V., and Natta, C.,** Preferential binding of Beta^s globin chains associated with stroma in sickle cell disorders, *J. Clin. Invest.,* 54, 805, 1974.

90. **Lessin, L. S., Kurantsin-Mills, J., Wallas, C., and Weems, H.,** Membrane alterations in irreversibly sickled cells: hemoglobin-membrane interaction, *J. Supramol. Struct.,* 9, 537, 1978.

91. **Asakura, T., Minakata, K., Adachi, K., Russell, M. O., and Schwartz, E.,** Denatured hemoglobin in sickle erythrocytes, *J. Clin. Invest.,* 59, 633, 1977.

92. **Sears, D. A., Friedman, J. M., and White, D. R.,** Binding of intracellular protein to the erythrocyte membrane during incubation: the production of Heinz bodies, *J. Lab. Clin. Med.,* 86, 722, 1975.

93. **Gourley, D. R. H.,** The role of adenosine triphosphate in the transport of phosphate in the human erythrocyte, *Arch. Biochem. Biophys.,* 40, 1, 1952.

94. **Prankerd, T. A. J. and Altman, K. I.,** A study of the metabolism of phosphorus in mammalian red cells, *Biochem. J.,* 58, 622, 1954.

95. **Gerlach, E., Fleckenstein, A., Gross, E., and Lübben, K.,** Der intermediäre Phosphat-Stoffwechsel des Menschen-Erythrocyten, *Pfluegers Arch.,* 266, 528, 1958.

96. **Schrier, S. L.,** Transfer of inorganic phosphate across human erythrocyte membranes, *J. Lab. Clin. Med.,* 75, 422, 1970.

97. **Rose, I. A. and Warms, J. V. B.,** Control of red cell glycolysis. The cause of triose phosphate accumulation, *J. Biol. Chem.,* 245, 4009, 1970.

98. **Till, U., Köhler, W., Ruschke, I., Köhler, A., and Lösche, W.,** Compartmentation of orthophosphate and adenine nucleotides in human red cells, *Eur. J. Biochem.,* 35, 167, 1973.

99. **Niehaus, W. G., Jr. and Hammerstedt, R. H.,** Mode of orthophosphate uptake and ATP labeling by mammalian cells, *Biochim. Biophys. Acta,* 443, 515, 1976.

100. **Latzkovits, L., Fajszi, Cs., and Szentistványi, I.,** Tracer kinetic analysis of phosphate incorporation into erythrocytes in vitro. II. Model analysis of the system with the ATP pool not in steady state, *Acta Biochim. Biophys. Acad. Sci. Hung.,* 7, 307, 1972.

101. **Shoemaker, D. G., Bender, C. A., and Gunn, R. B.,** Sodium-phosphate cotransport in human red blood cells. Kinetics and role of membrane metabolism, *J. Gen. Physiol.,* 92, 449, 1988.

102. **Schrier, S. L.,** Organization of enzymes in human erythrocyte membranes, *Am. J. Physiol.,* 210, 139, 1966.

103. **Schrier, S. L.,** ATP synthesis in human erythrocyte membranes, *Biochim. Biophys. Acta,* 135, 591, 1967.

104. **Steck, T. L.,** Preparation of impermeable inside-out and right-side-out vesicles from erythrocyte membranes, in *Methods in Membrane Biology,* Vol. 2, Korn, E. D., Ed., Plenum Press, New York, 1974, 245.

105. **Steck, T. L., Fairbanks, G., and Wallach, D. F. H.,** Disposition of the major proteins in the isolated erythrocyte membrane. Proteolytic dissection, *Biochemistry,* 10, 2617, 1971.

106. **Carraway, K. L. and Shin, B. C.,** Specific modification, isolation, and partial characterization of an erythrocyte membrane protein, *J. Biol. Chem.,* 247, 2102, 1972.

107. **Solti, M. and Friedrich, P.,** Partial reversible inactivation of enzymes due to binding to the human erythrocyte membrane, *Mol. Cell. Biochem.,* 10, 145, 1976.

108. **Strapazon, E. and Steck, T. L.,** Binding of rabbit muscle aldolase to band 3, the predominant polypeptide of the human erythrocyte membrane, *Biochemistry,* 15, 1421, 1976.

109. **Strapazon, E. and Steck, T. L.,** Interaction of the aldolase and the membrane of human erythrocytes, *Biochemistry,* 16, 2966, 1977.

110. **Karadsheh, N. S. and Uyeda, K.,** Changes in allosteric properties of phosphofructokinase bound to erythrocyte membranes, *J. Biol. Chem.,* 252, 7418, 1977.

111. **Higashi, T., Richards, C. S., and Uyeda, K.,** The interaction of phosphofructokinase with erythrocyte membranes, *J. Biol. Chem.,* 254, 9542, 1979.

112. **Jenkins, J. D., Kezdy, F. J., and Steck, T. L.,** Mode of interaction of phosphofructokinase with the erythrocyte membrane, *J. Biol. Chem.,* 260, 10426, 1985.

113. **Michalak, K., Gutowicz, J., and Modrzycka, T.,** Fluorescent probe studies on binding of glyceraldehyde-3-phosphate dehydrogenase to phosphatidylinositol liposomes, *FEBS Lett.,* 219, 233, 1987.

114. **Jay, D. G.,** Characterization of the chicken erythrocyte anion exchange protein, *J. Biol. Chem.,* 258, 9431, 1983.

115. **Wooster, M. S. and Wrigglesworth, J. M.,** Modification of glyceraldehyde 3-phosphate dehydrogenase activity by adsorption on phospholipid vesicles, *Biochem. J.,* 159, 627, 1976.

116. **Wrigglesworth, J. M., Keokitichai, S., Wooster, M. S., and Millar, F. A.,** Modification of glyceraldehyde 3-phosphate dehydrogenase activity by adsorption to erythrocyte membranes and phospholipid vesicles, *Biochem. Soc. Trans.,* 4, 637, 1976.

117. **Eby, D. and Kirtley, M. E.,** Isolation and characterization of glyceraldehyde-3-phosphate dehydrogenase from human erythrocyte membranes, *Arch. Biochem. Biophys.,* 198, 608, 1979.

118. **Tsai, I.-H., Prasanna Murthy, S. N., and Steck, T. L.,** Effect of red cell membrane binding on the catalytic activity of glyceraldehyde-3-phosphate dehydrogenase, *J. Biol. Chem.,* 257, 1438, 1982.

119. **Shulman, R. G.,** High resolution NMR *in vivo, Trends Biochem. Sci.,* 13, 37, 1988.

120. **Calissano, P., Alema, S., and Rusca, G.,** Effect of haemoglobin on liposome permeability to Rb⁺ and other solutes, *Biochim. Biophys. Acta,* 255, 1009, 1972.

121. **Fromherz, P., Peters, J., Müldner, H. G., and Otting, W.,** An infrared spectroscopic study on the lipid-protein interaction in an artificial lamellar system, *Biochim. Biophys. Acta,* 274, 644, 1972.

122. **Papahadjopoulos, D., Cowden, M., and Kimelberg, H.,** Role of cholesterol in membranes. Effects on phospholipid-protein interactions, membrane permeability and enzymatic activity, *Biochim. Biophys. Acta,* 330, 8, 1973.

123. **Papahadjopoulos, D., Moscarello, M., Eylar, E. H., and Isac, T.,** Effects of proteins on thermotropic phase transitions of phospholipid membranes, *Biochim. Biophys. Acta,* 401, 317, 1975.

124. **Bossi, L., Alema, S., Calissano, P., and Marra, E.,** Interaction of different forms of haemoglobin with artificial lipid membranes, *Biochim. Biophys. Acta,* 375, 477, 1975.

125. **Szundi, I., Szelényi, J. G., Breuer, J. H., and Bérczi, A.,** Interactions of haemoglobin with erythrocyte membrane phospholipids in monomolecular lipid layers, *Biochim. Biophys. Acta,* 595, 41, 1980.

126. **Shviro, Y., Zilber, I., and Shaklai, N.,** The interaction of hemoglobin with phosphatidylserine vesicles, *Biochim. Biophys. Acta,* 687, 63, 1982.

127. **Szebeni, J., Hauser, H., Eskelson, C. D., Watson, R. R., and Winterhalter, K. H.,** Interaction of hemoglobin derivatives with liposomes. Membrane cholesterol protects against the changes of hemoglobin, *Biochemistry,* 27, 6425, 1988.

128. **Shaklai, N., Yguerabide, J., and Ranney, H. M.,** Interaction of hemoglobin with red blood cell membranes as shown by a fluorescent chromophore, *Biochemistry,* 16, 5585, 1977.

129. **Shaklai, N., Yguerabide, J., and Ranney, H. M.,** Classification and localization of hemoglobin binding sites on the red blood cell membrane, *Biochemistry,* 16, 5593, 1977.

130. **Salhany, J. M., Cordes, K. A., and Gaines, E. D.,** Light-scattering measurements of hemoglobin binding to the erythrocyte membrane. Evidence for transmembrane effects related to a disulfonic stilbene binding to band 3, *Biochemistry,* 19, 1447, 1980.

131. **Shaklai, N. and Sharma, V. S.,** Kinetic study of the interaction of oxy- and deoxyhemoglobins with the erythrocyte membrane, *Proc. Natl. Acad. Sci U.S.A.,* 77, 7147, 1980.

132. **Salhany, J. M. and Shaklai, N.,** Functional properties of human hemoglobin bound to the erythrocyte membrane, *Biochemistry,* 18, 893, 1979.

133. **Cordes, K. A. and Salhany, J. M.,** Cytosolic protein binding to band-3 protein inhibits endocytosis of isolated human erythrocyte membranes, *Biochem. J.,* 207, 595, 1982.

134. **Low, P. S., Allen, D. P., Zioncheck, T. F., Chari, P., Willardson, B. M., Geahlen, R. L., and Harrison, M. L.,** Tyrosine phosphorylation of band 3 inhibits peripheral protein binding, *J. Biol. Chem.,* 262, 4592, 1987.

135. **Rauenbuehler, P. B., Cordes, K. A., and Salhany, J. M.,** Identification of the hemoglobin binding sites on the inner surface of the erythrocyte membrane, *Biochim. Biophys. Acta,* 692, 361, 1982.

136. **Chaimanee, P. and Yuthavong, Y.,** Binding of haemoglobin to spectrin of human erythrocytes, *FEBS Lett.,* 78, 119, 1977.

137. **Cassoly, R.,** Evidence against the binding of native hemoglobin to spectrin of human erythrocytes, *FEBS Lett.,* 85, 357, 1978.

138. **Liu, S.-C. and Palek, J.,** Hemoglobin enhances the self-association of spectrin heterodimers in human erythrocytes, *J. Biol. Chem.* 259, 11556, 1984.

139. **Wiedenmann, B. and Elbaum, D.,** Effect of hemoglobin A and S on human erythrocyte ghosts, *J. Biol. Chem.* 258, 5483, 1983.

140. **Lebbar, I., Stetzkowski-Marden, F., Mauffret, O., and Cassoly, R.,** Interactions of actin and tubulin with human deoxyhemoglobin. Their possible occurrence within erythrocytes, *Eur. J. Biochem.,* 170, 273, 1987.

141. **Podolski, J. L. and Steck, T. L.,** Association of deoxyribonuclease I with the pointed ends of actin filaments in human red blood cell membrane skeletons, *J. Biol. Chem.,* 263, 638, 1988.

142 **Prasanna-Murthy, S. N., Kaul, R. K., and Köhler, H.,** Hemoglobin binds to the amino-terminal 23-residue fragment of human erythrocyte band 3 protein, *Hoppe Seyler's Z. Physiol. Chem.,* 365, 9, 1984.

143. **Eaton, J. W., Tsai, M. Y., Leida, M. N., and Branda, R.,** Red cell anion channel blockade: extracellular modulation of internal membrane function, *Prog. Clin. Biol. Res.,* 55, 409, 1981.

144. **Olson, J. S., Andersen, M. E., and Gibson, Q. H.,** The dissociation of the first oxygen molecule from some mammalian oxyhemoglobins, *J. Biol. Chem.,* 246, 5919, 1971.

145. **Allen, D. W., Cadman, S., McCann, S. R., and Finkel, B.,** Increased membrane binding of erythrocyte catalase in hereditary spherocytosis and in metabolically stressed normal cells, *Blood,* 49, 113, 1977.

146. **Snyder, L. M., Liu, S. C., Palek, J., Bulat, P., Edelstein, L., Srivastava, S. K, and Fortier, N. L.,** Partition of catalase and its peroxidase activities in human red cell membrane. Effect of ATP depletion, *Biochim. Biophys. Acta,* 470, 290, 1977.

147. **Deas, J. E., Lee, L. T., and Howe, C.,** Peripheral proteins of human erythrocytes, *Biochem. Biophys. Res. Commun.,* 82, 296, 1978.

148. **Aviram, I. and Shaklai, N.,** The association of human erythrocyte catalase with the cell membrane, *Arch. Biochem. Biophys.,* 212, 329, 1981.

149. **Habib-Mohamed, A. and Steck, T. L.,** Band 3 tyrosine kinase. Association with the human erythrocyte membrane, *J. Biol. Chem.,* 261, 2804, 1986.

150. **Waugh, S. M. and Low, P. S.,** Hemichrome binding to band 3: nucleation of Heinz bodies on the erythrocyte membrane, *Biochemistry,* 24, 34, 1985.

151. **Waugh, S. M., Walder, J. A., and Low, P. S.,** Partial characterization of the copolymerization reaction of erythrocyte membrane band 3 with hemichromes, *Biochemistry,* 26, 1777, 1987.

152. **Low, P. S., Waugh, S. M., Zinke, K., and Drenckhahn, D.,** The role of hemoglobin denaturation and band 3 clustering in red blood cell aging, *Science,* 227, 531, 1985.

153. **Waugh, S. M., Willardson, B. M., Kannan, R., Labotka, R. J., and Low, P.S.,** Heinz bodies induce clustering of band 3 glycophorin and ankyrin in sickle cell erythrocytes, *J. Clin. Invest.,* 78, 1155, 1986.

154. **Kannan, R., Labotka, R., and Low, P. S,** Isolation and characterization of the hemichrome-stabilized membrane protein aggregates from sickle erythrocytes. Major site of autologous antibody binding. *J. Biol. Chem.,* 263, 13766, 1988.

155. **Schlüter, K. and Drenckhahn, D.,** Co-clustering of denatured hemoglobin with band 3: its role in binding of autoantibodies against band 3 to abnormal and aged erythrocytes, *Proc. Natl. Acad. Sci. U.S.A.,* 83, 6137, 1986.

156. **Mueller, T. J., Jackson, C. W., Dockter, M. E., and Morrison, M.,** Membrane skeletal alterations during *in vivo* mouse red cell aging. Increase in the band 4.1a and 4.1b ratio, *J. Clin. Invest.,* 79, 492, 1987.

157. **Fischbeck, K. H., Bonilla, E., and Schotland, D. L.,** Freeze-fracture characterization of "young" and "old" human erythrocytes, *Biochim. Biophys. Acta,* 685, 207, 1982.

158. **Gaczynska, M. and Bartosz, G.,** Crosslinking of membrane proteins during erythrocyte ageing, *Int. J. Biochem.* 18, 377, 1986.

159. **Kay, M. M. B., Bosman, G. J. C. G. M., Shapiro, S. S., Bendich, A., and Bassel, P. S.,** Oxidation as a possible mechanism of cellular aging: vitamin E deficiency causes premature aging and IgG binding to erythrocytes, *Proc. Natl. Acad. Sci. U.S.A.,* 83, 2463, 1986.

160. **Bartosz, G. and Gwozdzinski, K.,** Aging of the erythrocyte. Changes in the permeation of spin-labeled electrolytes, *Am. J. Hematol.,* 14, 377, 1983.

161. **Zanner, M. A. and Galey, W. R.,** Aged human erythrocytes exhibit increased anion exchange, *Biochim. Biophys. Acta,* 818, 310, 1985.

162. **Aminoff, D., Ghalambor, M. A., and Henrich, C. J.,** GOST, galactose oxidase and sialyl transferase, substrate and receptor sites in erythrocyte senescence, *Prog. Clin. Biol. Res.,* 56, 269, 1981.

163. **Kay, M. M. B.,** Mechanism of removal of senescent cells by human macrophages *in situ, Proc. Natl. Acad. Sci., U.S.A.,* 72, 3521, 1975.

164. **Lelkes, G., Fodor, I., Lelkes, G., Hollán, S. R., and Verkleij, A. J.,** The distribution and aggregatability of intramembrane particles in phenylhydrazine-treated human erythrocytes, *Biochim. Biophys. Acta,* 945, 105, 1988.

165. **Gahmberg, C. G., Myllyla, G., Leikola, J., Pirkola, A., and Nordling, S.,** Absence of the major sialoglycoprotein in the membrane of human En(a-) erythrocytes and increased glycosylation of band 3, *J. Biol. Chem.,* 251, 6108, 1976.

166. **Lorand, L., and Michalska, M.,** Altered response of stored red cells to Ca^{2+} stress, *Blood,* 65, 1025, 1985.

167. **Morison, M., Au, K. S., and Hsu, L.,** Are the red cell proteases a clock mechanism which turns on a signal of senescence? *Biomed. Biochim. Acta,* 46, S79, 1987.

168. **Passow, H., Fasold, H., Gärtner, E. M., Legrum, B., Ruffing, W., and Zaki, L.,** Anion transport across the red blood cell membrane and the conformation of the protein in band 3, *Ann. N.Y. Acad. Sci.,* 341, 361, 1980.

169. **Low, P. S.,** Specific cation modulation of anion transport across the human erythrocyte membrane, *Biochim. Biophys. Acta,* 514, 264, 1978.

170. **Wilson, J. E., Reid, S., and Masters, C. J.,** A comparative study of the binding of aldolase and glyceraldehyde-3-phosphate dehydrogenase to the human erythrocyte membrane, *Arch. Biochem. Biophys.,* 215, 610, 1982.

171. **Prasanna-Murthy, S. N., Liu, T., Kaul, R. K., Köhler, H., and Steck, T. L.,** The aldolase-binding site of the human erythrocyte membrane is at the NH_2 terminus of band 3, *J. Biol. Chem.,* 256, 11203, 1981.

172. **Kirschner-Zilber, I. and Shaklai, N.,** The interaction of hemoglobin with isolated band 3 cytoplasmic fragments, *Biochem. Int.,* 4, 297, 1982.

173. **Moriyama, R. and Makino, S.,** Interaction of glyceraldehyde-3-phosphate dehydrogenase with the cytoplasmic pole of band 3 from bovine erythrocyte membrane: the mode of association and identification of the binding site of band 3 polypeptide, *Arch. Biochem. Biophys.,* 256, 606, 1987.

174. **Kaul, R. K., Prasanna-Murthy, S. N., Reddy, A. G., Steck, T. L., and Kohler, H.,** Amino acid sequence of the N-alpha-terminal 201 residues of human erythrocyte membrane band 3, *J. Biol. Chem.,* 258, 7981, 1983.

175. **Kirschner-Zilber, I. and Shaklai, N.,** The specificity of hemoglobin for band 3 membrane sites, *Biochem. Int.,* 5, 309, 1982.

176. **Cassoly, R. and Salhany, J. M.,** Spectral and oxygen release kinetic properties of human hemoglobin bound to the cytoplasmic fragment of band 3 protein in solution, *Biochim. Biophys. Acta,* 745, 134, 1983.

177. **Sayare, M. and Fikiet, M.,** Cross-linking of hemoglobin to the cytoplasmic surface of human erythrocyte membranes. Identification of band 3 as a site for hemoglobin binding in Cu^{2+}-*o*-phenanthroline catalyzed cross-linking, *J. Biol. Chem.,* 256, 13152, 1981.

178. **Salhany, J. M., Cordes, K. A., Gaines, E. D., and Rauenbuehler, P. B.,** Interaction of hemoglobin with the anion transport protein of the erythrocyte membrane, in *Hemoglobin and Oxygen Binding,* Chien, H., Ed., Elsevier, New York, 1982, 283.

179. **Beth, A. H., Balasubramanian, K., Wilder, R. T., Venkataramu, S. D., Robinson, B. H., Dalton, L. R., Pearson, D. E., and Park, J. H.,** Structural and motional changes in glyceraldehyde-3-phosphate dehydrogenase upon binding to the band 3 protein of the erythrocyte membrane examined with [^{15}N,^{2}H] maleimide spin label and electron paramagnetic resonance, *Proc. Natl. Acad. Sci. U.S.A.,* 78, 4955, 1981.

180. **Cassoly, R.,** Interaction of hemoglobin with the red blood cell membrane. A saturation transfer electron paramagnetic resonance study, *Biochim. Biophys. Acta,* 689, 203, 1982.

181. **Walder, J. A., Chatterjee, R., Steck, T. L., Low, P. S., Musso, G. F., Kaiser, E. T., Rogers, P. H., and Arnone, A.,** The interaction of hemoglobin with the cytoplasmic domain of band 3 of the human erythrocyte membrane, *J. Biol. Chem.,* 259, 10238, 1984.

182. **Phan-Dinh-Tuy, F., Henry, J., and Kahn, A.,** Characterization of human red blood cell tyrosine kinase, *Biochem. Biophys. Res. Commun.,* 126, 304, 1985.

183. **Tsuneshige, A., Imai, K., and Tyuma, I.,** The binding of hemoglobin to red cell membrane lowers its oxygen affinity, *J. Biochem. (Tokyo),* 101, 695, 1987.

184. **Cassoly, R.,** Quantitative analysis of the association of human hemoglobin with the cytoplasmic fragment of band 3 protein, *J. Biol. Chem.,* 258, 3859, 1983.

185. **Grinstein, S., Ship, S., and Rothstein, A.,** Anion transport in relation to proteolytic dissection of band 3 protein, *Biochim. Biophys. Acta,* 507, 294, 1978.

186. **Ducis, I., Kandrach, A., and Racker, E.,** Stimulation of ^{32}P$_i$ transport into human erythrocyte ghosts and reconstituted vesicles by Mg^{2+} and hemoglobin, *J. Biol. Chem.,* 263, 8544, 1988.

187. **Rao, A., Reinhart, P. M., Reithmeier, R. A. F., and Cantley, L. C.,** Location of the stilbenedisulfonate binding site of the human erythrocyte anion-exchange system by resonance energy transfer, *Biochemistry,* 18, 4505, 1979.

188. **Jánosházi, Á., Ojcius, D. M., and Solomon, A. K.,** Possible role for the cytoskeleton in coupling anion exchange and cation transport proteins in human red cells, *J. Gen. Physiol.,* 90, 22a, 1987.

189. **Verkman, A. S., Dix, J. A., and Solomon, A. K.,** Anion transport inhibitor binding to band 3 in red blood cell membranes, *J. Gen. Physiol.,* 81, 421, 1983.

190. **Appell, K. C. and Low, P. S.,** Evaluation of structural interdependence of membrane-spanning and cytoplasmic domains of band 3, *Biochemistry,* 21, 2151, 1982.

191. **Premachandra, B. R.,** Interaction of hemoglobin and its component alpha and beta chains with band 3 protein, *Biochemistry,* 25, 3455, 1986.

192. **Shaklai, N. and Abrahami, H.,** The interaction of deoxyhemoglobin with the red cell membrane, *Biochem. Biophys. Res. Commun.,* 95, 1105, 1980.

193. **Salhany, J. M. and Cassoly, R.,** Kinetics of *p*-mercuribenzoate binding to the sulfhydryl groups on the isolated cytoplasmic fragment of band 3 protein. Effect of hemoglobin binding on the conformation, *J. Biol. Chem.,* 264, 1399, 1989.

194. **Solti, M., Bartha, F., Halász, N., Tóth, G., Sirokmán, F., and Friedrich, P.,** Localization of glyceraldehyde-3-phosphate dehydrogenase in intact human erythrocytes. Evaluation of membrane adherence in autoradiographs at low grain density, *J. Biol. Chem.,* 256, 9260, 1981.

195. **Yeltman, D. R. and Harris, B. G.,** Localization and membrane association of aldolase in human erythrocytes, *Arch. Biochem. Biophys.,* 199, 186, 1980.

196. **Keokitichai, S. and Wrigglesworth, J. M.,** Association of glyceraldehyde 3-phosphate dehydrogenase with the membrane of the intact human erythrocyte, *Biochem. J.,* 187, 837, 1980.

197. **Kliman, H. J. and Steck, T. L.,** Association of glyceraldehyde 3-phosphate dehydrogenase with the human red cell membrane. A kinetic analysis, *J. Biol. Chem.,* 255, 6314, 1980.

198. **Jenkins, J. D., Madden, D. P., and Steck, T. L.,** Association of phosphofructokinase and aldolase with the membrane of the intact erythrocyte, *J. Biol. Chem.,* 259, 9374, 1984.

199. **Szabolcsi, G. and Cseke, E.,** On the molecular sieving property of the human erythrocyte membrane. Localization of some proteins within the cell, *Acta Biol. Med. Ger.,* 40, 471, 1981.

200. **Rich, G. T., Pryor, J. S., and Dawson, A. P.,** Lack of binding of glyceraldehyde-3-phosphate dehydrogenase to erythrocyte membranes under *in vivo* conditions, *Biochim. Biophys. Acta,* 817, 61, 1985.

201. **Brindle, K. M., Campbell, I. D., and Simpson, R. J.,** A ^{1}H n.m.r. study of the kinetic properties expressed by glyceraldehyde phosphate dehydrogenase in the intact human erythrocyte, *Biochem. J.,* 208, 583, 1982.

202. **Fossel, E. T. and Solomon, A. K.,** Membrane mediated link between ion transport and metabolism in human red cells, *Biochim. Biophys. Acta,* 464, 82, 1977.

203. **Fossel, E. T. and Solomon, A. K.,** Ouabain-sensitive interaction between human red cell membrane and glycolytic enzyme complex in cytosol, *Biochim. Biophys. Acta,* 510, 99, 1978.

204. **Fossel, E. T. and Solomon, A. K.,** Effect of the sodium/potassium ratio on glyceraldehyde 3-phosphate dehydrogenase interaction with red cell vesicles, *Biochim. Biophys. Acta,* 553, 142, 1979.

205. **Fossel, E. T. and Solomon, A. K.,** Relation between red cell membrane ($Na^+ + K^+$)-ATPase and band 3 protein, *Biochim. Biophys. Acta,* 649, 557, 1981.

206. **Friedrich, P., Apró-Kovács, V.A., and Solti, M.,** Study of metabolite compartmentation in erythrocyte glycolysis, *FEBS Lett.,* 84, 183, 1977.

207. **Eisinger, J., Flores, J., and Salhany, J. M.,** Association of cytosol hemoglobin with the membrane in intact erythrocytes, *Proc. Natl. Acad. Sci. U.S.A.,* 79, 408, 1982.

208. **Eisinger, J. and Flores, J.,** Cytosol-membrane interface of human erythrocytes. A resonance energy transfer study, *Biophys. J.,* 41, 367, 1983.

209. **Fung, L. W.-M.,** Spin-label detection of hemoglobin-membrane interaction at physiological pH, *Biochemistry,* 20, 7162, 1981.

210. **Chetrite, G. and Cassoly, R.,** Affinity of hemoglobin for the cytoplasmic fragment of human erythrocyte membrane band 3. Equilibrium measurements at physiological pH using matrix-bound proteins: the effects of ionic strength, deoxygenation and of 2,3-diphosphoglycerate, *J. Mol. Biol.,* 185, 639, 1985.

211. **Salhany, J. M., Pingerelli, P., Baxter, P., and Mizukami, H.,** unpublished observations.

212. **Rogalski, A. A., Steck, T. L., and Waseem, A.,** Association of Glyceraldehyde-3-phosphate dehydrogenase with the plasma membrane of intact human red blood cells, *J. Biol.Chem.,* 264, 6438, 1989.

213. **Davis, L., Lux, S. E., and Bennett, V.,** Mapping the ankyrin-binding site of the human erythrocyte anion exchanger, *J. Biol. Chem.,* 264, 9665, 1989.

214. **Clague, M. J., Harrison, J. P., and Cherry, R. J.,** Cytoskeletal restraints of band 3 rotational mobility in human erythrocyte membranes, *Biochim. Biophys. Acta,* 981, 43, 1989.

Chapter 5

BAND 3 PORTER: GENERAL CONSIDERATIONS

I. INTRODUCTION

The inclination to generalize knowledge gained from the study of the red cell to other cell systems (of which Eric Ponder spoke over 40 years ago; see the Preface) has been a successful one in certain notable instances. The work with hemoglobin is one example. Although hemoglobin is a very specialized protein, much has been learned about allosteric protein structure and function by its study. Perutz's structural work[1] laid important foundations for the interpretation of function, while the allosteric theory of Monod and co-workers[2] and Koshland and co-workers[3] gave models illustrating how spatially separated active sites on "working" proteins could communicate through changes in subunit conformation and quaternary structure. It is in this spirit that we may hope that a study of the band 3 porter mechanism will teach us general laws for porter function. Because of its abundance and the increasing interest in this function, band 3 may contribute to porter molecular biology what hemoglobin contributed to the study of allosteric proteins in solution.

In this chapter three topics will be considered. One is whether there are other functions for band 3. Potentially important functions which have been assigned to band 3 include water and organic anion transport. There is some indication that band 3 could transport glucose (although this is not currently in favor). A second topic is whether band 3 exists in other cell membranes or whether it may even be an ubiquitous protein. Considering the ubiquity of carbonic anhydrase and the related need to transport bicarbonate for chloride, band 3 ubiquity seems plausible. The third and final topic for consideration is whether the allosteric homotropic dimer hypothesis for porter function can be generally applied to all membrane proteins which show porter functional characteristics.

II. OTHER TRANSPORT FUNCTIONS OF BAND 3

A. ORGANIC ACID TRANSPORT

The range of anions which can be transported by the band 3 system is rather unbelievable.[4] These include a wide variety of organic anions.[5-8] Organic anions may penetrate the red cell as either the dissociated or undissociated acid.[6] Aromatic and aliphatic sulfonic acids have very low pKs and penetrate the membrane as anions, as do dicarboxylic acids.[4] Aliphatic and aromatic monocarboxylic acids (except formic acid) primarily penetrate in the uncharged form. Anions which penetrate in the ionic form largely use the chloride-bicarbonate system (band 3) of the red cell.[6] Giebel and Passow[9] and Aubert and Motais[10] have studied variation of the penetration rates of various organic acids as a function of the chemical characteristics of the substrate. The evidence suggested that the intercharge distance may not exceed 3.7 Å.[10] Larger molecules with hydrophobic character in addition to an anionic moiety may be transported by using hydrophobic parts of the molecule normally not accessible to physiological anions, while the anionic moiety somehow continues to make contact with the transport site. There are certain specific structural features of organic anion transport which are important.[6,10] For example, the penetration of amino substituted benzene sulfonates is sensitive to the relative position of the amino and the sulfonic groups. Para amino sulfonic acid penetrates much faster than the 3-amino derivative, while the 2-amino derivative does not enter at all. On this basis Aubert and Motais[10] suggested a three-point attachment of electronegative oxygen atoms to binding sites of the transport system.

Monocarboxylic acids penetrate by using band 3[5,7,8] and by using a specific porter in the membrane.[11-14] Rabbit erythrocytes seem to have more copies of this carrier than human red cells, and the specific protein responsible for transport has been identified.[13,14] This porter is important because the major pathway for energy metabolism in the red cell is glycolysis which produces monocarboxylic acids as products. It is also possible that the red cell porter could participate in the clearance of monocarboxylic acids produced by muscles during exercise (a speculation).

B. WATER AND UREA TRANSPORT

In 1957, Paganelli and Solomon[15] measured water diffusion across the human red cell membrane and proposed that the membrane was traversed by an "equivalent pore" of radius 3.5 Å. Several kinetic studies of water transport further characterized this function of the red cell membrane.[16-19] The involvement of a protein sulfhydryl in water transport inhibition was established by Macey and Farmer[20] using *p*-chloromercuribenzenesulfonate (pCMBS). pCMBS can induce a large cation leak in human red cells, but it has little effect on anion exchange.[21] Addition of SITS (4-acetamido-4′-isothiocyano-2,2′-stilbene disulfonate) to cells can block the uptake of pCMBS, yet SITS does not affect the pCMBS-induced leak of cations.[22] pCMBS inhibits water transport by binding to a "cryptic" sulfhydryl group on CH17 of band 3.[23-25]

When Macey[26] reviewed the evidence, he pointed out that the kinetics of pCMBS inhibition of urea transport was much faster than the kinetics of inhibition of water transport. Toon and Solomon[27] were able to determine the constants of binding to the functional urea site and the functional water site. On the basis of this and other kinetic arguments, Toon and Solomon[27] suggested that the urea inhibition site is also on band 3. However, Benga and co-workers[28,29] suggested the involvement of band 4.5 protein after using gel electrophoresis to assign sites. There is, unfortunately, a major problem in the use of pCMBS in site-assignment studies with gel electrophoresis. Rao[30] discovered that bound pCMBS is labile. Radioactivity can be slowly lost during electrophoresis and staining procedures.

Ojcius and co-workers[31,32] have presented evidence which appears to clarify the use of pCMBS in gel electrophoresis experiments. These papers support a band 3 location for the urea and water pCMBS inhibitory sites. The binding stoichiometries for each site show one urea inhibition site and three water inhibition sites for every four band 3 molecules. Such stoichiometries suggest that a band 3 tetramer may form the aqueous pore, in agreement with previous suggestions for both water[25] and urea[33] transport. New cross-linking evidence of Salhany and Sloan[34] suggests that band 3 can exist as a tetramer in the intact red cell, making Solomon's functional tetrameric arguments somewhat more tenable. On the other hand, Fröhlich and Jones[35] have recently added 4,4′-dinitrostibene-2,2′-disulfonate (DNDS) to band 3 and showed that urea transport was unaffected. They suggest that the absence of an effect means that urea uses another protein. It is somewhat difficult to see how a negative result on urea transport using an anion transport inhibitor leads to a conclusion that band 3 is not involved in urea transport. If the band 3 tetrameric state exists before and after addition of DNDS (albeit in a different anion functional state), an effect of DNDS would not be expected.

One interesting observation of Ojcius and co-workers[32] was that hemolysis and gradual removal of hemoglobin caused a severe attenuation in the ability of pCMBS to inhibit both water and urea transport. This effect would fit with the view developed in Chapter 4 that cytoskeletal and perhaps cytosolic protein associations can modulate band 3 function. Although water transport per se was not changed, urea transport was drastically reduced. This indicates that pCMBS binding to band 3 allosterically inhibits water transport. The pCMBS inhibition site should be located either on a domain of band 3 separate from the parts of the protein intimate to the water channel or on an adjacent protein.

It is worth noting that the location of the pCMBS water inhibitory site is thought to be on the CH17 subdomain of band 3.[25] Salhany and co-workers[36] have identified a very subtle conformational change in CH17 which occurs upon hemolysis. Evidence exists that hemolysis changes the rotational mobility of band 3,[37] presumably by disrupting cytoskeletal contacts. There is a CH17 mutant form of band 3 which shows a higher anion transport rate and lower ankyrin-binding capacity.[38] The mechanism involved may be related to changes in the state of band 3 association. Dix and co-workers[33] reported a radiation inactivation target size for urea transport consistent with the tetramer. However, in similar studies Verkman and co-workers[39] found that pCMBS inhibition of water transport yields a target size of 31 kDa which is inconsistent with an oligomeric functional unit. Could the pCMBS inhibition effect be associated with changes in the association state of band 3 in the membrane? Benz and co-workers[40] have tested this possibility and state that incubation of 4,4′-diisothiocyano-1,2-diphenylethane-2,2′-disulfonate (H_2DIDS) or pCMBS with band 3 does not influence the self-association state of the protein. However, Makino and co-workers[41] have recently reported that stilbene disulfonates do change the association state of band 3 in detergent solutions. *In situ* tests are needed. Other papers on the measurement and properties of the water and urea transport system of red cells should be consulted.[42-61]

C. GLUCOSE TRANSPORT

The glucose transporter of the red cell has been among one of the most widely studied transport systems.[62-64] One of the major controversies in this field has been the identification of the protein responsible for glucose transport in the red cell. The two candidates are band 3 and band 4.5. Langdon and co-workers[65-68] presented evidence, that band 3 is the glucose carrier, from experiments using the glucose affinity probe maltosylisothiocyanate (MITC) and from reconstitution studies. However, there is much evidence to suggest that a distinct protein in band 4.5 contains the glucose transport activity.[69-83] Reconstitution studies show that band 4.5 has glucose transport activity. Recombinant DNA techniques show that the protein in this region has a completely different amino acid sequence than band 3.[84] Yet, in recent studies, May[85] showed that MITC was specifically bound to band 3. It irreversibly inhibited both DIDS labeling of band 3 and sulfate uptake. Enough DIDS to completely inhibit anion transport was not sufficient to significantly inhibit glucose transport, but inhibitors of glucose transport significantly inhibited dihydro-DIDS binding to band 3. On the other hand, it is worth pointing out that Lowe and Walmsley[86] have made "half-turnover" studies with the human erythrocyte glucose transport system, and the number of glucose carriers so determined was between 124,000 and 190,000. This stoichiometry would not be consistent with the number of band 3 monomers present (10^6), but it could be consistent with a band 3 tetramer functional unit.

In recent reviews, the consensus opinion is that band 4.5 is the glucose porter.[87,88] But the issue does not seem to be settled. Langdon and Holman[89] present some new and apparently persuasive evidence to support their hypothesis that band 3 transports glucose as one of its many functions. They found that monoclonal and polyclonal antibodies to epitopes on band 3 specifically remove band 3 and with it more than 90% of the reconstitutable glucose transport activity from unfractionated octylglucoside extracts of erythrocyte membranes. Western blots to whole-membrane extracts showed that the polyclonal antibody to band 4.5 used to isolate the cDNA clones[84] reacts with several bands in the band 4.5 region. One band may be a proteolyzed integral domain of band 3.[89] Langdon's basic argument is that although band 4.5 contains a protein with glucose transport activity, that activity is only a small fraction of the total and that 90% of the activity is associated with band 3. One unresolved fact is that when band 3 is reconstituted into vesicles, the glucose transport activity is not inhibitable by cytochalasin B. Since cytochalasin B is a potent inhibitor of glucose transport *in situ,* some explanation for its failure to inhibit glucose transport in the band 3 reconstituted system must be found.

III. IS BAND 3 AN UBIQUITOUS PROTEIN?

So much attention has been given to the movement of cations across plasma membranes that any associated anion transport was taken for granted. Yet, it is becoming apparent that a basic anion-exchange activity is also probably ubiquitous. Whether band 3 is ubiquitous or whether it is part of a family of such porters responsible for anion exchange is only now being studied in earnest. The evidence for the existence of a band 3-like anion-exchange function in other cells usually involves functional evidence for chloride-bicarbonate exchange,[90-96] immunological evidence,[97-103] evidence based on the use of stilbene disulfonates as potent inhibitors of anion exchange,[103-117] and more recently, genetic evidence.[118,119] The anion-transport function tends to be found in those locations where regulation of intracellular pH is important.[116,120-123] The control of intracellular pH seems regulated by the tight coupling of a sodium-proton antiport with the chloride-bicarbonate exchange function. There is also evidence that cellular volume regulation may involve these coupled antiports. For example, swelling of *Amphiuma* red cells seems to be associated with the combined effects of the sodium-proton and chloride-bicarbonate antiports.[124] The process is inhibitable by the sodium-proton inhibitor amiloride, while SITS inhibition of anion exchange unmasks a 1:1 exchange of sodium for hydrogen, also amiloride inhibitable. Although there is evidence that nonerythroid band 3-like proteins exist which have highly similar sequence homology to the integral domain of erythroid band 3,[118,119] there is also evidence that one band 3 homologue found in K562 cells (which lack band 3) has a very different mechanism.[125] The selectivity ratio of chloride to sulfate is quite considerably lower than erythrocyte band 3, and the exchanger is much less sensitive to a list of inhibitors which are potent inhibitors of band 3 anion exchange.[125]

The case for the existence of erythrocyte band 3 in the kidney seems good.[103,118,119,126] Proton is secreted in the medullary collecting duct by a proton-ATPase on the luminal membrane. Concomitant with proton release is the equivalent formation of bicarbonate within the cell which is excreted to the circulation through a chloride-bicarbonate exchange mechanism at the basolateral face of the tubular segment.[127,128] Bicarbonate reabsorption is SITS inhibitable.[127] Kopito and co-workers[118] have shown that the erythroid band 3 gene is expressed in the kidney. The erythroid and renal transcripts share a common 5' upstream nucleotide sequence, although they initiate at different sites on the sequence. The characteristics of the gene suggest tissue-specific expression mechanisms rather than overt expression of the gene in all cells. The functional characteristics of renal band 3 with regard to reversible DBDS (4,4'-dibenzamido-2,2'-disulfonic stilbene) binding seem virtually identical to the erythrocyte porter, suggesting structural similarity.[117] Finally, there has been some suggestion in a recent paper[103] that a fetal isoform of band 3 exists in the apical and basal plasma membranes of the human placental syncytiotrophoblasts. There is also evidence for DIDS inhibition of anion exchange in human placental microvillous membrane vesicles.[129]

In summary, band 3 or a family of band 3-like porters may be widely placed. However, based on the genetic analysis, tissue specificity in the expression of the gene rather than overt expression seems to be extant.

IV. IS AN ALLOSTERIC HOMOTROPIC DIMER MODEL A GENERAL MECHANISM FOR ALL PORTERS?

A. INTRODUCTION

The current general view of porter function is interesting to consider. It seems to suggest that despite the fact that most (if not all) porters are oligomeric,[130] and despite the fact that all investigators agree that some type of porter conformational change is involved, one porter monomer is considered energetically insulated from the function of its neighbor within the oligomer. What are the reasons for this view? One reason may be that there is a tendency to picture integral membrane proteins as rigidly held. Yet receptor proteins seem to respond to small ligands by changing global conformation.[131] The essence of porter function is, in the last analysis, one of linkage.[62] Solute movement in one direction is coupled to or catalyzed by solute movement in the other direction for exchange porters. Simple porter models can recycle without the assistance of the *trans* solute, but to be seen in one notable case, solute exchange is faster than net transport. Do these facts mean that two allosterically coupled active sites are involved? Do all porters use hemoglobin-like[1] or receptor-like[131] global conformational changes to link transmembrane events or activities at distinct sites on the porter? Why should the laws of protein physical chemistry (such as homotropic allosterism) somehow not be seriously considered when studying protein oligomers in a membrane? These are important questions. Of course, the ultimate answer may require the determination of the complete structure of at least one porter. The best three-dimensional structure of a transport protein is that of bacteriorhodopsin.[132] However, that protein is unique and does not follow the classic porter functionality.

If the homotropic dimer model is common to all porters, then we should look for three characteristics based on the band 3 study. We should first seek evidence that the porter is an oligomer. We should then investigate its transport kinetic patterns. Finally, we should see if a single substrate site exists in direct binding studies or if complex multisite behavior is evident. The two best-characterized porters besides band 3 porter are the ATP/ADP exchanger and the glucose porter.

B. PORTERS WHICH MAY USE A HOMOTROPIC ALLOSTERIC DIMER MECHANISM

1. ADP/ATP Exchanger of the Mitochondria

The ADP/ATP exchange porter (AEP) is a 1:1 exchanger found in mitochondria. It is part of a family of mitochondrial porters including the phosphate carrier and the uncoupling protein.[133] AEP is a dimer in the membrane and in detergent solutions. The functional binding stoichiometry of the inhibitor carboxyatractylate or the substrate ATP is 0.5 mol per mole of porter monomer. One ligand binding center requires two polypeptides. This would fit the central two-fold structure for the active site shown in Figure 5B of Chapter 1. On the other hand, the kinetics of AEP exchange show negative cooperativity, as was illustrated in Figure 12 of Chapter 1. This would be consistent with the existence of two interacting ligand binding sites, one on each porter monomer. If there were tight half-site reactivity, half-site stoichiometry could be understood, but the transport kinetics should be hyperbolic if two half-sites are tightly coupled. The observation of negative cooperativity suggests the existence of two interacting sites, one on each monomer. The inability to see a low-affinity binding site may be due to the use of relatively low ligand or inhibitor concentrations. One may need to study higher ligand concentrations to search for the expected negative cooperativity in binding.

In summary, AEP is one of the best-characterized anion-exchange porters. It has two of the properties we might expect for the allosteric homotropic dimer porter model; it exists as a dimer and shows negative cooperativity in transport. However, binding stoichiometry does not appear consistent with that model or with the observation of negative cooperativity.

2. The General Properties of the Glucose Porter

The glucose porter is one of the best-characterized porters and many reviews exist.[62-64,134-139] The monomeric structure of this porter has been deduced from the amino acid sequence.[84] The motif for structure is very similar to band 3. Hydrophobicity plots suggest 12 transmembrane helices and a 55-kDa monomer molecular weight. Freeze-fracture electron microscopic studies of the reconstituted porter show 62-Å particles, suggesting a dimeric state of association.[136] The dimeric state of association is also supported by gradient centrifugation in Triton X-100.[136] Radiation inactivation studies suggest a functional unit of 185,000, which would indicate a tetrameric state of association.[139]

What do the transport kinetics indicate? Stein is very clear in his discussion of the transport kinetics of the glucose porter.[62] He states on page 255 of his book (after showing extensive kinetic data) that "The simple carrier model must be rejected... However, the immense amount of data that has accumulated…justify their further deep study." Why does the simple carrier model fail? The analysis of the simple carrier requires that when transport is studied from both directions the ratio of the K_m for the two directions must equal the ratio of V_{max}s.[62,136] The problem arises in that the asymmetry for K_m is much greater than that for V_{max}. In addition, there seems to be a "high-affinity" site at the inner surface. This is unexpected in the simple model since that model does not explain the observation of two Michaelis constants for sugar exit and one for sugar entrance. Some authors reject the simple model based on this evidence.[62] Others propose "modifier sites".[137] But what if two porter monomers are conformationally coupled? Could the "modifier site" be a low-affinity state of the other monomer? It is interesting that glucose self-exchange is much faster than glucose net transport. Although a single site model can explain this, considering the failure of that model to explain the other features of the kinetics, perhaps two coupled monomers of a homotropic allosteric dimer is the answer. Holman[140] has suggested an allosteric pore model involving two sugar binding sites. Yet the kinetics seem hyperbolic over ranges studied. Perhaps higher sugar concentrations need to be explored.

Recently, Carruthers[141] and Helgerson and Carruthers[142] have presented clear direct binding evidence that there are two sugar binding sites per porter unit and that ATP can, by binding to a different site, modulate sugar binding. This is the evidence needed to support an allosteric interpretation of the complex kinetics. It is interesting to note that recent measurements of the kinetics of binding of an impermeant sugar analogue have shown results inconsistent with a single-site porter model.[143] The only way to make them consistent was to propose that this impermeant reagent binds to the single porter site when it faces inward. However, the loosening of model constraints to such an extent seems equivalent to discarding the model altogether. What if the low affinity second binding site is an allosterically coupled monomer, the affinity of which has been allosterically lowered due to binding of the substrate to the first monomer? Could this suggestion explain the kinetics?

Despite the evidence just discussed, there is much evidence that there is a transmembrane conformational change in the glucose porter.[137] Furthermore, nuclear magnetic resonance data show that ligand binding to one side of the membrane lowers ligand affinity at the other side.[144] Although this effect is consistent with the single site model, it would also be consistent with two allosterically coupled sites "moving back and forth" across the membrane together as in an ordered sequential model.[145] One site could be active and ligand bound, while the other would be low affinity and less active or inactive. The two sites could alternate activity during the transport cycle. Such an ordered sequential model is a mechanistically asymmetric model and has the potential to explain the mechanistic asymmetries observed.

V. CONCLUDING REMARKS

Allosteric interpretations are often at the fringe of the porter literature because a single-site monomeric model has such strong appeal owing to its simplicity. Yet, porters exist as dimeric or tetrameric structures with one or more substrate binding sites per monomer. How can we consider that there is no communication of energies between monomers when most data show complexities in substrate binding and transport? We have seen examples of transport site ligands (PLP or DNDS) which change the quaternary structure of band 3 (reversibly in the case of DNDS, see Chapter 2). Intermonomeric allosteric interaction energies must be included in any model, even if the monomer is inherently capable of transport. Allosteric effects may (and in our view probably do) dominate *in situ*. If stilbene disulfonates stop allosteric interactions while allowing unlabeled monomers to function, it does not mean that monomeric independence is the natural state. Based on our analysis, it may be argued that stilbene disulfonates create an artifactual (but interesting and historically important) condition for band 3. As work with other inhibitors progresses, we feel that stilbene disulfonates will be placed in their proper perspective as important, but unnatural ligands. Finally, we may ask why allosteric theory should be so foreign to membrane transport.

Although the mere existence of oligomers does not provide per force evidence for homotropic allosterism, allosteric models should be preferred when the kinetic and binding data are complex. Ultimately of course, more detailed structural information is needed so that the functional studies can be interpreted. Only then will it be possible to settle some of these issues.

REFERENCES

1. **Perutz, M. F.,** The haemoglobin modecule, *Proc. R. Soc. London, Ser. B,* 173, 113, 1969.
2. **Monod, J., Wyman, J., and Changeux, J.-P.,** On the nature of allosteric transitions: a plausible model, *J. Mol. Biol.,* 12, 88, 1965.
3. **Koshland, D. E., Jr., Némethy, G., and Filmer, D.,** Comparison of experimental binding data and theoretical models in proteins containing subunits, *Biochemistry,* 5, 365, 1966.
4. **Knauf, P. A.,** Erythrocyte anion exchange and the band 3 protein: transport kinetics and molecular structure, *Curr. Top. Membr. Transp.,* 12, 249, 1979.
5. **Deuticke, B.,** Properties and structural basis of simple diffusion pathways in the erythrocyte membrane, *Rev. Physiol. Biochem. Pharmacol.,* 78, 1, 1977.
6. **Motais, R.,** Organic anion transport in red blood cells, in *Membrane Transport in Red Cells,* Ellory, J.C. and Lowe, V.L., Eds., Academic Press, New York, 1977, 197.
7. **Deuticke, B.,** Kinetic properties and substrate specificity of the monocarboxylate carrier in the human erythrocyte membrane, in *Membrane Transport in Erythrocytes, Alfred Benzon Symp.* 14, Lassen, U.V., Ussing, H.H. and Wieth, J.O., Eds., Munksgaard, Copenhagen, 1980, 539.
8. **Rice, W. R. and Steck, T. L.,** Pyruvate flux into resealed ghosts from human erythrocytes, *Biochim. Biophys. Acta,* 433, 39, 1976.
9. **Giebel, O. and Passow, H.,** Die Permeabilität der Erythrocytenmembran für organishe Anionen. Zur Frage der Diffusion durch Poren, *Pfluegers Arch. Gesamte Physiol. Menschen Tiere,* 271, 378, 1960.
10. **Aubert, L. and Motais, R.,** Molecular features of organic anion permeability in ox red blood cell, *J. Physiol. (London),* 246, 159, 1975.
11. **Halestrap, A. P.,** Transport of pyruvate and lactate into human erythrocytes. Evidence for the involvement of the chloride carrier and a chloride-independent carrier, *Biochem. J.,* 156, 193, 1976.
12. **Dubinsky, W. P. and Racker, E.,** The mechanism of lactate transport in human erythrocytes, *J. Membr. Biol.,* 44, 25, 1978.
13. **Jennings, M. L. and Adams-Lackey, M.,** A rabbit erythrocyte membrane protein associated with l-lactate transport, *J. Biol. Chem.,* 257, 12866, 1982.
14. **Donovan, J. A. and Jennings, M. L.,** N-hydroxysulfosuccinimido active esters and the L-(+)-lactate transport protein in rabbit erythrocytes, *Biochemistry,* 25, 1538, 1986.
15. **Paganelli, C. V. and Solomon, A. K.,** The rate of exchange of tritiated water across the human red cell membrane, *J. Gen. Physiol.,* 41, 259, 1957.
16. **Sidel, V. W. and Solomon, A. K.,** Entrance of water into human red cells under an osmotic pressure gradient, *J. Gen. Physiol.,* 41, 243, 1957.
17. **Goldstein, D. A. and Solomon, A. K.,** Determination of equivalent pore radius for human red cells by osmotic pressure measurement, *J. Gen. Physiol.,* 44, 1, 1960.
18. **Solomon, A. K.,** Characterization of biological membranes by equivalent pores, *J. Gen. Physiol.,* 51, 335s, 1968.
19. **Solomon, A. K. and Gary-Bobo, C. M.,** Aqueous pores in lipid bilayers and red cell membranes, *Biochim. Biophys. Acta,* 255, 1019, 1972.
20. **Macey, R. I. and Farmer, R. E. L.,** Inhibition of water and solute permeability in human red cells, *Biochim. Biophys. Acta.,* 211, 104, 1970.
21. **Knauf, P. A. and Rothstein, A.,** Chemical modification of membranes. I. Effects of sulfhydryl and amino reactive reagents on anion and cation permeability of the human red blood cell, *J. Gen. Physiol.,* 58, 190, 1971.
22. **Knauf, P. A. and Rothstein, A.,** Chemical modification of membranes. II. Permeation paths for sulfhydryl agents, *J. Gen. Physiol.,* 58, 211, 1971.
23. **Sha'afi, R. I. and Feinstein, M. B.,** Membrane water channels and SH-groups, *Adv. Exp. Med. Biol.,* 84, 67, 1977.

24. **Brown, P. A., Feinstein, M. B., and Sha'afi, R. I.,** Membrane proteins related to water transport in human erythrocytes, *Nature (London),* 254, 523, 1975.

25. **Solomon, A. K., Chasan, B., Dix, J. A., Lukacovic, M. F., Toon, M. R., and Verkman, A. S.,** The aqueous pore in the red cell membrane: band 3 as a channel for anions, cations nonelectrolytes, andwater, *Ann.N.Y.Acad.Sci.,* 414, 97, 1983.

26. **Macey, R. I.,** Transport of water and urea in red blood cells, *Am. J. Physiol.,* 246, C195, 1984.

27. **Toon, M. R. and Solomon, A. K.,** Control of red cell urea and water permeability by sulfhydryl reagents, *Biochim. Biophys. Acta,* 860, 361, 1986.

28. **Benga, G., Popescu, O., Pop, V. I., and Holmes, R. P.,** p-(Chloromercuri) benzenesulfonate binding by membrane proteins and the inhibition of water transport in human erythrocytes, *Biochemistry,* 25, 1535, 1986.

29. **Benga, G., Popescu, O., Borza, V., Pop, V. I., Muresan, A., Mocsy, I., Brain, A., and Wrigglesworth, J. M.,** Water permeability in human erythrocytes: identification of membrane proteins involved in water transport, *Eur. J. Cell Biol.,* 41, 252, 1986.

30. **Rao, A.,** Ph.D. thesis, Harvard University, Cambridge, MA, 1978.

31. **Ojcius, D. M. and Solomon, A. K.,** Sites of p-chloromercuri-benzenesulfonate inhibition of red cell urea and water transport, *Biochim. Biophys. Acta,* 942, 73, 1988.

32. **Ojcius, D. M., Toon, M. R., and Solomon, A. K.,** Is an intact cytoskeleton required for red cell urea and water transport?, *Biochim. Biophys. Acta,* 944, 19, 1988.

33. **Dix, J. A., Ausiello, D. A., Jung, C. Y., and Verkman, A. S.,** Target analysis studies of red cell water and urea transport, *Biochim. Biophys. Acta,* 821, 243, 1985.

34. **Salhany, J. M. and Sloan, R. L.,** Partial covalent labeling with pyridoxal 5'-phosphate induces bis(sulfosuccinimidyl)-suberate crosslinking of band 3 protein tetramers in intact human red blood cells, *Biochem. Biophys. Res. Commun.,* 156, 1215, 1988.

35. **Fröhlich, O. and Jones, S. C.,** Kinetic independence between red cell anion exchange and urea transport, *Biochim. Biophys. Acta,* 943, 531, 1988.

36. **Salhany, J. M., Rauenbuehler, P. B., and Sloan, R. L.,** Alterations in pyridoxal 5'-phosphate inhibition of human erythrocyte anion transport associated with osmotic hemolysis and resealing, *J. Biol. Chem.,* 262, 15974, 1987.

37. **Beth, A. H., Conturo, T. E., Venkataramu, S. D., and Staros, J. V.,** Dynamics and interactions of the anion channel in intact human erythrocytes: an electron paramagnetic resonance spectroscopic study employing a new membrane-impermeant bifunctional spin-label, *Biochemistry,* 25, 3824, 1986.

38. **Kay, M. M. B., Bosman, G. J. C. G. M., and Lawrence, C.,** Functional topography of band 3: specific structural alteration linked to functional aberrations in human erythrocytes, *Proc. Natl. Acad. Sci. U.S.A.,* 85, 492, 1988.

39. **Verkman, A. S., Skorecki, K. L., Jung, C. Y., and Ausiello, D. A.,** Target molecular weights for red cell band 3 stilbene and mercurial binding sites, *Am. J. Physiol.,* 251, C541, 1986.

40. **Benz, R., Tosteson, M. T., and Schubert, D.,** Formation and properties of tetramers of band 3 protein from human erythrocyte membranes in planar lipid bilayers, *Biochim. Biophys. Acta,* 775, 347,1984.

41. **Tomida, M., Kondo, Y., Moriyama, R., Machida, H., and Makino, S.,** Effect of stilbenedisulfonate binding on the state of association of the membrane-spanning domain of band 3 from bovine erythrocyte membrane, *Biochim. Biophys. Acta,* 943, 493, 1988.

42. **Lukacovic, M. F., Toon, M. R., and Solomon, A. K.,** Site of red cell cation leak induced by mercurial sulfhydryl reagents, *Biochim. Biophys. Acta,* 772, 313, 1984.

43. **Dorogi, P. L. and Solomon, A. K.,** Interaction of thiourea with band 3 in human red cell membranes, *J. Membr. Biol.,* 85, 37, 1985.

44. **Ashley, D. L. and Goldstein, J. H.,** Nuclear magnetic resonance evidence for abnormal water transport in duchenne muscular dystrophy erythrocytes, *Biochem. Biophys. Res. Commun.,* 100, 364, 1981.

45. **Toon, M. R. and Solomon, A. K.,** Relation between red cell anion exchange and urea transport, *Biochim. Biophys. Acta,* 821, 502, 1985.

46. **Toon, M. R., Dorogi, P.L., Lukacovic, M. F., and Solomon, A. K.,** Binding of DTNB to band 3 in the human red cell membrane, *Biochim. Biophys. Acta,* 818, 158, 1985.

47. **Reithmeier, R. A. F.,** Inhibition of anion transport in human red blood cells by 5,5'-dithiobis(2-nitrobenzoic acid), *Biochim. Biophys. Acta,* 732, 122, 1983.

48. **Morariu, V. V. and Benga, G.,** Evaluation of a nuclear magnetic resonance technique for the study of water exchange through erythrocyte membranes in normal and pathological subjects, *Biochim. Biophys. Acta,* 469, 301, 1977.

49. **Sutherland, R. M., Rothstein, A., and Weed, R. I.,** Erythrocyte membrane sulfhydryl groups and cation permeability, *J. Cell. Physiol.,* 69, 185, 1967

50. **Naccache, P. and Sha'afi, R. I.,** Effect of PCMBS on water transfer across biological membranes, *J. Cell. Physiol.,* 83, 449, 1974.

51. **Chasan, B., Lukacovic, M. F., Toon, M. R., and Solomon, A. K.,** Effect of thiourea on PCMBS inhibition of osmotic water transport in human red cells, *Biochim. Biophys. Acta,* 778, 185, 1984.

52. **Benga, G., Pop, V. I., Ionescu, M., Holmes, R. P., and Popescu, O.,** Irreversible inhibition of water transport in erythrocytes by fluoresceinmercuric acetate, *Cell Biol. Int. Rep.,* 6, 775, 1982.

53. **Conlon, T. and Outhred, R.,** Water diffusion permeability of erythrocytes using an NMR technique, *Biochim. Biophys. Acta,* 288, 354, 1972.

54. **Lukacovic, M. F., Verkman, A. S., Dix, J. A., and Solomon, A. K.,** Specific interaction of the water transport inhibitor, pCMBS, with band 3 in red blood cell membranes, *Biochim. Biophys. Acta,* 778, 253, 1984.

55. **Yoon, S. C., Toon, M. R., and Solomon, A. K.,** Relation between red cell anion exchange and water transport, *Biochim. Biophys. Acta,* 778, 385, 1984.

56. **Toon, M. R. and Solomon, A. K.,** Interrelation of ethylene glycol, urea and water transport in the red cell, *Biochim. Biophys. Acta,* 898, 275, 1987.

57. **Craescu, C. T., Cassoly, R., Galacteros, F., and Prehu, C.,** Kinetics of water transport in sickle cells, *Biochim. Biophys. Acta,* 812, 811, 1985.

58. **Brahm, J. and Wieth, J. O.,** Separate pathways for urea and water, and for chloride in chicken erythrocytes, *J. Physiol. (London),* 266, 727, 1977.

59. **Karan, D. M. and Macey, R. I.,** The permeability of the human red cell to deuterium oxide (heavy water), *J. Cell. Physiol.,* 104, 209, 1980.

60. **Solomon, A. K., Toon, M. R., and Dix, J. A.,** Osmotic properties of human red cells, *J. Membr. Biol.,* 91, 259, 1986

61. **Brahm, J.,** Diffusional water permeability of human erythrocytes and their ghosts, *J.Gen. Physiol.,* 79, 791, 1982.

62. **Stein, W. D.,** *Transport and Diffusion across Cell Membranes,* Academic Press, New York, 1986.

63. **Widdas, W. F.,** The asymmetry of the hexose transfer system in the human red cell membrane, *Curr. Top. Membr. Transp.,* 14, 165, 1980.

64. **Carruthers, A.,** Sugar transport in animal cells: the passive hexose transfer system, *Prog. Biophys. Mol. Biol.,* 43, 33, 1984.

65. **Taverna, R. D. and Langdon, R. G.,** D-Glucosyl isothiocyanate, an affinity label for the glucose transport proteins of the human erythrocyte membrane, *Biochem. Biophys. Res. Commun.,* 54, 593, 1973.

66. **Mullins, R. E. and Langdon, R. G.,** Maltosyl isothiocyanate: an affinity label for the glucose transporter of the human erythrocyte membrane. I. Inhibition of glucose transport. *Biochemistry,* 19, 1199, 1980.

67. **Mullins, R. E. and Langdon, R. G.,** Maltosyl isothiocyanate: an affinity label for the glucose transporter of the human erythrocyte membrane. II. Identification of the transporter, *Biochemistry,* 19, 1205, 1980.

68. **Shelton, R. L. and Langdon, R. G.,** Reconstitution of glucose transport using human erythrocyte band 3, *Biochim. Biophys. Acta,* 733, 25, 1983.

69. **Lienhard, G. E., Gorga, F. R., Orasky, J. E., Jr., and Zoccoli, M. A.,** Monosaccharide transport system of the human erythrocyte. Identification of the cytochalasin B binding component, *Biochemistry,* 16, 4921, 1977.

70. **Shanahan, M. F. and Jacquez, J. A.,** Differential labeling of components in human erythrocyte membranes associated with the transport of glucose, *Membr. Biochem.,* 1, 239, 1978.

71. **Batt, E. R., Abbott, R. E., and Schachter, D.,** Impermeant maleimides. Identification of an exofacial component of the human erythrocyte hexose transport mechanism, *J. Biol. Chem.,* 251, 7184, 1976.

72. **Sogin, D. C. and Hinkle, P. C.,** Characterization of the glucose transporter from human erythrocytes, *J. Supramol. Struct.,* 8, 447, 1978.

73. **Baldwin, S. A., Baldwin, J. M., Gorga, F. R., and Lienhard, G. E.,** Purification of the cytochalasin B binding component of the human erythrocyte monosaccharide transport system, *Biochim. Biophys. Acta,* 552, 183, 1979.

74. **Shanahan, M. F.,** Cytochalasin B. A natural photoaffinity ligand for labeling the human erythrocyte glucose transporter, *J. Biol. Chem.,* 257, 7290, 1982.

75. **Carter-Su, C., Pessin, J. E., Mora, R., Gitomer, W., and Czech, M. P.,** Photoaffinity labeling of the human erythrocyte D-glucose transporter, *J. Biol. Chem.,* 257, 5419, 1982.

76. **Weber, T. M. and Eichholz, A.,** Characterization of a photosensitive glucose derivative. A photoaffinity reagent for the erythrocyte hexose transporter, *Biochim. Biophys. Acta,* 812, 503, 1985.

77. **Shanahan, M. F., Wadzinski, B. E., Lowndes, J. M., and Ruoho, A. E.,** Photoaffinity labeling of the human erythrocyte monosaccharide transporter with an aryl azide derivative of D-glucose, *J. Biol. Chem.,* 260, 10897, 1985.

78. **Holman, G. D., Parkar, B. A., and Midgley, P. J. W.,** Exofacial photoaffinity labelling of the human erythrocyte sugar transporter, *Biochim. Biophys. Acta,* 855, 115, 1986.

79. **Kasahara, M. and Hinkle, P. C.,** Reconstitution and purification of the D-glucose transporter from human erythrocytes, *J. Biol. Chem.,* 252, 7384, 1977.

80. **Kahlenberg, A. and Zala, C. A.,** Reconstitution of D-glucose transport in vesicles composed of lipids and intrinsic protein (zone 4.5) of the human erythrocyte membrane, *J. Supramol. Struct.,* 7, 287, 1977.

81. **Baldwin, J. M., Gorga, J. C., and Lienhard, G. E.,** The monosaccharide transporter of the human erythrocyte. Transport activity upon reconstitution. *J. Biol. Chem.,* 256, 3685, 1981.

82. **Baldwin, S. A. and Lienhard, G. E.,** Immunological identification of the human erythrocyte monosaccharide transporter, *Biochem. Biophys. Res. Commun.,* 94, 1401, 1980.

83. **Sogin, D. C. and Hinkle, P. C.,** Immunological identification of the human erythrocyte glucose transporter, *Proc. Natl. Acad. Sci. U.S.A.,* 77, 5725, 1980.

84. **Mueckler, M., Caruso, C., Baldwin, S. A., Panico, M., Blench, I., Morris, H. R., Allard, W. J., Lienhard, G. E., and Lodish, H. F.,** Sequence and structure of a human glucose transporter, *Science,* 229, 941, 1985.

85. **May, J. M.,** Labeling of human erythrocyte band 3 with maltosylisothiocyanate. Interaction with the anion transporter, *J. Biol. Chem.,* 262, 3140, 1987.

86. **Lowe, A. G. and Walmsley, A. R.,** A single half-turnover of the glucose carrier of the human erythrocyte, *Biochim. Biophys. Acta,* 903, 547, 1987.

87. **Baly, D. L. and Horuk, R.,** The biology and biochemistry of the glucose transporter, *Biochim. Biophys. Acta,* 947, 571, 1988.

88. **Walmsley, A. R.,** The dynamics of the glucose transporter, *Trends Biochem. Sci.,* 13, 226, 1988.

89. **Langdon, R. G. and Holman, V. P.,** Immunological evidence that band 3 is the major glucose transporter of the human erythrocyte membrane, *Biochim. Biophys. Acta,* 945, 23, 1988.

90. **Heintze, K., Petersen, K.-U., Olles, P., Saverymuttu, S. H., and Wood, J. R.,** Effects of bicarbonate on fluid and electrolyte transport by the guinea pig gallbladder: a bicarbonate-chloride exchange, *J. Membr. Biol.,* 45, 43, 1979.

91. **Hoffmann, E. K., Simonsen, L. O., and Sjøholm, C.,** Membrane potential, chloride exchange, and chloride conductance in Ehrlich mouse ascites tumour cells, *J. Physiol. (London),* 296, 61, 1979.

92. **Page, E., Polimeni, P. I., and Macchia, D. D.,** Chloride distribution and exchange in vertebrate heart and skeletal muscle, *Ann. N.Y. Acad. Sci.,* 341, 524, 1980.

93. **Skydsgaard, J. M.,** Saturation kinetics of chloride exchange across the cell membrane of frog muscle, *Proc. Int. Union Physiol. Sci.,* 13, 703, 1977.

94. **Friedman, P. A. and Andreoli, T. E.,** CO_2-stimulated NaCl absorption in the mouse renal cortical thick ascending limb of Henle, *J. Gen. Physiol.,* 80, 683, 1982.

95. **Reuss, L., Costantin, J. L., and Bazile, J. E.,** Diphenylamine-2-carboxylate blocks Cl^--HCO_3^- exchange in Necturus gallbladder epithelium, *Am. J. Physiol.,* 253, C79, 1987.

96. **Tønnessen, T. I., Ludt, J., Sandvig, K., and Olsnes, S.,** Bicarbonate/chloride antiport in Vero cells. I. Evidence for both sodium-linked and sodium-independent exchange, *J. Cell. Physiol.,* 132, 183, 1987.

97. **Edwards, P. A. W.,** Monoclonal antibodies that bind to the human erythrocyte-membrane glycoproteins glycophorin A and band 3, *Biochem. Soc. Trans.,* 8, 334, 1980.

98. **Kay, M. M. B., Tracey, C. M., Goodman, J. R., Cone, J. C., and Bassel, P. S.,** Polypeptides immunologically related to band 3 are present in nucleated somatic cells, *Proc. Natl. Acad. Sci. U.S.A.,* 80, 6882, 1983.

99. **Cox, J. V., Moon, R. T., and Lazarides, E.,** Anion transporter: highly cell-type-specific expression of distinct polypeptides and transcripts in erythroid cells, *J. Cell Biol.,* 100, 1548, 1985.

100. **Drenckhahn, D., Oelmann, M., Schaaf, P., Wagner, M., and Wagner, S.,** Band 3 is the basolateral anion exchanger of dark epithelial cells of turtle urinary bladder, *Am. J. Physiol.,* 252, C570, 1987.

101. **Hazen-Martin, D. J., Pasternack, G., Hennigar, R. A., Spicer, S. S., and Sens, D. A.,** Immunocytochemistry of band 3 protein in kidney and other tissues of control and cystic fibrosis patients, *Pediatr. Res.,* 21, 235, 1987.

102. **Schuster, V. L., Bonsib, S. M., and Jennings, M. L.,** Two types of collecting duct mitochondria-rich (intercalated) cells: lectin and band 3 cytochemistry, *Am. J. Physiol.,* 251, C347, 1986.

103. **Vanderpuye, O. A., Kelley, L. K., Morrison, M. M., and Smith, C. H.,** The apical and basal plasma membranes of the human placental syncytiotrophoblast contain different erythrocyte membrane protein isoforms. Evidence for placental forms of band 3 and spectrin, *Biochim. Biophys. Acta,* 943, 277, 1988.

104. **Liedtke, C. M. and Hopfer, U.,** Mechanism of Cl^- translocation across small intestinal brush-border membrane. II. Demonstration of CL^--OH^- exchange and CL^- conductance, *Am. J. Physiol.,* 242, G272, 1982.

105. **Jentsch, T. J., Schwartz, P., Schill, B. S., Langner, B., Lepple, A. P., Keller, S. K., and Wiederholt, M.,** Kinetic properties of the sodium bicarbonate (carbonate) symport in monkey kidney epithelial cells (BSC-1). Interactions between Na^+, HCO_3^-, and pH, *J. Biol. Chem.,* 261, 10673, 1986.

106. **Jessen, F., Sjøholm, C., and Hoffmann, E. K.,** Identification of the anion exchange protein of Ehrlich Cells: a kinetic analysis of the inhibitory effects of 4,4'-diisothiocyano-2,2'-stilbene-disulfonic acid (DIDS) and labeling of membrane proteins with ^{3}H-DIDS, *J. Membr. Biol.,* 92, 195, 1986.

107. **Talor, Z., Gold, R. M., Yang, W. -C., and Arruda, J. A. L.,** Anion exchanger is present in both luminal and basolateral renal membranes, *Eur. J. Biochem.,* 164, 695, 1987.

108. **Madshus, I. H. and Olsnes, S.,** Selective inhibition of sodium-linked and sodium-independent bicarbonate/chloride antiport in Vero cells, *J. Biol. Chem.,* 262, 7486, 1987.

109. **Skydsgaard, J. M.,** Inhibition of chloride self-exchange with stilbene disulfonates in depolarized skeletal muscle of *Rana Temporaria, J. Physiol. (London),* 397, 433, 1987.

110. **Elgavish, A., DiBona, D. R., Norton, P., and Meezan, E.,** Sulfate transport in apical membrane vesicles isolated from tracheal epithelium, *Am. J. Physiol.,* 253, C416, 1987.

111. **Paradiso, A. M., Tsien, R. Y., Demarest, J. R., and Machen, T. E.,** Na-H and Cl⁻/HCO₃ exchange in rabbit oxyntic cells using fluorescence microscopy, *Am. J. Physiol.,* 253, C30, 1987.

112. **Ruetz, S., Fricker, G., Hugentobler, G., Winterhalter, K., Kurz, G., and Meier, P. J.,** Isolation and characterization of the putative canalicular bile salt transport system of rat liver, *J. Biol. Chem.,* 262, 11324, 1987.

113. **Olsnes, S., Ludt, J., Tønnessen, T. I., and Sandvig, K.,** Bicarbonate/chloride antiport in Vero cells. II. Mechanisms for bicarbonate-dependent regulation of intracellular pH, *J. Cell. Physiol.,* 132, 192, 1987.

114. **Nord, E. P., Brown, S. E. S., and Crandall, E. D.,** Cl⁻/HCO₃⁻ exchange modulates intracellular pH in rat type II alveolar epithelial cells, *J. Biol. Chem.,* 262, 5599, 1988.

115. **Pazoles, C. J. and Pollard, H. B.,** Evidence for stimulation of anion transport in ATP-evoked transmitter release from isolated secretory vesicles, *J. Biol. Chem.,* 253, 3962, 1978.

116. **Reinertsen, K. V., Tønnessen, T. I., Jacobsen, J., Sandvig, K., and Olsnes, S.,** Role of chloride/bicarbonate antiport in the control of cytosolic pH. Cell-line differences in activity and regulation of antiport. *J. Biol. Chem.* 263, 11117, 1988.

117. **Janoshazi, A., Ojcius, D. M., Kone, B., Seifter, J. L., and Solomon, A. K.,** Relation between the anion exchange protein in kidney medullary collecting duct cells and red cell band 3, *J. Membr. Biol.,* 103, 181, 1988.

118. **Kopito, R. R., Andersson, M. A., and Lodish, H. F.,** Multiple tissue-specific sites of transcriptional initiation of the mouse anion antiport gene in erythroid and renal cells, *Proc. Natl. Acad. Sci. U.S.A.,* 84, 7149, 1987.

119. **Alper, S. L., Kopito, R. R., Libresco, S. M., and Lodish, H. F.,** Cloning and characterization of a murine band 3-related cDNA from kidney and from a lymphoid cell line, *J. Biol. Chem.,* 263, 17092, 1988.

120. **Wieth, J. O. and Brahm, J.,** Cellular anion transport, in *The Kidney: Physiology and Pathophysiology,* Seldin, D.W. and Giebisch, G., Eds., Raven Press, New York, 1985, 49.

121. **Lowe, A. G. and Lambert, A.,** Chloride-bicarbonate exchange and related transport processes, *Biochim. Biophys. Acta,* 694, 353, 1983.

122. **Hoffmann, E. K.,** Anion transport systems in the plasma membrane of vertebrate cells, *Biochim. Biophys. Acta,* 864, 1, 1986.

123. **Shennan, D. B. and Boyd, C. A. R.,** Ion transport by the placenta: a review of membrane transport systems, *Biochim. Biophys. Acta,* 906, 437, 1987.

124. **Kregenow, F. M.,** Osmoregulatory salt transporting mechanisms: control of cell volume in anisotonic media, *Annu. Rev. Physiol.,* 43, 493, 1981.

125. **Law, F.-Y., Steinfeld, R., and Knauf, P. A.,** K 562 cell anion exchange differs markedly from that of mature red blood cells, *Am. J. Physiol.,* 244, C68, 1983.

126. **Drenckhahn, D., Schlüter, K., Allen, D. P., and Bennett, V.,** Colocalization of band 3 with ankyrin and spectrin at the basal membrane of intercalated cells in the rat kidney, *Science,* 230, 1287, 1985.

127. **Stone, D. K., Seldin, D. W., Kokko, J. P., and Jacobson, H. R.,** Anion dependence of rabbit medullary collecting duct acidification, *J. Clin. Invest..,* 71, 1505, 1983.

128. **Koeppen, B. M.,** Conductive properties of the rabbit outer medullary collecting duct: inner stripe, *Am. J. Physiol.,* 248, F500, 1985.

129. **Shennan, D. B., Davis, B., and Boyd, C. A. R.,** Chloride transport in human placental microvillus membrane vesicles. I. Evidence for anion exchange, *Pfluegers Arch.,* 406, 60, 1986.

130. **Klingenberg, M.,** Membrane protein oligomeric structure and transport function, *Nature (London),* 290, 449, 1981.

131. **Falke, J. J. and Koshland, D. E., Jr.,** Global flexibility in a sensory receptor: a site-directed cross-linking approach, *Science,* 237, 1596, 1987.

132. **Henderson, R. and Unwin, P. N. T.,** Three-dimensional model of purple membrane obtained by electron microscopy, *Nature (London),* 257, 28, 1975.

133. **Aquila, H., Link, T. A., and Klingenberg, M.,** Solute carriers involved in energy transfer of mitochondria form a homologous protein family, *FEBS Lett.,* 212, 1, 1987.

134. **Jones, M. N. and Nickson, J. K.,** Monosaccharide transport proteins of the human erythrocyte membrane, *Biochim. Biophys. Acta,* 650, 1, 1981.

135. **Pessin, J. E. and Czech, M. P.,** Hexose transport and its regulation in mammalian cells. in *The Enzymes of Biological Membranes, Vol. 3, Membrane Transport,* 2nd ed., Martonosi, A.N., Ed., Plenum Press, New York, 1985, 497.

136. **Wheeler, T. J. and Hinkle, P. C.,** The glucose transporter of mammalian cells, *Annu. Rev. Physiol.,* 47, 503, 1985.

137. **Widdas, W. F.,** Old and new concepts of the membrane transport for glucose in cells, *Biochim. Biophys. Acta,* 947, 385, 1988.

138. **Zoccoli, M. A., Baldwin, S. A., and Lienhard, G. E.,** The monosaccharide transport system of the human erythrocyte. Solubilization and characterization on the basis of cytochalasin B binding, *J. Biol. Chem.,* 253, 6923, 1978.

139. **Cuppoletti, J., Jung, C. Y., and Green, F. A.,** Glucose transport carrier of human erythrocytes. Radiation target size measurement based on flux inactivation. *J. Biol.Chem.* 256, 1305, 1981.

140. **Holman, G. D.,** An allosteric pore model for sugar transport in human erythrocytes, *Biochim. Biophys. Acta,* 599, 202, 1980.

141. **Carruthers, A.,** ATP regulation of the human red cell sugar transporter, *J. Biol. Chem.,* 261, 11028, 1986.

142. **Helgerson, A. L. and Carruthers, A.,** Equilibrium ligand binding to the human erythrocyte sugar transporter. Evidence for two sugar-binding sites per carrier, *J. Biol. Chem.,* 262, 5464, 1987.

143. **Appleman, J. R. and Lienhard, G. E.,** Rapid kinetics of the glucose transporter from human erythrocytes. Detection and measurement of a half-turnover of the purified transporter, *J. Biol. Chem.,* 260, 4575, 1985.

144. **Wang, J.-F., Falke, J. J., and Chan, S. I.,** A proton NMR study of the mechanism of the erythrocyte glucose transporter, *Proc. Natl. Acad. Sci. U.S.A.,* 83, 3277, 1986.

145. **Salhany, J. M. and Rauenbuehler, P. B.,** Kinetics and mechanism of erythrocyte anion exchange, *J. Biol. Chem.* 258, 245, 1983.

ADDENDUM

Since submission of this manuscript, several important papers have appeared which should be noted. One of the single most important advances for future research is the determination of the complete amino acid sequence of human erythrocyte band 3 protein by Prof. Michael J. A. Tanner, P. G. Martin and Stephen High.[1] We have translated the sequence into an easily readable table for study (Table 1). Some important facts about the sequence are the existence of exactly five cysteine residues (in agreement with Rao's biochemical study[2]), two of which are on the cytoplasmic domain (in agreement with p-mercuribenzoate titration studies[3]). Furthermore, there are 27 lysine residues in the whole molecule. If the intracellular chymotryptic cleavage site is taken as residue 359 (tyr) and the extracellular chymotryptic site as 553 (tyr), then the integral subdomain delineated by residues 360 to 553 contains 5 lysine residues. This subdomain is CH17. The presence of 5 lysine residues more than accounts for those titratable by pyridoxal 5'-phosphate on CH17.[4] Lysines 539 and 542 are the ones which can be covalently reacted with one isothiocyanate group of DIDS. Finally, the sequence of the human N-terminus, determined earlier,[5] has an aspartic acid at residue 11 (Chapter 2), while according to the gene sequence, the residue is a methionine (Table 1).

Also relevant is the publication of the primary structure[6] and some functional properties[7] of the major kidney band 3 gene. The 848 amino acid sequence of rat kidney band 3 protein is nearly identical to mouse erythrocyte band 3. They differ in that the kidney protein lacks the first 79 amino acids of the N-terminal cytoplasmic domain, which is known to bind hemolglobin and the glycolytic enzymes in human erythrocyte band 3. This truncated form of band 3 is capable of exchanging anions, showing that the acidic N terminus is not essential for the anion-exchange function as expected from the proteolytic digestion studies (Chapter 3). Whether or not that domain is involved in modulation of the anion exchange rate was not tested. The observed exchange rates based on 10 oocytes infected with kidney band 3 RNA, were significantly faster than those infected with the complete mouse band 3 protein RNA. Unfortunately, what was not known was whether there were more or fewer copies of the truncated protein in the membrane. The truncated band 3 consistently exchanged anions 1.5 times faster than the fully extended protein. If there are fewer copies of the truncated porter in the oocyte membrane, then the "turn over number" could be quite considerably larger. Future studies of the transport properties and the ankyrin binding characteristics of this truncated porter will be of great interest.

Passow's group has presented some temperature dependence studies which have implications for the conformational flexibility of band 3 porter.[8] They found that the internal energy required to transport anions over the rate-limiting barrier is largely compensated for by an increase in the entropy of the system (i.e., protein and surroundings). This result suggests a great degree of conformational flexibility associated with the function of band 3 protein. That ligand binding energies can in fact be felt at the subunit interface, was demonstrated by Makino's group.[9] They showed that when the cytoplasmic domain of band 3 is removed, the integral domain exists in an equilibrium mixture of dimers and tetramers in octylglucoside. This equilibrium is totally shifted to the dimeric form by pretreatment with DIDS. Since the DIDS binding sites on each monomer are now thought to be greater than16 Å apart (see Chapter 3), simple charge repulsion seems unlikely as an explanation. It seems more probable that DIDS stabilizes one quaternary structure of the porter. These findings, like those of Salhany and Sloan[10,11] indicate that transport site ligands modulate global changes in the quaternary structure.

Makino's results with bovine band 3 in detergents do not necessarily contradict the studies of Salhany and Sloan,[10,11] carried out with intact human red cells. In the latter studies, partial covalent modification with PLP or addition of DNDS induced an increase in the tetramer crosslinkable state.[10,11] Suppose that ankyrin stabilizes a band 3 tetramer due to interactions at the cytosolic extension.[12] Suppose further that two quaternary structures exist for the integral domain within the tetrameric state of association. Without ligands bound, the integral domains

TABLE 1
Human Erythrocyte Band 3

MET	GLU	GLU	LEU	GLN	ASP	ASP	TYR	GLU	ASP	MET	MET	GLU	GLU	ASN	15
LEU	GLU	GLN	GLU	GLU	TYR	GLU	ASP	PRO	ASP	ILE	PRO	GLU	SER	GLN	30
MET	GLU	GLU	PRO	ALA	ALA	HIS	ASP	THR	GLU	ALA	THR	ALA	THR	ASP	45
TYR	HIS	THR	THR	SER	HIS	PRO	GLY	THR	HIS	GLU	VAL	TYR	VAL	GLU	60
LEU	GLN	GLU	LEU	VAL	MET	ASP	GLU	LYS	ASN	GLN	GLU	LEU	ARG	TRP	75
MET	GLU	ALA	ALA	ARG	TRP	VAL	GLN	LEU	GLU	GLU	ASN	LEU	GLY	GLU	90
ASN	GLY	ALA	TRP	GLY	ARG	PRO	HIS	LEU	SER	HIS	LEU	THR	PHE	TRP	105
SER	LEU	LEU	GLU	LEU	ARG	ARG	VAL	PHE	THR	LYS	GLY	THR	VAL	LEU	120
LEU	ASP	LEU	GLN	GLU	THR	SER	LEU	ALA	GLY	VAL	ALA	ASN	GLN	LEU	135
LEU	ASP	ARG	PHE	ILE	PHE	GLU	ASP	GLN	ILE	ARG	PRO	GLN	ASP	ARG	150
GLU	GLU	LEU	LEU	ARG	ALA	LEU	LEU	LEU	LYS	HIS	SER	HIS	ALA	GLY	165
GLU	LEU	GLU	ALA	LEU	GLY	GLY	VAL	LYS	PRO	ALA	VAL	LEU	THR	ARG	180
SER	GLY	ASP	PRO	SER	GLN	PRO	LEU	LEU	PRO	GLN	HIS	SER	SER	LEU	195
GLU	THR	GLN	LEU	PHE	**CYS**	GLU	GLN	GLY	ASP	GLY	GLY	THR	GLU	GLY	210
HIS	SER	PRO	SER	GLY	ILE	LEU	GLU	LYS	ILE	PRO	PRO	ASP	SER	GLU	225
ALA	THR	LEU	VAL	LEU	VAL	GLY	ARG	ALA	ASP	PHE	LEU	GLU	GLN	PRO	240
VAL	LEU	GLY	PHE	VAL	ARG	LEU	GLN	GLU	ALA	ALA	GLU	LEU	GLU	ALA	255
VAL	GLU	LEU	PRO	VAL	PRO	ILE	ARG	PHE	LEU	PHE	VAL	LEU	LEU	GLY	270
PRO	GLU	ALA	PRO	HIS	ILE	ASP	TYR	THR	GLN	LEU	GLY	ARG	ALA	ALA	285
ALA	THR	LEU	MET	SER	GLU	ARG	VAL	PHE	ARG	ILE	ASP	ALA	TYR	MET	300
ALA	GLN	SER	ARG	GLY	GLU	LEU	LEU	HIS	SER	LEU	GLU	GLY	PHE	LEU	315
ASP	**CYS**	SER	LEU	VAL	LEU	PRO	PRO	THR	ASP	ALA	PRO	SER	GLU	GLN	330
ALA	LEU	LEU	SER	LEU	VAL	PRO	VAL	GLN	ARG	GLU	LEU	LEU	ARG	ARG	345
ARG	TYR	GLN	SER	SER	PRO	ALA	LYS	PRO	ASP	SER	SER	PHE	TYR	LYS	360
GLY	LEU	ASP	LEU	ASN	GLY	GLY	PRO	ASP	ASP	PRO	LEU	GLN	GLN	THR	375
GLY	GLN	LEU	PHE	GLY	GLY	LEU	VAL	ARG	ASP	ILE	ARG	ARG	ARG	TYR	390
PRO	TYR	TYR	LEU	SER	ASP	ILE	THR	ASP	ALA	PHE	SER	PRO	GLN	VAL	405
LEU	ALA	ALA	VAL	ILE	PHE	ILE	TYR	PHE	ALA	ALA	LEU	SER	PRO	ALA	420
ILE	THR	PHE	GLY	GLY	LEU	LEU	GLY	GLU	LYS	THR	ARG	ASN	GLN	MET	435
GLY	VAL	SER	GLU	LEU	LEU	ILE	SER	THR	ALA	VAL	GLN	GLY	ILE	LEU	450
PHE	ALA	LEU	LEU	GLY	ALA	GLN	PRO	LEU	LEU	VAL	VAL	GLY	PHE	SER	465
GLY	PRO	LEU	LEU	VAL	PHE	GLU	GLU	ALA	PHE	PHE	SER	PHE	**CYS**	GLU	480
THR	ASN	GLY	LEU	GLU	TYR	ILE	VAL	GLY	ARG	VAL	TRP	ILE	GLY	PHE	495
TRP	LEU	ILE	LEU	LEU	VAL	VAL	LEU	VAL	VAL	ALA	PHE	GLU	GLY	SER	510
PHE	LEU	VAL	ARG	PHE	ILE	SER	ARG	TYR	THR	GLN	GLU	ILE	PHE	SER	525
PHE	LEU	ILE	SER	LEU	ILE	PHE	ILE	TYR	GLU	THR	PHE	SER	LYS	LEU	540
ILE	LYS	ILE	PHE	GLN	ASP	HIS	PRO	LEU	GLN	LYS	THR	TYR	ASN	TYR	555
ASN	VAL	LEU	MET	VAL	PRO	LYS	PRO	GLN	GLY	PRO	LEU	PRO	ASN	THR	570
ALA	LEU	LEU	SER	LEU	VAL	LEU	MET	ALA	GLY	THR	PHE	PHE	PHE	ALA	585
MET	MET	LEU	ARG	LYS	PHE	LYS	ASN	SER	SER	TYR	PHE	PRO	GLY	LYS	600
LEU	ARG	ARG	VAL	ILE	GLY	ASP	PHE	GLY	VAL	PRO	ILE	SER	ILE	LEU	615
ILE	MET	VAL	LEU	VAL	ASP	PHE	PHE	ILE	GLN	ASP	THR	TYR	THR	GLN	630
LYS	LEU	SER	VAL	PRO	ASP	GLY	PHE	LYS	VAL	SER	ASN	SER	SER	ALA	645
ARG	GLY	TRP	VAL	ILE	HIS	PRO	LEU	GLY	LEU	ARG	SER	GLU	PHE	PRO	660
ILE	TRP	MET	MET	PHE	ALA	SER	ALA	LEU	PRO	ALA	LEU	LEU	VAL	PHE	675
ILE	LEU	ILE	PHE	LEU	GLU	SER	GLN	ILE	THR	THR	LEU	ILE	VAL	SER	690
LYS	PRO	GLU	ARG	LYS	MET	VAL	LYS	GLY	SER	GLY	PHE	HIS	LEU	ASP	705
LEU	LEU	LEU	VAL	VAL	GLY	MET	GLY	GLY	VAL	ALA	ALA	LEU	PHE	GLY	720
MET	PRO	TRP	LEU	SER	ALA	THR	THR	VAL	ARG	SER	VAL	THR	HIS	ALA	735
ASN	ALA	LEU	THR	VAL	MET	GLY	LYS	ALA	SER	THR	PRO	GLY	ALA	ALA	750
ALA	GLN	ILE	GLN	GLU	VAL	LYS	GLU	GLN	ARG	ILE	SER	GLY	LEU	LEU	765
VAL	ALA	VAL	LEU	VAL	GLY	LEU	SER	ILE	LEU	MET	GLU	PRO	ILE	LEU	780
SER	ARG	ILE	PRO	LEU	ALA	VAL	LEU	PHE	GLY	ILE	PHE	LEU	TYR	MET	795
GLY	VAL	THR	SER	LEU	SER	GLY	ILE	GLN	LEU	PHE	ASP	ARG	ILE	LEU	810
LEU	LEU	PHE	LYS	PRO	PRO	LYS	TYR	HIS	PRO	ASP	VAL	PRO	TYR	VAL	825
LYS	ARG	VAL	LYS	THR	TRP	ARG	MET	HIS	LEU	PHE	THR	GLY	ILE	GLN	840
ILE	ILE	**CYS**	LEU	ALA	VAL	LEU	TRP	VAL	VAL	LYS	SER	THR	PRO	ALA	855
SER	LEU	ALA	LEU	PRO	PHE	VAL	LEU	ILE	LEU	THR	VAL	PRO	LEU	ARG	870

TABLE 1 (continued)
Human Erythrocyte Band 3

ARG	VAL	LEU	LEU	PRO	LEU	ILE	PHE	ARG	ASN	VAL	GLU	LEU	GLN	**CYS**	885
LEU	ASP	ALA	ASP	ASP	ALA	LYS	ALA	THR	PHE	ASP	GLU	GLU	GLU	GLY	900
ARG	ASP	GLU	TYR	ASP	GLU	VAL	ALA	MET	PRO	VAL					

are crosslinked to dimers *in situ* by BS[3], despite the fact that the tetrameric form of this state is stable in detergents.[9] In other words, even though the tetramer is stable, the lysines needed to make the interdimeric crosslinks are either not exposed or they are not in the correct position to form a crosslink. When DNDS is added, the quaternary structure of the integral domain changes to a less stable state. But because ankyrin is still bound and is holding the two band 3 dimers together, they do not rapidly dissociate *in situ*. In this destabilized quaternary structure of the integral domain of the porter, either the lysines are exposed to the extracellular surface (consequent to a change in conformation[4]), or they are always exposed but due to the conformational change are now in the correct position to be crosslinked by BS[3]; and we see an increase in the population of the crosslinked tetrameric product.[11] Exposure of nonoverlapping lysines consequent to DNDS binding, has been observed previously.[4]

Renee Sloan and I have further characterized the DNDS-induced effect on BS[3] crosslinking, and have shown that it is highly specific with an apparent half effect constant of 150 μM in the presence of 5 mM BS[3]. In addition, we have ruled out complex non-specific mechanisms by showing that the crosslinked products do indeed represent *in situ* structures, since they are observed without the use of NaOH to "strip" the membranes of peripheral proteins. Finally, Legrum and Passow[13] have shown that the stilbene DBDS does not directly compete with sulfate for the transport site, despite the fact that DIDS can totally inhibit sulfate transport. It is possible that DNDS reaches the transport site and that DBDS does not. But, as Legrum and Passow point out, the effects of DNDS on the chloride binding[14] seem extremely small. The results suggesting that stilbene disulfonates can change band 3 quaternary structure[9-11] support the allosteric interpretation for band 3 structure-function.[15]

For a ping-pong mechanism, Lineweaver-Burk plots constructed at various constant *trans* anion concentrations will show parallel lines (Chapter 3). On the other hand, for any mechanism involving a ternary complex, intersecting lines will be observed. It is often supposed that intersecting lines mean that a simple sequential model is extant. But this is not true. Salhany and Rauenbuehler[16] found that human erythrocyte band 3 had intersecting Lineweaver-Burk plots in dithionite-sulfate exchange, while at the same time there was clear evidence for site recruitment. Thus, some model needs to be proposed which can account for both effects. The authors suggested an ordered sequential model, where ternary complexes occur at both membrane surfaces, but where binary complexes move across the membrane. That is, two sites (one empty and one loaded) "move back and forth" together.[16] As we discussed in Chapter 3, Hautmann and Schnell[17] found intersecting lines in chloride self-exchange studies with human red cells. This result supports the findings of Salhany and Rauenbuehler.[16] New work from Knauf's lab[18] has shown that a human nonerythroid band 3 also shows intersecting Lineweaver-Burk plots. Since there is greater than 70% sequence homology in the integral domain of human erythroid and nonerythroid band 3 (Chapter 2), the likelihood that one protein uses one mechanism and the other a completely different mechanism seems small. It seems more likely that all band 3 proteins use the same basic transport mechanism but that the interaction constants between the two sites or classes of sites (or channels) are different. For example, it is not uncommon to find enzymes which follow an ordered sequential model while having very nearly parallel lines in Lineweaver-Burk plots. I believe this is the situation with human erythroid band 3 for chloride transport. The lines of the ordered sequential model are nearly, but not exactly parallel.[16,17] A two site ordered sequential model[16] with both sites "moving back and forth" together, may be able to account for all of the data in the literature. Further tests of this model seem warranted.

Some additional references are given below.[12,19-22] The paper by Kunimoto and co-workers[12] is particularly interesting in that it shows that the ankyrin-bound form of band 3 is tetrameric. This finding supports the *in situ* crosslinking results of Salhany and Sloan.[10,11] The demonstration that cadmium promotes band 3 binding to the cytoskeleton, while *p*-mercuribenzoate breaks those links, is interesting and worth further investigation as to the mechanism(s) involved. The paper by Knauf and co-workers[21] shows what may be a clear example of band 3 allosterism. The authors demonstrate that addition of iodine to an internal transport site alters the apparent affinity of flufenamate to an exofacial noncompetitive inhibitory site. In a strict ping-pong model, the transport site should not affect the affinity of an exofacial noncompetitive inhibitory site. This type of linkage falls in the province of protein allosterism. Evidence has been published showing that inhibitors of anion transport can alter interactions of the protein with the immediate lipid environment.[20] This type of interaction may be expected as a consequence of global conformational changes in the porter.

Bjerrum and co-workers[22] have published a detailed study of the inhibition of anion exchange by an impermeant carbodiimide (EAC, see Chapter 3). They found that EAC (which modifies exofacial carboxyl groups) inhibits transport biphasically and that the biphasicity results from *intramonomeric* effects. It is interesting that addition of DNDS leads to the elimination of the biphasicity even though the sites do not seem to be mutually exclusive. This is reminiscent of what Salhany and co-workers[4] saw with PLP inhibition of anion exchange. The difference is that PLP biphasicity was shown to be due to *intermonomeric* interactions. At 50% PLP saturation, both subdomains of the integral domain of band 3 were nearly equally labeled and DIDS crosslinked 50% of the band 3 monomers (which were devoid of PLP; see Chapter 3). Apparently, the global nature of the DNDS conformational change affects both intermonomeric and intramonomeric allosteric interactions on band 3. In addition to these effects, modification of the exofacial carboxyl groups by EAC caused the elimination of an *intracellular* anion transport titration with a pK of 5.4.[22] Since the carboxyl groups which caused this change are exofacial and different than those modified by Woodward's reagent K (see Chapter 3), and since both cause the same transmembrane effect, Bjerrum and co-workers[22] suggest that the exofacial and endofacial sites are allosterically linked. These results support our interpretation of the pH dependence of anion exchange given in Chapter 3.

In summary, there is an increasing amount of evidence to support the view presented in this book that protein allosterism contributes major energies to the anion exchange mechanism. The exact manner in which allosteric interactions accomplish anion exchange is unknown, but seems to involve at least two sites which interact. The interactions seem to be predominantly intermonomeric, but intramonomeric effects have also been documented in this book. With this evidence we begin to see what may be called a "paradigm shift" from the concept of a single site "moving back and forth" to the view that at least two allosterically interacting sites or classes of sites (channels?) are involved.

REFERENCES

1. **Tanner, M. J. A., Martin, P. G., and High, S.,** The complete amino acid sequence of the human erythrocyte membrane anion-transport protein deduced from the cDNA sequence, *Biochem. J.,* 256, 703, 1989.
2. **Rao, A.,** Disposition of the band 3 polypeptide in the human erythrocyte membrane, The reactive sulfhydryl groups. *J. Biol. Chem.,* 254, 3503, 1979.

3. **Salhany, J. M. and Cassoly, R.,** Kinetics of *p*-mercuribenzoate binding to sulfhydryl groups on the isolated cytoplasmic fragment of band 3 protein, *J. Biol. Chem.,* 264, 1399, 1989.

4. **Salhany, J. M., Rauenbuehler, P. B., and Sloan, R. L.,** Characterization of pyridoxal 5'-phosphate affinity labeling of band 3 protein. Evidence for allosterically interacting transport inhibitory subdomains, *J. Biol. Chem.,* 262, 15965, 1987.

5. **Kaul, R. K., Murthy, S. N. P., Reddy, A. G., Steck, T. L., and Kohler, H.** Amino acid sequence of the N-alpha-terminal 201 residues of human erythrocyte membrane band 3, *J. Biol. Chem.,* 258, 7981, 1983.

6. **Kudrycki, K. and Shull, G. E.,** Primary structure of the rat kidney band 3 anion exchange protein deduced from cDNA, *J. Biol. Chem.,* 264, 8185, 1989.

7. **Brosius III, F. C., Alper, S. L., Garcia, A. M., and Lodish, H. F.,** The major kidney band 3 gene transcript predicts amino-terminal truncated band 3 polypeptide, *J. Biol. Chem.,* 264, 7784, 1989.

8. **Glibowicka, M., Winckler, B., Aranibar, N., Schuster, M., Hanssum, H., Ruterjans, H., and Passow, H,** Temperature dependence of anion transport in the human red blood cell, *Biochem. Biophys. Acta,* 946, 345, 1988.

9. **Tomida, M., Kondo, Y., Moriyama, R., Machida, H., and Makino, S.,** Effect of stilbene disulfonate binding on the state of association of the membrane-spanning domain of band 3 form bovine erythrocyte membrane, *Biochim. Biophys. Acta,* 943, 493, 1988.

10. **Salhany, J. M. and Sloan, R. L.,** Partial covalent labeling with pyridoxal 5'-phosphate induces bis(sulfosuccinimidyl)suberate crosslinking of band 3 protein tetramers in intact human red blood cells, *Biochem. Biophys. Res. Commun.,* 156, 1215, 1988.

11. **Salhany, J. M. and Sloan, R. L.,** Direct evidence for modulation of porter quaternary structure by transport site ligands, *Biochem. Biophys. Res. Commum.,* 159, 1337, 1989.

12. **Kunimoto, M., Shibata, K., and Miura, T.,** Comparison of the cytoskeleton fractions of rat red blood cells prepared with non-ionic detergents, *J. Biochem. (Tokyo),* 105, 190, 1989.

13. **Legrum, B. and Passow, H.,** Inhibition of inorganic anion transport across the human red blood cell membrane by chloride-dependent association of dipyridamole with a stilbene disulfonate binding site on the band 3 protein, *Biochim. Biophys. Acta,* 979, 193, 1989.

14. **Frohlich, O.,** The external anion binding site of the human erythrocyte anion transporter: DNDS binding and competition with chloride, *J. Membr. Biol.,* 65, 111, 1982.

15. **Salhany, J. M. and Swanson, J. C.,** Kinetics of passive anion transport across the human erythrocyte membrane, *Biochemistry,* 17, 3354, 1978.

16. **Salhany, J. M. and Rauenbuehler, P. B.,** Kinetics and mechanism of erythrocyte anion exchange, *J. Biol. Chem.,* 258, 245, 1983.

17. **Hautmann, E. K. and Schnell, K. F.,** Concentration dependence of the chloride selfexchange and homoexchange fluxes in human red cell ghosts, *Pflugers Arch.,* 405, 193, 1985.

18. **Knauf, P. A., Spinelli, L. J., Mann, N. A., Diefenback, B. L., Kozody, D. J., and Restrepo, D.,** Use of Noncompetitive Inhibitors to sense transport-related conformational changes and asymmetry in band 3, in *Recent Advances in Molecular Mechanisms of Anion Transport,* Hamasaki, N. and Jennings, M. L., Eds., Elsievier, New York 1989, in press.

19. **Raida, M., Wendel, J., Kojro, E., Fahrenholz, F., Fasold, H., Legrum, B., and Passow, H.,** Major proteolytic fragments of the murine band 3 protein as obtained after *in situ* proteolysis, *Biochim. Biophys Acta,* 980, 291, 1989.

20. **Wyse, J. W., Blank, M. E., Maynard, C. L., Diedrich, D. F., and Butterfield, D. A.,** Electron spin resonance investigation of the interaction of the anion and glucose transport inhibitor, p-azidobenzylphlorizin with the human red cell membrane, *Biochim. Biophys. Acta,* 979, 127, 1989.

21. **Knauf, P. A., Spinelli, L. J., and Mann, N. A.,** Flufenamic acid senses conformation and asymmetry of the band 3 protein, *Am. J. Physiol. (Cell Physiol.),* in press.

22. **Bjerrum, P. J., Andersen, C. L., Borders C. L., Jr., and Wieth, J. O.,** Functional Carboxyl Groups in the Red Cell Anion Exchange Protein. Modification with an impermeant carbodiimide, *J. Gen. Physiol.,* 93, 813, 1989.

INDEX